SUICIDE PREVENTION

SUICIDE PREVENTION

An Ethically and Scientifically Informed Approach

SAMUEL J. KNAPP

AMERICAN PSYCHOLOGICAL ASSOCIATION
Washington, DC

Published by
American Psychological Association
750 First Street, NE
Washington, DC 20002
https://www.apa.org

Order Department
https://www.apa.org/pubs/books
order@apa.org

In the U.K., Europe, Africa, and the Middle East, copies may be ordered from Eurospan
https://www.eurospanbookstore.com/apa
info@eurospangroup.com

Typeset in Meridien and Ortodoxa by Circle Graphics, Inc., Reisterstown, MD

Printer: Sheridan Books, Chelsea, MI
Cover Designer: Beth Schlenoff, Bethesda, MD

Library of Congress Cataloging-in-Publication Data

Names: Knapp, Samuel, author.
Title: Suicide prevention : an ethically and scientifically informed approach/
  Samuel J. Knapp.
Description: Washington, DC : American Psychological Association, [2020] |
  Includes bibliographical references and index.
Identifiers: LCCN 2019010442 (print) | LCCN 2019011829 (ebook) |
  ISBN 9781433831409 (eBook) | ISBN 1433831406 (eBook) |
  ISBN 9781433830808 (hardcover) | ISBN 1433830809 (hardcover)
Subjects: LCSH: Suicide—Psychological aspects. | Suicidal behavior. |
  Suicide—Prevention.
Classification: LCC HV6545 (ebook) | LCC HV6545 .K537 2020 (print) |
  DDC 362.28/7—dc23
LC record available at https://lccn.loc.gov/2019010442

http://dx.doi.org/10.1037/0000145-000

Printed in the United States of America

10 9 8 7 6 5 4 3 2 1

To Jane Marie Heesen Knapp

CONTENTS

ACKNOWLEDGMENTS

I thank James Dirks, Frank Hertzel, Richard Kocher, Dennis Kojsza, Susan Krause, Frances Manning, Jean McClung, Denise Adams Newman, Ronald Sharp, Sharon Sharp, Cynthia Stauffer, Mary Lee Webb, William C. Work, and other coworkers for their support and assistance while I delivered crisis intervention and psychotherapy services in community mental health centers in Indiana, Pennsylvania (Indiana County), and Millersburg, Pennsylvania (Dauphin County). They demonstrated the importance of a supportive community when dealing with suicidal patients.

I have a special debt to Dr. Leon VandeCreek for our collaborative work in applying principle-based ethics to life-endangering and other clinical situations.

I have benefited greatly from my ongoing associations with Drs. Michael Gottlieb, Mitchell Handelsman, and Rachael Baturin, and also Molly Haas Cowan, Randy Fingerhut, John Gavazzi, Peter Keller, Linda Knauss, John Lemoncelli, Donald McAleer, Jeanne Slattery, Richard Small, Jeff Sternlieb, Allan M. Tepper, Alan Tjeltveit, and the late Patricia M. Bricklin. Drs. Brett Schur and Ron Sherman have helped me clarify my thinking about suicide prevention.

I thank Judy Smith Huntley, Ann Marie Frakes, and Erin Brady for supporting my work in providing continuing education programs on suicide prevention through the Pennsylvania Psychological Association. I also thank the Pennsylvania Psychological Association for permitting me to adapt materials that were first published in the *Pennsylvania Psychologist* or presented as continuing education programs.

I acknowledge the contributions of the American Association of Suicidology and the numerous researchers, clinicians, and authors who have contributed so much to improve the quality of services provided to persons at risk to die from suicide. I have never met most of them, but I want them to know that their contributions are appreciated.

Most of all, I want to express appreciation to my wife, closest friend, and life companion, Jane Marie Heesen Knapp, PsyD, an extraordinary psychologist in her own right, for all that she has done in many many ways. I dedicate this book to her.

SUICIDE PREVENTION

Introduction

Those who belong to a community in which they feel loved and valued are much less likely to die from suicide. Unfortunately, many people lack that sense of connection. Often, they end up in the offices of psychotherapists who must help them build or reestablish the social connections and resources needed to make life worth living.

I wrote this book to help psychotherapists become better at assessing, managing, and treating patients who are suicidal. This topic is important to me. During the 1970s and 1980s, I delivered emergency services in two community mental health centers in rural Pennsylvania. I remember the faces and the stories of many of my patients. I remember the young man who shot himself in the head with a pistol (and lived); the young woman who took an overdose of drugs, came into my office the next day, and refused to talk; and the middle-aged mother who hated herself because she had neglected her children years ago during a depressive episode. These memories evoke strong emotions even 40 years later. The emotional quality to these stories is hard to capture fully in written text.

I also worked with the survivors of suicide. They often stated that their lives were shattered by guilt and loneliness. Suddenly they questioned basic assumptions about themselves as good parents or good spouses. Their expectations for the future changed for the worse.

During those years, my colleagues and I tried to deliver effective and respectful services (see Knapp, Dirks, & Magee, 1982). Most patients were cooperative and received outpatient treatment. But some seriously suicidal

http://dx.doi.org/10.1037/0000145-001
Suicide Prevention: An Ethically and Scientifically Informed Approach, by S. J. Knapp
Copyright © 2020 by the American Psychological Association. All rights reserved.

patients resisted treatment. Although I was not yet well-versed in bioethical concepts such as beneficence, nonmaleficence, or respect for patient autonomy, my colleagues and I worked hard to get reluctant patients to "buy into" treatment. We believed that we should not force treatment without exhausting efforts to secure the patient's cooperation.

I made many mistakes during those years, but fortunately none of my patients died from suicide. In part, it was because I had some basic competence in evaluating and managing suicidal patients. I never discounted the possibility of suicide. It is a frightening enemy, and I never underestimated its power. But at the same time, I was lucky. I have known psychotherapists, far more competent than I, who have had patients die from suicide. Since the time that I worked in crisis intervention, I have conducted many workshops on suicide prevention, consulted with many psychologists on suicidal patients, and written articles and book chapters dealing with suicide.

INTENDED READERSHIP

This book is intended for professional psychologists and other psychotherapists who deal with adult outpatients with suicidal behavior. In selecting the content, I ask, "What will psychotherapists with suicidal patients in front of them need to know?" To reach this goal, this book links its recommendations both to science and to the real-life experiences of patients and psychotherapists. It incorporates the most recent research findings on suicide that the well-established books on suicide intervention have not had the opportunity to cover. It emphasizes a caring attitude that is neither alarmist nor dismissive. It identifies competencies that effective psychotherapists need to acquire, including emotional competence and the ability to make ethical decisions.

Suicide is caused by many factors embedded in the personal histories and experiences of every patient. Nonetheless, research has generated some commonalities that can guide effective interventions. I relied on that evidence to inform the recommendations made in this book. I explain suicidal behavior primarily through the lens of the ideation-to-action theories of suicide such as the interpersonal theory of suicide (e.g., Joiner, Van Orden, Witte, & Rudd, 2009), and I justify treatment decisions through the lens of principle-based ethics (e.g., Knapp, VandeCreek, & Fingerhut, 2017). I inserted personal experiences when they illustrated or supported important concepts.

In addition to making specific recommendations, this book also explains why these recommendations were made. No book, no matter how comprehensive, can predict all the contingencies that psychotherapists will face when treating suicidal patients. Therefore, effective psychotherapists will need to modify, discard, or adapt some of the recommendations made herein. Psychotherapists will make better decisions if they understand why the recommendations were made.

Roush et al. (2018) found that psychotherapists who felt the most anxiety around suicidal patients were most likely to endorse interventions lacking in evidence. Ideally, this book will give psychotherapists more confidence in assessing, managing, and treating suicidal patients; keep them from exaggerated fears of liability; and lead them to study and learn evidence-informed interventions.

OVERVIEW OF THE BOOK[1]

Chapter 1 ("Facts, Theories, and Perspectives on Suicide") describes the public health importance of suicide; attitudes toward suicide in society and among psychotherapists; and essential competencies needed to assess, manage, and treat suicidal patients. Later chapters expand on each of these competencies. Finally, it reviews the ideation-to-action theories of suicide, including the interpersonal theory of suicide and the role of principle-based ethics in informing treatment.

Chapter 2 ("Screening and Assessment") reviews the steps in screening and assessing suicidal risk, including learning about the patient's suicide ideation, suicide plans, and past suicide attempts. Also, Chapter 2 expands on the psychological states that often precede suicide attempts. The emotional or behavioral symptoms expressed by the patient in these crisis states can be viewed as warning signs that will help predict the immediate risk of suicide. Also, Chapter 2 emphasizes the importance of establishing and maintaining a good treatment alliance with the patient.

In addition, Chapter 2 describes additional information that psychotherapists need in assessing their patients. It describes certain topics that should be explored, including the patient's history, recent stressors, social network, physical health, religious or spiritual values, and mental health diagnosis. The ideation-to-action theories of suicide can guide psychotherapists on what patient factors to look for in these evaluations.

Chapter 3 ("Interventions Part One: Including Managing Suicide Risk") presents recommendations for the first stages of treatment, which emphasize informed consent, establishment of a good treatment relationship, and suicide management. Chapter 3 describes how psychotherapists can use the fluid vulnerability theory to integrate patient information and determine the appropriate level of service. The goal of suicide management is to keep patients alive until psychotherapy has a chance to work. Psychotherapists can manage suicidal risk by motivating patients (and creating a crisis–response plan), restricting access to lethal means, monitoring patients, and other options to reduce risk.

Chapter 4 ("Interventions Part Two: Suicide-Informed Psychotherapy") describes how psychotherapists can adapt their interventions to address

---

[1]All case examples in this book are either composites of several real patients or single patients whose identifying characteristics have been changed to protect confidentiality.

issues that arise in the treatment of suicidal patients. It does not endorse any one treatment approach but rather recommends that any treatment approach for suicidal patients should consider how to respond when suicide attempts happen during treatment, and so on. Finally, Chapter 4 identifies trans-theoretical interventions that can address the symptoms commonly associated with suicidal behavior and considers how psychotherapists can integrate religion and value perspectives into psychotherapy.

Chapter 5 ("Professional Liability, Quality Enhancement, and Emotional Competence") describes how to reduce the risk of professional liability. It covers ethically based quality enhancement (risk management) strategies and documentation. Finally, it highlights the importance of emotional competence as an essential quality for doing good clinical work.

1

Facts, Theories, and Perspectives on Suicide

The goal of this book is to present an evidence-informed approach to evaluating, managing, and treating suicidal patients. The opening vignette describes several of the real-life problems that psychotherapists face in trying to estimate the risk of suicide among patients, building productive treatment relationships, and developing effective interventions. The rest of the book addresses these and other issues.

This chapter describes the public health importance of suicide, attitudes toward suicide in society and among psychotherapists, the ideation-to-action theories of suicide, and the role of principle-based ethics in informing treatment. Also, it identifies 10 essential competencies needed to assess, manage, and treat suicidal patients. Later chapters expand on each of these competencies; describe how psychotherapists can use the ideation-to-action theories of suicide to guide the assessment, management, and treatment of suicidal patients; and explain how psychotherapists can use principle-based ethics to guide treatment decisions and resolve ethical conflicts. Before moving into those topics, consider the following example that will illustrate some themes found in this book.

One Tuesday afternoon, an apparently ordinary intake interview suddenly became less routine when the 28-year-old patient, Miguel, said that he was having thoughts of killing himself. The psychotherapist adopted an attitude of alert concern in which she implemented the protocols that she had learned about suicide prevention. In the interview the psychotherapist learned that

- Miguel has been unemployed for 6 months and believes that the likelihood of getting a good job is poor.

http://dx.doi.org/10.1037/0000145-002
Suicide Prevention: An Ethically and Scientifically Informed Approach, by S. J. Knapp

- He has little energy to get work done around the house.

- He is married and has a daughter.

- Miguel's wife does not know of his suicidal thoughts, but she knows he is depressed and insisted that he get treatment. His family physician made the referral.

- Miguel had a suicide attempt about 10 years ago but says he will not kill himself because he could never do that to his family.

- Miguel has access to guns in his house and likes to hunt, but he has agreed to put his guns into a secure locker and give his wife the key.

- Miguel has trouble sleeping and shows symptoms of a major depression. He has been drinking more in the last month, although there was no long-term history of alcohol misuse.

Following is some more information that may be relevant.

Although the psychotherapist asked some questions to get basic information, she made sure that Miguel had a chance to tell his story and tried to show concern for him. In the informed-consent process, the psychotherapist went over some fundamentals of psychotherapy, including the role of confidentiality and the importance of his involvement in treatment goals. The psychotherapist promised to go over psychotherapy procedures in more detail later to ensure that Miguel understood why certain recommendations were being made. His most immediate goal was improving his sleep, and the psychotherapist promised that they would work on that. They also agreed that they would discuss ways to involve his wife in treatment at their next meeting.

Looking at a totality of factors, including Miguel's baseline of distress, access to means of harm, and other factors, the psychotherapist determined that he did not need to be in a hospital but that he would need close monitoring as an outpatient (see the levels of service chart in Chapter 3). She made an appointment for him to see her in 2 days and for him to call her tomorrow to tell her how he was doing. An appointment was made with their agency psychiatrist later that week. They went over a safety plan. Miguel promised to have his wife call the psychotherapist the next day to confirm that the guns were locked away and that she had the key.

Later that day the psychotherapist spoke to her colleague about this patient. When reviewing her intervention, a colleague asked the psychotherapist why she had not notified the wife immediately. It was a good question. Although involving family members is the preferred intervention, the psychotherapist sensed that Miguel was getting fatigued, and she did not want to overwhelm him with too much in the first session. Besides, she was going to be talking to the wife on the following day. Perhaps she was wrong, but so many decisions needed to be made on the spur of the moment.

Her long-term goal is to get Miguel over this episode of depression characterized by suicidal thoughts. If he gets over this episode, then the likelihood is that he will live a relatively productive and meaningful life. Her short-term goal is to ensure Miguel's safety until psychotherapy has a chance to work.

If Miguel dies from suicide, then his wife would be a secondary victim of the suicide, and it is likely that she would suffer a severe emotional trauma that far exceeds what she would experience if he were to die from natural causes. If Miguel dies from suicide, then it is likely that the psychotherapist would also be a secondary victim of the suicide and would suffer self-doubt and anguish, although not to the extent that the wife would.

This brief description includes several themes that reappear throughout this book. The first theme is the attitude of the psychotherapist. Suicide is an emotionally charged event that could create excessive worry. The optimal reaction is to show alert concern without being too paternalistic or too protective.

The second theme is that the effective treatment of suicidal patients requires both good professional habits and good decision-making skills. This includes knowing facts about suicide, having an ability to form meaningful relationships with patients, and being able to think through difficult decisions carefully.

A final theme is that effective treatments need to be based on overarching ethical principles such as beneficence (promoting the well-being of patients) and respect for patient autonomy. Although the description in the vignette was brief, it noted that she intended to ask Miguel for his permission to involve his wife more in the treatment later and to tell him that they would work on treatment goals together.

The themes in the vignette reflect the major points identified in this and later chapters: the importance of a caring attitude that is neither dismissive nor alarmist, the importance of professional competencies, and the role of values in guiding treatment decisions and making treatment decisions.

THE PUBLIC HEALTH IMPORTANCE OF SUICIDE

In 2016, nearly 45,000 Americans died from suicide (Stone et al., 2018), and it regularly ranks as the 10th or 11th leading cause of death. Twice as many people die from suicide in the United States as die from homicide. The age-adjusted suicide rate in the United States was 14.0 per 100,000 in 2017 (22.4 for men and 6.1 for women; Hedegaard, Curtin, & Warner, 2018). Whereas the rates of death from most diseases have decreased over the last 20 years, the rate of suicide has increased 33% from 1999 to 2017 (Hedegaard et al., 2018).

The rates of suicide and suicide ideation vary according to age, gender, ethnicity, education level, and socioeconomic status. Throughout their lifespans, about 15% of Americans will think about suicide, 4% will have a suicide plan, 4.6% will attempt suicide (Kessler, Borges, & Walters, 1999), and less than 1% will die from suicide. Since that study was published in 1999, the rates of suicidal ideation, planning, and attempts have likely increased.

TABLE 1.1. Suicide Rates per 100,000 by Gender and Age in the United States, 2017

Age (years)	Female	Male
10–14	1.7	3.3
15–24	5.8	22.7
25–44	7.8	27.5
45–64	9.7	30.1
65–74	6.2	26.2
75 and older	4.0	39.7
All ages	6.1	22.4

Note. Data from Hedegaard, Curtin, and Warner (2018).

Within 1 year, about 3.7% of Americans will think about suicide (B. Han, McKeon, & Gfroerer, 2014), 1% will have a suicide plan, and 0.3% will attempt suicide (Liotta, Mento, & Settineri, 2015). The frequency of suicidal ideation varies by age and education. About 6.6% of Americans between the ages of 18 and 25 had thought of suicide in the last year, compared with 4% for those between the ages of 26 and 40, and 2.5% for those who are 50 or older. Suicidal ideation is higher among those who have a high school education (compared with those who went to college), who are a disabled or unemployed adult under 65, or who are unmarried or live in poverty (B. Han et al., 2014).

The rate of suicide varies by age. Rates are highest for men who are 75 or older (Hedegaard, Curtin, & Warner, 2016). Suicide is the second leading cause of death among Americans ages 10 through 34, although the absolute number of suicides in this age group is far less than that of older adults (Centers for Disease Control, 2016).

The rates of suicidal ideation are about the same for men and women (1-year rates are 3.5% for men and 3.9% for women; B. Han et al., 2014). Women attempt suicide more often than men, but men are four times more likely to die from suicide than women (Liotta et al., 2015). Table 1.1 presents the rates of suicide according to gender and age.

The rate of suicide varies by race, with Native Americans, Native Alaskans, and Pacific Islanders having the highest rates, followed by Whites and then Hispanics and African Americans (National Institute of Mental Health, 2018). Table 1.2 presents the rates of suicide according to gender and ethnicity.

TABLE 1.2. Suicide Rates per 100,000 by Gender and Ethnicity in the United States, 2016

Ethnicity	Females	Males
Non-Hispanic, White	7.9	26.5
Non-Hispanic, Black	2.4	10.5
Asian, Pacific Islander	3.6	10.2
American Indian, Alaskan Native	10.2	32.8
Hispanic	2.8	11.6
All races	6.1	22.4

Note. Data from the National Institute of Mental Health (2018).

The differences in suicide rates by race and ethnicity need to be viewed critically because suicide rates can vary considerably within these large designations of ethnic groups. For example, suicide among different groups of Asian Americans (Chinese, Filipino, Indian, Japanese, Korean, and Vietnamese) vary considerably (Wong, Vaughan, Liu, & Chang, 2014). Because of shame, suicides among Asian Americans may be underreported.

The rate of suicide is lower for African Americans than for White Americans. The reasons for this finding are not clear. Cultural attitudes, such as having strong moral objections to suicide, may be a factor (Morrison & Downey, 2000). Also, suicides may be underreported among African Americans (Rockett et al., 2010).

The rate of suicide varies geographically. Suicides are increasingly more common in rural areas compared with urban areas, perhaps because of social isolation, lower educational levels, an increase in opioid misuse (Kegler, Stone, & Holland, 2017), easier access to guns, or attitudes of self-reliance that discourage seeking help from others.

The rate of suicide also varies by educational level. Those over the age of 25 who had a college education had a rate of suicide half that of those over the age of 25 who had only a high school education. Perhaps those with less education have more mental health or job-related problems (Phillips & Hempstead, 2017) or less access to health care.

Education is often used as a proxy for socioeconomic status (SES) in epidemiological research. One robust finding is that mental illness is more common among persons of lower SES, although the reasons are not entirely clear. Part of the link may be due to social causation in that persons with lower SES have more stressors, fewer financial resources to buffer the impact of those stressors, and less access to health care. In addition, stressful environments at an early age may predispose some individuals to react poorly to stressful events later in life. But part of the link may be due to social selection in that some persons with mental or physical illnesses may experience a decline in their SES because they are less likely to perform well in school or on the job or may not even be able to work.

SES, suicide, and ethnicity interact in complex ways. As one would predict from SES, White Americans have lower rates of suicide than Native American/ Alaskan/Pacific Islander Americans. Also, one would predict that social discrimination would additionally increase the risk of suicide not only because it restricts access to educational and employment opportunities but also because of the stress caused by overt discrimination and microaggressions. Nonetheless, African Americans have lower rates of suicide than White Americans, suggesting that other factors can mitigate the impact of stress.

In the United States, firearms accounted for 51% of all suicides, followed by suffocation (27%) and poisoning (including overdoses; 16%), while falls, cutting, drowning, and other causes accounted for the other 6% (National Center for Health Statistics, 2017).

B. Han et al. (2016) estimated that 3% of attempted suicides resulted in death, although other studies have found that the percentage of suicide attempts to suicides was as high as 10% (Bongar & Sullivan, 2013). But males over the age of 65, who are more likely to shoot themselves, will have 25% of attempts result in death. Nonetheless, the data on suicide attempts are also imprecise because about half of suicide attempters do not seek out medical attention.

The low ratio of attempts to suicides may reflect the difficulty in effectuating a plan while in the throes of strong negative emotions or the patient's lack of knowledge about the lethality of certain techniques (Bryan, Stone, & Rudd, 2011). Perhaps a greater knowledge of the lethality of medications partially explains the high rate of suicide among physicians (Austin, van den Heuvel, & Byard, 2013), veterinarians (Fink-Miller & Nestler, 2018), and nurses (Alderson, Parent-Rocheleau, & Mishara, 2015).

Among those who disclosed an event that precipitated the attempt, 53% reported it was due to intimate partner, family, or interpersonal problems; 22%, physical health problems; 11%, job or financial problems; and 9%, a recent criminal charge (K. A. Fowler, Jack, Lyons, Betz, & Petrosky, 2018). Interpersonal conflicts may be especially important precipitants in collectivist cultures.

The data on suicides are imprecise because suicide is often underreported or misclassified, especially among African Americans, who have a larger number of death certificates with undetermined causes (Rockett et al., 2010). In addition, suicides from drug overdoses may be substantially underreported (Rockett et al., 2014). As discussed in more detail in Chapter 2 of this volume, it can be hard to distinguish accidental from deliberate overdoses, and even the dichotomy of deaths into either accidental or deliberate has controversies associated with it. Even without adjusting for this possible under reporting, suicides have increased faster than the national average in the areas of the country especially hit by the widespread misuse of opioids ("U.S. Suicide Rates Display Growing Geographic Disparity," 2017).

Of course, deaths from suicides represent only a fraction of the public health costs because nonfatal attempts often result in psychiatric hospitalizations, medical office visits, or emergency room encounters. The Substance Abuse and Mental Health Services Administration (2013) estimated that 729,000 adults received medical attention for suicide attempts in 2012, and 500,000 adults stayed at least one night in an inpatient facility following a suicide attempt. Given the prevalence of suicide as a major cause of death, one would think that research on suicide would be funded at the levels comparable to other causes of death. This is not the case, however. Although research on liver disease (the 12th leading cause of death) and hypertension (the 13th leading cause of death) is well funded, research on suicide is not (Hewer, 2015). Furthermore, federally funded studies of mental health treatment usually exclude suicidal patients.

PSYCHOTHERAPISTS AND SUICIDE

Treating suicidal patients is technically difficult because suicidal behavior is complex and multidetermined. Treating suicidal patients is emotionally difficult because so much is at stake. The threat of a patient suicide is the emergency most frequently experienced by psychotherapists, and a patient suicide is the professional event most feared by psychotherapists (Roush et al., 2018). Almost every psychologist has this fear (Pope & Tabachnick, 1993). In addition, treating suicidal patients involves uncertainty because even the best predictive models have a high rate of false positives.

Psychotherapists who treat suicidal patients know that things could suddenly go terribly wrong. Having a patient die from suicide is an occupational hazard. Although skilled psychotherapists are less likely to have had a patient die from suicide, many highly competent psychotherapists have had patients die from suicide even when they delivered good care. About 50% of psychiatrists and 25% of psychologists have had a patient die from suicide (Kleespies & Dettmer, 2000). A survey found that 4% of the members of the Pennsylvania Psychological Association had at least one patient die from suicide in the last year (Leitzel & Knapp, 2017).

A suicide[1] represents a tragic loss of a sacred life. Spouses lose their partners, children lose their parents, parents lose their children, and siblings and friends lose loved ones. According to the 2016 General Social Survey, 51% of Americans reported knowing someone who died from suicide, and one third reported being bereaved by a suicide (Feigelman, Cerel, McIntosh, Brent, & Gutin, 2018). For close friends or relatives of suicide victims, the scars can last a lifetime. Often the survivors blame themselves or ask what they could have done differently. They also endure the social stigma that surrounds suicide. One can imagine that neighbors might think "What kind of parent drives his child to suicide?" or "A good friend would never have let him kill himself," and so on.

Over the years, I have consulted with many psychologists[2] who have just lost a patient to suicide. The first thing I say to them is, "I am sorry for your loss," because I view them as secondary victims of the suicide. Although a suicide does not impact them as much as it does the immediate family, they are victims nonetheless. Often, they will develop an *International Classification of Diseases* diagnosis such as an adjustment disorder, although some will develop more severe mental illnesses (Rothes, Scheerder, Van Audenhove, & Henriques, 2013). The emotional strain of a patient suicide on psychotherapists is discussed in more detail in Chapter 5.

---

[1] It is common to say that an individual "committed" suicide or that an individual had a "successful suicide attempt." However, the phrase "committed suicide" implies that the suicide was a crime akin to committing robbery or committing murder. Instead, suicide almost always occurs when an individual's judgment is compromised by extreme negative emotions. Consequently, this book refers to persons who died from suicide, as opposed to persons who committed suicide. In addition, the phrase "successful suicide" implies that the suicide represented an accomplishment, an assumption that should be challenged because the real accomplishment comes from staying alive. Consequently, this book refers to suicides, as opposed to successful suicides. Notwithstanding, even I, who knows better, have been known to slip into inappropriate language.

[2] This book usually uses the word *psychotherapists* because the discussions apply to all who are giving psychotherapy to suicidal patients, regardless of their professional affiliation. At times, however, the book uses the term *psychologists* to refer specifically to those who are licensed psychologists.

State of the Field When Working With Suicidal Patients

Over the years, I have consulted with hundreds of psychologists working with suicidal patients, and I believe that most delivered adequate, good, or excellent care. At times, I have finished a consultation with the impression that this psychotherapist is far more skilled than I would have been under the same circumstances. They might not have read the latest article on suicide, but they knew how to develop caring relationships with their patients, take the suicidal thoughts seriously without overreacting, and develop effective suicide management strategies and interventions.

My positive evaluation, however, is qualified by several sources of data that suggest shortcomings in the quality of treatment of suicidal patients. First, those who seek out consultation might represent a more conscientious population of psychologists who understand the importance of consultations. Also, I have consulted in a few cases where suicidal patients have received less-than-optimal (in one case, poor) care. Typically, these poorly performing professionals knew that their skills were deficient.

Although outcome studies rarely include suicidal behavior as a dependent variable, some outcome data reveal shortcomings in the treatment for suicidal patients. For example, Kraus, Castonguay, Boswell, Nordberg, and Hayes (2011) found that about 15% of patients with suicidal thoughts got worse throughout the course of psychotherapy, and almost 50% showed no significant improvement. Almost two thirds failed to improve! Also, Kraus et al. (2016) found that those psychotherapists who were effective with suicidal patients tended to remain effective with suicidal patients over time, whereas those who performed poorly with suicidal patients tended to perform poorly with suicidal patients over time. However, both studies by Kraus and his colleagues ceased to measure progress past 16 weeks and used a sample of mental health professionals with limited experience wherein only a few held doctoral degrees. Therefore, their results might not generalize to more experienced and better trained psychotherapists. However, the findings of Kraus et al. should not be dismissed entirely and show that many psychotherapists get poor outcomes with suicidal patients.

Furthermore, many psychotherapists reported that their training programs inadequately prepared them to work with suicidal patients (Bongar & Sullivan, 2013). Presumably, they learned it on the job or not at all. For example, Jahn, Quinnett, and Ries (2016) found that 21% of psychotherapists reported that their training and expertise in working with suicidal patients was inadequate. Leitzel and Knapp (2017) found that 10% of the members of the Pennsylvania Psychological Association did not believe that they were proficient in working with suicidal patients.

Jobes, Rudd, Overholser, and Joiner (2008) opined that many suicidal patients received less-than-optimal care because clinicians often failed to use proven interventions. Some data have suggested that they are correct. For example, Roush et al. (2018) found that 30% of the mental health professionals did not routinely ask patients about suicidal behavior, even though professional standards for psychiatrists hold that they should be routinely screened (J. J. Silverman et al., 2015). The 30% figure from Roush et al. approximates that 30% to 40% of students seen by mental health professionals were not asked about suicidality (Hom, Stanley, Podlogar, & Joiner, 2017).

Also, Roush et al. (2018) found that 18% of their sample of psychotherapists routinely used no-suicide contracts, despite the lack of evidence of their effectiveness (this is discussed in more detail in Chapter 3). Also, Roush et al. found that 5% of their sample of psychotherapists commonly referred patients with suicidal thoughts to inpatient facilities or emergency departments. However, hospitalizations are seldom the first line of treatment for suicidal patients, and emergency rooms often lack the resources or qualified staff to help suicidal patients. (Hospitalizations and use of emergency departments are discussed in more detail in Chapter 3.) In addition, some psychotherapists give inadequate attention to the management of suicide risk and assume that treating an underlying mental disorder is sufficient to reduce the risk of suicide (Weissberg, 2011).

Therefore, it appears that a noticeable minority of psychotherapists lack the skills to work effectively with suicidal patients. One could argue that those psychotherapists who do not feel competent working with suicidal patients will simply refuse to take suicidal patients into their practices or refer them out. However, that option has problems associated with it. First, suicidal behavior occurs across diagnoses, and any professional who purports to treat mental illnesses should expect to encounter some suicidal patients eventually. Second, any communication by a health care professional that they do not treat patients with suicidal thoughts encourages the patients to be silent about their suicidal thoughts and reinforces a stereotype of suicidal thoughts as shameful or embarrassing. In reality, those psychotherapists are not saying that they do not treat patients with suicidal thoughts, what they are really saying is that they do not treat patients who tell them that they have suicidal thoughts.

Standards of Competence When Working With Suicidal Patients

It is worth asking what steps psychotherapists can take to ensure that they are competent to treat suicidal patients.[3] The American Psychological Association (e.g., Rubin et al., 2007) and the Association of State and Provincial Psychology Boards (2017) have developed generic competencies required of psychologists delivering health care services, but neither group defined *competence* with sufficient specificity to include behavioral emergencies as one of the core competencies. Nonetheless, all psychotherapists should be competent in working with behavioral emergencies (Kleespies, 2017).

---

[3]This section is from "Competence with Suicidal Patients," by S. Knapp, 2017, *The Pennsylvania Psychologist*, 77, pp. 1, 7. Copyright 2017 by the Pennsylvania Psychological Association. Adapted with permission.

The definition of competence by physicians Epstein and Hundert (2002) may be relevant. Their well-regarded definition of competence is as follows:

> the habitual and judicious use of communication, knowledge, technical skills, clinical reasoning, emotions, values, and reflection in daily practice for the benefit of the individuals and communities being served. (p. 226)

This definition includes some of the "whats" of competence, including knowledge, technical skills, clinical reasoning, and so on within its definition. This definition also involves both habits of practice ("habitual") and the use of judgment ("judicious"). Finally, it requires that competence occur in daily practice, implying that it cannot be obtained simply by attending workshops or reading books.

Epstein and Hundert's (2002) process of defining the "whats" of competence is relevant in determining competence in treating suicidal patients. The "whats" of competencies are "clusters of integrated knowledge, skills, and abilities that enable an individual to fully perform a task" (Kleespies, 2017, p. 31). To help promote competence when working with suicidal patients, suicidologists and suicide prevention organizations have developed lists of skills specific to the treatment of suicidal patients. For example, the American Association of Suicidology identified seven domains and 24 statements related to competence (American Association of Suicidology, n.d.; Rudd, Cukrowicz, & Bryan, 2008), although Cramer, Johnson, McLaughlin, Rausch, and Conroy (2013) modified them to make 10 domains of competence.

This book relies on the competence domains developed by Cramer et al. (2013), which appears to better organize and consolidate the 24 statements of the American Association of Suicidology. Their 10 core competencies are (a) knowing and managing attitudes and reactions to suicide, (b) developing and maintaining a collaborative stance with the patients, (c) knowing and eliciting evidence-based risk and protective factors, (d) focusing on current suicide plans and intent of suicidal ideation, (e) determining level of risk, (f) developing and implementing a collaborative and evidence-based treatment plan, (g) notifying and involving other persons, (h) documenting risk plans, (i) knowing the laws dealing with suicide, and (j) ensuring self-care (emotional competence). All of these core competencies are interrelated. For example, understanding one's personal reaction to suicidal patients may make the psychotherapists better able to develop a caring and collaborative relationship with the patient.

Epstein and Hundert's (2002) process of identifying both habitual and judicious aspects of competence is also relevant. Most of the competencies identified by Cramer et al. (2013) require practice habits that should be routine with suicidal patients, such as knowing how to elicit risk and protective factors from patients, knowing how to maintain a collaborative and nonadversarial stance with patients, and so on. Other competencies identified by Cramer et al. require judgment or decision-making skills, such as how to develop treatment or safety plans and so on. This book will highlight areas in which judgment becomes especially important, and the steps that psychotherapists can take to

TABLE 1.3. Core Competencies and Suicide Addressed in This Book

Competencies	Primarily addressed in chapter/heading
1. Knowing and managing attitudes and reactions to suicidal patients	Chapter 1: Psychotherapists and Suicide Chapter 5: Ensuring Emotional Competence
2. Developing an empathic and collaborative stance toward the patient	Chapter 2: The Relationship in the Screening and Assessment Process Chapter 3: The Psychotherapeutic Relationship Chapter 4: (entire chapter)
3. Knowing and eliciting evidence-based risk factors	Chapter 2: (entire chapter)
4. Learning about current plan and suicidal ideation[a]	Chapter 2: Screening for Suicide; Assessment Step One: Asking About Suicide
5. Determining levels of risk	Chapter 3: Levels of Service
6. Developing [and implementing] a collaboratively based treatment plan[b]	Chapter 3: Patient Empowerment (Informed Consent) Chapter 5: Effective and False Risk-Management Strategies
7. Notifying and involving other persons	Chapter 3: The Three Ms of Managing Suicide Risk Chapter 5: Effective and False Risk-Management Strategies
8. Documenting risk, plans, and reasoning	Chapter 5: Effective and False Risk-Management Strategies
9. Knowing and applying ethical principles, laws concerning suicide[c]	Chapter 1: Values That Guide Professional Behavior Chapter 3: Other Options for Managing Suicide Risk Chapter 5: Effective and False Risk-Management Strategies
10. Engaging in debriefing, self-reflection, and self-care[d]	Chapter 5: Ensuring Emotional Competence

Note. [a]The original phrase was "focusing on current plan. . . ." [b]"Implementing" was added to this core competency. [c]"Ethical principles" and "applying" were added to this core competency. [d]"Self-reflection" was added to this core competency.

improve the quality of their decision making. Table 1.3 lists the competencies and the locations where they are addressed in this book and notes where the wording in some of the domains has been modified slightly.

Cultural competence and ethical decision making are metaskills that should be embedded in all these categories. Cultural competence related to suicide includes understanding cultural idioms of distress, the impact of minority stress, cultural attitudes toward suicide, and the role of social factors in precipitating suicide attempts (J. P. Chu, Goldblum, Floyd, & Bongar, 2010).

Psychotherapist Attitudes Toward Suicidal Patients

Cramer et al.'s (2013) first core competency is that psychotherapists should manage their reactions to suicide and suicidal patients. Ideally, psychotherapists will take the same accepting and nonjudgmental attitude toward their suicidal patients that they take with their other patients. However, that is not always the case. Maltsberger and Buie (1974) noted that psychotherapists often dislike suicidal patients. This finding makes intuitive sense, is consistent with the anecdotal reports of many clinicians, and has some research supporting it. For example, Westgate, Shiner, Thompson, and Watts (2015) looked at the content of clinician notes for VA patients who died from suicide and compared them with the notes for patients who did not die from suicide. The notes about patients who died from suicide included more language suggesting emotional distance from patients, perhaps as an effort of clinicians outside of their conscious awareness to protect themselves emotionally from the expected death of the patient. These negative feelings may degrade the quality of treatment if they lead psychotherapists to withhold empathic statements, make unkind or untherapeutic comments, or otherwise act in a manner that diminished the likelihood of a successful treatment.

Also, the personal experiences of psychotherapists may influence their feelings toward suicidal patients. Almost half of Americans have known someone who has died from suicide (Feigelman et al., 2018), and there is no reason to think that psychotherapists differ from those of other Americans in this regard. The suicide decedent might have been a family member, friend, or a more casual acquaintance. Perhaps the suicide occurred long before the individual started training as a psychotherapist. Any feelings of anger, hurt, or compassion arising from the suicides encountered in their personal lives may influence how psychotherapists respond to a patient with suicidal thoughts.

Negative feelings toward suicidal patients may also be driven by pernicious prejudices that appear common in society. Historically, persons who died from suicide were vilified. Within the Christian tradition, they were denied burials in Christian cemeteries until the modern era. Dante assigned victims of suicide to a special place in Hell. In early Massachusetts, a stake was often driven through the hearts of suicide victims, and their property was confiscated. In parts of Europe, the bodies of suicide victims were mutilated. As the Enlightenment came and the education level of the population increased, these reactions to suicidal behavior began to change. In Colonial America, some juries refused to enforce the property confiscation rule against suicide decedents, representing the start of a societal shift toward more humane reactions to persons who died from suicide (Snyder, 2015).

Although today most religious leaders view suicide as evidence of mental illness and not moral culpability, negative attitudes toward suicidal patients continue, albeit in a less public or pernicious form. For example, Corrigan, Sheehan, Al-Khouja, and the Stigma of Suicide Research Team (2017) found that many members of the public viewed suicidal persons as weak, selfish, or cowardly. They often felt fear or anger toward them and would prefer to avoid them or use coercive methods to control them.

The belief that suicidal patients are cowardly is belied by the evidence. Some extremely valiant and courageous war heroes or law enforcement officers have died from suicide. The belief that suicidal patients are selfish is also belied by the evidence. Most of those who attempt suicide perceive themselves as a burden on others and believe that they are acting selflessly (Joiner, 2010).

The belief that no one can stop a patient "who *really* wants to die" assumes that the patient has a clear and consistent mental state, which is almost never the case. Every patient with suicidal thoughts that I ever saw in treatment was ambivalent about dying.

No well-trained psychotherapist would consider suicide (or any other mental illness) to be a manifestation of a moral weakness. Nevertheless, few of us are completely immune from the myths or negative stereotypes that pervade society. It is possible that some of us may still hold such views, at least on some level.

Myths about suicide may degrade the quality of care. The belief that suicidal patients are selfish cowards would appear to interfere with effective and compassion driven interventions. It is better to view suicidal individuals as worthy of compassion and assistance, the same as any other patient who seeks help.

The belief that no one can stop a patient who "really wants to die" could also degrade the quality of treatment. Psychotherapists can use this belief to absolve themselves from blame in case something goes wrong and a patient attempts suicide. Although the motive to avoid guilt is understandable, this belief may undercut the psychotherapists' confidence in their ability to help suicidal patients. As the noted suicidologist David Jobes (2016) stated, "While I cannot guarantee a nonfatal outcome, I can nevertheless provide *the best possible clinical care* to the suicidal patient" (p. 49, italics in the original).

On the one hand, some psychotherapists may over react to suicidal patients with fear and anxiety. This may be driven, in part, by a fear that the psychotherapists could be liable if a patient died or was hurt during a suicide attempt. But "concerns about responsibility could lead to repressive management decisions" (Waern, Kaiser, & Renberg, 2016, p. 1). Anxious psychotherapists may, for example, adopt a "better-safe-than-sorry" approach and select the most restrictive or conservative treatment options, such as a hospitalization, to reduce their own anxiety, even when a hospitalization might be clinically contraindicated. The problem is that the procedures identified as "safe" in the better-safe-than-sorry approach are not necessarily safe and may be iatrogenic.

On the other hand, some psychotherapists may overreact to suicidal patients with benevolent feelings. They may assume more responsibility for the patient than is warranted and overextend themselves. They may, for example, impulsively offer additional sessions at no charge, allow sessions to extend beyond the normal time limit with no clinical rationale for doing so, become lax at enforcing ordinary office policies concerning no-shows, and so on. Of course, nothing is inherently wrong with offering pro bono services or being flexible in scheduling, but these decisions need to be based on patient need, not on fear-driven impulses.

At times psychotherapists have even gone to patients' homes for psychotherapy sessions or allowed patients to visit them at their homes (Freedenthal,

2018). It is possible that sometimes these behaviors could be justified. But psychotherapists should identify a clinical reason why they loosened the boundaries. These behaviors can be clinically contraindicated if the psychotherapists have a "savior mentality" ("only I can save the patient") or assume total responsibility for the recovery of the patient. Although psychotherapists must assume the responsibility to offer competent treatment, no psychotherapist can assume full responsibility for whether a patient lives or dies.

Psychotherapists have told me that when they let go of a sense of total responsibility for the life of their patients, they felt less tense, more objective, and more effective with their patients. This is not an attitude of indifference; these psychotherapists never stopped caring for their patients. They only stopped concentrating on the areas where they had no control and concentrated more on the areas where they had some control.

Although it is harmful to overreact to suicidal patients, it is also harmful to underreact. Suicidal concerns need to be taken very seriously. Consider this case.

A Highly Suicidal Patient

A depressed woman made an emergency visit with a psychiatrist who dismissed her suicidal thoughts with a perfunctory statement that she "did not have the guts to do it." No follow-up appointment was made. The woman went home and took an overdose of drugs. Fortunately, her roommate came home unexpectedly and got the medical intervention needed to save her life.

Perhaps the dismissive reaction came from negative feelings toward the patient. As detailed in Chapter 5, it is inevitable that some psychotherapists will develop some negative feelings toward some patients. The optimal response is to acknowledge these feelings and try to understand their origins. These feelings may alert psychotherapists to changes that they may need to make in themselves, or they may alert psychotherapists to the dynamics of the patients that can help them better understand the case.

IDEATION-TO-ACTION THEORIES OF SUICIDE

Effective psychotherapists know what to do and why they are doing it. The "why-I-am-doing-it" is often as important as the "what-to-do." No textbook, no matter how comprehensive, can anticipate all the circumstances that may occur with suicidal patients. When I conduct workshops on suicide prevention, I tell the participants that if they always do everything that I recommend, they are probably doing something wrong. The same principle applies here. Readers will likely encounter situations where patient characteristics or contexts will require them to deviate from the usual protocol. But they should have a clinical rationale for their decisions, and the theories of suicide may help guide those decisions.

Over the years many theories have been proposed to explain suicide, including those that focus primarily on one factor such as psychache (Schneidman), despair (Maltsberger), or escape from self (Baumeister; see the review by Bongar & Sullivan, 2013). However, recent work has focused on more complex models that consider the interaction of several factors and that address the finding that the factors associated with suicidal thoughts may not necessarily be the same factors that are associated with suicide attempts (Klonsky, Qiu, & Saffer, 2017).

Theories that consider the suicidal ideation/suicidal attempt distinction are called *ideation-to-action theories*. These theories help organize the vast amount of literature on suicide and guide the assessment, management, and treatment of suicidal patients. We should not draw too fine a line between the different ideation-to-action theories (Kleiman, Liu, & Riskind, 2014). They build on each other, include common elements, and all give high weight to the transition from suicidal ideation to suicide attempt. The three ideation-to-action theories are the interpersonal theory (IPT) of suicide (Joiner, 2005), the integrated motivational–volitional (IMV) theory (O'Connor & Portzky, 2018), and the three-step theory (3ST; Klonsky & May, 2015).

Interpersonal Theory of Suicide

The IPT has an intuitive appeal to it and has inspired much research on suicide. It postulates that suicide occurs when patients (a) have a desire to die and (b) have acquired the capability to kill themselves. The desire and capability distinction is meaningful from both a research and clinical perspective.

The Desire to Die

The desire to die, typically reflected in suicide ideation, occurs because of thwarted (failed) belongingness or perceived burdensomeness. These states of mind are linked to social relationships. Those with thwarted belongingness feel lonely and lack reciprocally caring relationships. It is the perception that "one does not belong—the feeling that one is alienated from others and not an integral part of a family, circle of friends, or other valued group" (Joiner, 2010, p. 8). Sometimes the social isolation occurs when loved ones have died or moved away. At other times, it may arise from family conflicts that patients regret but see little prospect of changing. In addition, they may not identify with a larger group, such as a social club, local neighborhood, or a religious group.

Those with perceived burdensomeness believe that family members or others would be happier if they were to die. They hate themselves and believe that they are a liability to others. It is the perception that "one's existence burdens family, friends, and society" (Joiner, 2010, p. 7). Perceived burdensomeness sometimes occurs among individuals with serious physical illnesses especially if they have chronic pain or limitations in performing activities of daily living. Sometimes the news of a serious medical condition, such as dementia among younger adults, can increase a person's perception that they would be a burden to others. Of course, the issue for the patient is the perception of burdensomeness, and patients often misconstrue the extent to which they are a burden. Those who report high levels of perceived burden-someness tend to have poor relationships with friends and family members (Christensen, Batterham, Mackinnon, Donker, & Soubelet, 2014).

Thwarted belongingness and perceived burdensomeness appear to have underlying qualities of hopelessness (helplessness) and self-disgust or self-hate. It could be argued that hopelessness and self-disgust are implicit in perceived burdensomeness and thwarted belongingness. Perhaps they are, but it is beneficial to make the implicit dimensions explicit.

Hopelessness "refers to a cognitive style characterized by a tendency to make negative attributions about the cause, consequences, and self-implications of future events" (Ribeiro, Bodell, Hames, Hagan, & Joiner, 2013, p. 208), and it resembles pessimism (Wingate et al., 2006). According to Van Orden et al. (2010), it is hopelessness about thwarted belongingness and perceived burden-someness that is linked to suicide.

Hopelessness and suicide are linked (Ribeiro et al., 2013). Some evidence suggests that hope is a moderator (a variable that qualifies the relationship) between thwarted belongingness, perceived burdensomeness, and suicide. For example, Hagan, Podlogar, Chu, and Joiner (2015) found that perceived burdensomeness and thwarted belongingness only predicted suicide risk when hopelessness was also present. This makes intuitive sense. All of us may feel thwarted belongingness or perceived burdensomeness at one time or another. The difference is that suicidal persons believe that these feelings would never end. Anestis, Moberg, and Arnau (2014) found that hopelessness incrementally increased the risk of suicidal behavior in addition to perceived burdensomeness and thwarted belongingness. The link is so strong that Kleiman, Law, and Anestis (2014) suggested that hopelessness may be a distal cause of suicidal behavior, whereas perceived burdensomeness and thwarted belongingness are the more proximal causes.

This need not be a global sense of hopelessness; it could be hopelessness in areas of importance to the individual. For example, Tucker et al. (2018) found that thwarted belongingness and perceived burdensomeness were related to interpersonal hopelessness and not just global feelings of hopelessness.

Self-hatred or self-disgust may be especially important features of perceived burdensomeness in that persons may view themselves as having qualities that make them unlovable or undesirable to others. Self-disgust has no universally agreed-on definition, and it is sometimes used synonymously with self-hate, which is defined as

> an enduring dysfunctional and destructive self-evaluation, characterized by attributions of undesirable and defective qualities, a failure to meet perceived standards and values leading to feelings of inadequacy, incompetency, and worth-lessness. High levels of self-hatred are marked by low self-esteem, shame, self-blame or guilt, as well as a mental state of agitation, creating an experience of substantial, often unbearable, psychological and emotional turmoil. (Turnell, Fassnacht, Batterham, Calear, & Kyrios, 2019, p. 780)

Often, those who feel self-hatred or self-disgust assume that others feel the same way, thus leading them to withdraw from others.

Self-forgiveness, the apparent anecdote for self-disgust, moderated the relationship (effected the direction and magnitude of the relationship) between perceived burdensomeness and suicide (Tucker, Michaels, Rogers, Wingate, & Joiner, 2016). Self-compassion, especially a sense of common humanity with others, influenced the connection between negative life events and suicidal behavior in college students (Chang et al., 2017). The relationship between perceived burdensomeness and suicidality was strongest when self-forgiveness was low (Cheavens, Cukrowicz, Hansen, & Mitchell, 2016).

Acquired Capability
Suicide attempts occur when individuals have both a desire to die and the acquired capacity to kill themselves. *Acquired capability* refers to fearlessness of death and habituation to pain and suffering. Although many people may want to die, they do not act on this desire unless they also have acquired the capacity to kill themselves. The acquired capability for death may not be pathological in and of itself and may even be adaptive in some cases. For example, emergency department physicians may work more effectively if they are habituated to pain because of repeated exposure to the suffering of their patients. Or soldiers, police, or firefighters may be more effective if they have a reduced fear of death (Anestis, Law, et al., 2017).

A portion of this acquired capability is likely genetic, and perhaps some people with a genetic predisposition to fearlessness select themselves into risky occupations such as corrections, police work, or the military. Nonetheless, social experiences appear to play a role as there is a process, usually gradual, by which individuals habituate themselves to pain, illness, or injury; increase their pain tolerance; and erode the natural inhibitions against self-harm. This could occur if the patient were exposed to violence either as victims, witnesses, or perpetrators of interpersonal violence or exposed to pain and suffering because of serious illness or injury.

The opponent process theory may help explain how acquired capability gets strengthened. According to the opponent process theory, repeated exposure to the feared stimulus leads to an increase in the secondary response, whereas the primary stimulus remains stable (Van Orden et al., 2010). For example, patients who cut themselves may experience only a small amount of relief following the first cutting, but the relief may become amplified after repeated cuttings.

Acquired capability may help explain why suicide rates are higher across a wide range of groups that, on the surface, may appear to have little in common. Physicians, correctional officers, anorexics, sex workers, and patients with nonsuicidal self-injuries all have an elevated risk of suicide: They are used to seeing or experiencing pain, thus habituating themselves to suffering. It may also partially explain why those who have had multiple suicide attempts are more likely to die from suicide. Previous exposures to near death experiences habituates them to their own death. Joiner believes that the acquired capability for harm is relatively stable and slow to modify.

Evaluating the Interpersonal Theory of Suicide

Although all of the ideation-to-action theories have data supporting them, the vast majority of research has been conducted on the IPT of suicide and especially the role of perceived burdensomeness and thwarted belongingness, two concepts that are also incorporated into the other ideation-to-action theories. C. Chu, Buchman-Schmitt, et al. (2017) found support for both thwarted belongingness and perceived burdensomeness in predicting suicide, although an earlier review by Ma, Batterham, Calear, and Han (2016) found weaker evidence for thwarted belongingness. C. Chu, Buchman-Schmitt, et al. also found that the interaction of thwarted belongingness and perceived burdensomeness predicted suicide attempts better than either did alone. Nonetheless, they concluded that suicide may occur through mechanisms other than thwarted belongingness and perceived burdensomeness. Suicidal behavior is complex and multidetermined, and it is possible that one theory may have "more explanatory power for certain subsets of individuals" (Ma et al., 2016, p. 40). Perhaps thwarted belongingness strongly predicts suicidal behavior in some subpopulations but fails to do so in others.

A natural consequence of the IPT is that interventions for suicide should focus on reducing thwarted belongingness and perceived burdensomeness presumably through activities that improve social relationships, social skills, and problem-solving skills and to address the beliefs and attitudes that allow, reinforce, or give rise to feelings of thwarted belongingness and perceived burdensomeness.

Integrated Motivational–Volitional Theory

The IMV theory of suicidal behavior, which was developed by Rory O'Connor and colleagues (e.g., R. C. O'Connor & Portzky, 2018), builds on the IPT but includes more factors and focuses more on the transition from suicidal thoughts to suicide attempts. The IMV postulates three stages: premotivational, motivational, and volitional. During the premotivational stage, the patient has characteristics that make them vulnerable to suicidal thoughts. During the motivational stage, the patient develops suicidal thoughts, and during the volitional stage, the patient acts on those suicidal thoughts.

During the first stage (the premotivational stage), an individual is influenced by his or her environment, life events, and interpretation of these events and experiences. Those who have certain vulnerabilities such as poor coping skills, defective thought processes, or poor problem-solving skills will be disproportionately impacted by these experiences and events.

During the second stage (the motivational stage), an individual develops suicidal thoughts. These may arise if patients have certain interpretive styles involving perceived burdensomeness, thwarted belongingness, defeat, humiliation—and most important—entrapment. Defeat occurs when an individual has lost a struggle, feels powerless, and has lost social rank. Entrapment occurs "when the usual psychological motivation to escape threat or stress is blocked" (Siddaway, Taylor, Wood, & Schulz, 2015, p. 150).

During the third stage (volitional stage), an individual moves from thoughts to attempts. The factors involving the transition from suicidal ideation to suicidal attempt include acquired capability, planning for suicide, exposure to the suicidal behavior of other persons, having access to the means of killing oneself, previous suicidal behavior, and mental imagery about death.

There is a distinct movement from suicidal ideation (found in the motivational stage) to suicidal attempts (found in the volitional stage). The desire to escape defeat and entrapment is what drives suicidal behavior, and it is often fueled by ruminations (R. C. O'Connor & Portzky, 2018).

The IMV theory differs from the IPT in that it considers defeat and entrapment to be the key components of emotional pain. Entrapment is like the hopelessness that is implicit in the IPT of suicide, but it differs in that hopelessness does not necessarily "involve a motivation to escape or a sense of diminished status" (Siddaway et al., 2015, p. 150). Also, the IMV theory recognizes that perceived burdensomeness and thwarted belongingness have a role, but their role is only in contributing to the sense of defeat and humiliation.

Finally, the IMV expands on factors that move an individual from suicidal desire to suicidal behavior. Although the IPT postulates that acquired capability is the factor that moves an individual from desire to action, the IMV theory also includes defeat and entrapment, impulsivity, access to lethal means, planning, and social contagion as factors (Klonsky, Saffer, & Bryan, 2018).

The Three-Step Theory

The 3ST is the last ideation-to-action theory (Klonsky & May, 2015; May & Klonsky, 2016). The three steps are (a) the patient feels pain and hopelessness, (b) the pain is greater than the patient's sense of connectedness, and (c) the patient has acquired the capability of attempting suicide.

In the first step of this theory, an individual feels pain and hopelessness. Although pain can come from many sources, it is so pervasive that the suicidal individual wants to withdraw from life. Depression, anxiety, perceived burdensomeness, and thwarted belongingness are important insofar as they increase hopelessness and pain. Pain alone is not sufficient to lead to suicidal thoughts; instead, pain must be combined with a sense of hopelessness.

In the second step, the pain and hopelessness exceed or overwhelm an individual's connectedness. Although many people will endure great pain to protect loved ones or a cherished ideal, the pain that the individual feels has no such redeeming justification. They do not see their pain as promoting any worthwhile social goal because they do not feel that they are sufficiently attached or connected to loved ones (or to a project or value system), and they believe that they and others would be better off if they were dead (Klonsky & May, 2015). However, the 3ST theory allows for the possibility that many people without connectedness may never have suicidal thoughts and that some people may have suicidal thoughts even if they feel connected.

In the third and last step, suicidal behavior occurs when an individual acquires the capability of killing him- or herself, which may involve (a) dispositional or long-term traits, such as a consistent fearlessness about pain or death; (b) acquired factors, such as decreased fear of pain and death as postulated by the IPT of suicide; and (c) practical issues, such as access and familiarity with lethal means.

The 3ST differs from the IPT in that pain and hopelessness are the primary drivers of suicidal desire, although thwarted belongingness and perceived burdensomeness may be important insofar as they contribute to pain. Nonetheless, the pain can come from other sources than those two. It also differs in that the movement from suicidal desire to suicidal behavior occurs when acquired capability is combined with dispositional factors (e.g., a high threshold for pain, fearlessness of death) and access to lethal means. However, this last difference may be more an artifact of specificity than a substantive difference. For example, Joiner's treatment of suicide based on the IPT (Joiner, Van Orden, Witte, & Rudd, 2009) addresses elements found in the other theories involving means restriction and monitoring.

The Suicidal Mode

All the ideation-to-action theories postulate a transition from the desire to die (idea) to an attempt (action). The psychological state that precedes or accompanies the transition thus becomes a focus of attention for researchers and clinicians. The term *suicidal mode* might best describe that transition state. The concept of the suicide mode derives from the cognitive theory of suicide, but it appears that it can be integrated into the ideation-to-action theories of suicide. Predictions of suicide require looking not only at the distal factors that are statistically linked to a suicide attempt but also at the proximal factors that are statistically linked to a suicide attempt, including the likelihood that patients will develop a suicidal mode of thinking (Wenzel, Brown, & Beck, 2009).

According to cognitive behavior therapy, a *mode* refers to "an amalgam of unified and functionally synchronous cognitive, affective, motivational and behavioral systems" (Ghahramanlou-Holloway, Neely, & Tucker, 2015, p. 96). These four systems interact in response to an external event or by some internal thought or interpretation of a past event. Modes become problematic if they allow the faulty processing of information through selective processing, cognitive distortion, or defective problem-solving. Emotions can be problematic if the individual lacks the skills necessary to regulate them. The lack of behavioral skills, such as the lack of social skills necessary to repair strained relationships, can facilitate a downward spiral.

A suicidal mode could lead to a crisis state and suicidal behavior. The acute suicidal affective disturbance (ASAD) state discussed by Tucker, Michaels, et al. (2016) and the suicide crisis syndrome (SCS) discussed by Galynker (2018) describe the presuicide psychological state. The symptoms in the SCS overlap with those found in the ASAD in many ways (see the review of these states in Chapter 2). One might say that the goal of suicide assessment is to identify when a patient will enter in a crisis state, and the goal of suicide management and treatment is to prevent or short-circuit the crisis states.

The behaviors, thoughts, or feelings that occur in these crisis states can be used as warning signs to alert patients and psychotherapists when the risk of a suicide attempt becomes especially high. Warning signs are an important part of the assessment of suicide risk and are discussed in Chapter 2.

Applications of the Ideation-to-Action Theories

How could these theories be applied in real life to patients? Consider the patient Miguel who was introduced at the start of this chapter. This 28-year-old man has had suicidal thoughts, an apparent major depression, and access to means to kill himself.

On a practical level, the actual behavior of the psychotherapist working from either of these perspectives might differ little. Using the IPT of suicide, a psychotherapist would want to know the extent to which the patient has thwarted belongingness or perceived burdensomeness and acquired capability of dying. A focus would be on interpersonal relationships and implicitly on hopelessness and self-disgust. One would want to know the extent to which his recent job loss has led to perceived burdensomeness. It would also be indicated to learn the extent to which he feels thwarted belongingness. A thorough social history would result in obtaining information about acquired capability such as by interviewing concerning past exposures to suffering or violence or other experiences that indicate a fearlessness of death or habituation to pain and suffering.

Using the IMV theory of suicide, a psychotherapist would still look at perceived burdensomeness and thwarted belongingness. But the psychotherapist would also be alert for Miguel's sense of humiliation, defeat, and entrapment, which is caused by unbearable pain and hopelessness, at least in the sense that there is no way out of the situation. A question before the psychotherapist would be if the recent job loss and frustrations in finding a new job are perceived as humiliations or give Miguel a sense of entrapment. The psychotherapist would also look at the cognitive processes of rumination, deficient problem-solving, and so on. Nothing in the IPT would preclude looking at those factors, but the IMV theory would give them greater prominence.

Using the 3ST, a psychotherapist would again still look at thwarted belongingness and perceived burdensomeness and related feelings of hopelessness but would be especially sensitive to other sources of emotional pain and Miguel's sense of connection to others. The psychotherapist would be alert to when pain and hopelessness would overwhelm Miguel's feeling of connectedness.

In estimating Miguel's risk of a suicide attempt, it would be important to look at the transition from suicidal ideation to suicide attempt. Working within the IMV theory, a psychotherapist would be especially open to impulsivity, access to lethal weapons, planning for suicide attempts, and any social contagion effect. A psychotherapist working within the 3ST would look at the same features but would also consider dispositional factors such as one would find through interviewing—for example, a history of fearlessness or habituation to suffering.

All theories recognize that there is a psychological state that precedes the suicide attempt. The nature of the transitional psychological states leading to suicide would overlap considerably in each of the theories, although a psychotherapist working from the IPT would look at acquired capability. The IPT does not specifically identify planning, access to weapons, and so forth as essential components of the theory, but a reasonable psychotherapist working from the IPT would consider those factors as well. A psychotherapist using the IMV theory would be more alert to Miguel's feelings of humiliation, defeat, and entrapment, whereas a psychotherapist using the 3ST would look for more sources of pain and hopelessness and would be especially alert if the pain appeared to overwhelm his connectedness.

VALUES THAT GUIDE PROFESSIONAL BEHAVIOR

Psychotherapists and other moral agents need an overarching ethical system or set of ethical principles to justify their day-to-day (habitual) behaviors and to guide their decision-making (judicious) behavior when a reasonable course of action is not obvious. Every professional behavior should be based on, justified by, or anchored on an overarching ethical principle. Although some psychotherapists dichotomize problems as either clinical or ethical, that distinction is misleading. Every behavior has an ethical dimension to it. Sometimes the ethical dimension is so obvious or noncontroversial that the ethical dimensions of the action are taken for granted and never questioned. For example, the use of a structured interviewed protocol with a suicidal patient is a clinical act, but it is also an ethical act to the extent that it promotes patient well-being (reflecting the principle of beneficence).

Principle-Based Ethics

This book looks at ethical issues through the standpoint of principle-based ethics. According to principle-based ethics, moral agents (such as psychotherapists) should generally follow several overarching ethical principles. W. D. Ross (1930/1998), the founder of principle-based ethics, identified numerous principles such as fidelity, gratitude, beneficence, or self-improvement, although he gave his list "without claiming completeness or finality for it" (p. 269). Later, Beauchamp and Childress (2009) identified the moral principles that appeared most relevant to health care: beneficence (working to promote the well-being of patients), nonmaleficence (avoiding harming patients), respect for patient autonomy, justice, and faithfulness to the professional

relationship.[4] Later, Knapp and VandeCreek (2004) identified general beneficence (obligations to the public in general) as being salient as well.

These overarching ethical principles can be combined or spliced in different
ways without losing their value. For example, the General (aspirational)
Principles found in the *Ethical Principles of Psychologists and Code of Conduct*
(APA, 2017) are based on principle-based ethics, but the ethical principles
are categorized slightly differently than previously described. For example,
beneficence and nonmaleficence are combined into one principle.

As it applies to the assessment, management, and treatment of suicidal
patients, psychotherapists should promote patient well-being (beneficence)
by conducting a thorough assessment, adopting helpful suicide management
strategies, and delivering effective treatments. Psychotherapists should also
avoid harming their patients (nonmaleficence) by refraining from legalistic and
off-putting no-suicide contracts or adopting alarmist or dismissive attitudes.

Psychotherapists respect their patient's autonomy by establishing the goals
of treatment collaboratively, explaining the reasoning behind their recommendations, and involving patients in other decisions throughout the course
of treatment, such as when or how to involve family members in psychotherapy. Psychotherapists honor the promises that they make to their patients
(veracity or fidelity) by being honest with them about the nature and limits
of confidentiality or other office policies. Psychotherapists treat all patients
fairly (justice), regardless of race, religion, ability level, ethnicity, and so on.

Psychotherapists show general or public beneficence by attending to the
interests of persons other than their patients. An example of general beneficence would be when a psychotherapist includes helpful and accurate information in a public lecture or article about suicide. Although the members
in the audience or the readers of the article are not patients, but members
of the public, psychotherapists nonetheless have obligations to promote their
well-being by presenting accurate information. As it applies to treating suicidal
patients, general beneficence could refer to the obligations that psychotherapists
might have toward nonpatients such as family members or close friends of the
suicidal patient. Although psychotherapists need to show primary concern for
the well-being of their patients, they may consider the well-being of others in
their work with their patients.

Most of the applications of these principles are so obvious that psychotherapists seldom think about them. Rarely do psychotherapists say to themselves, "I am going to do a thorough assessment because the overarching
principle of beneficence requires me to do so." However, psychotherapists can
improve the quality of patient care if they strive to base their professional
behavior on the overarching ethical principles.

Considerations of overarching ethical principles appear to have been a factor,
at least implicitly, in the development of newer interventions. For example,

---

[4]Early works by Beauchamp and Childress (e.g., 1994) did not identify faithfulness
to the relationship, although Kitchener (1984) proposed this principle earlier.

Jobes (2016) based the Collaborative Assessment and Management of Suicide approach, an evidence-based protocol to assess and manage suicide, on certain overarching ethical principles such as respect for patient autonomy (through its emphasis on a collaborative approach and "directly solicit[ing] patient input into their treatment plan" [p. 4]), fidelity (through its emphasis on "direct and respectful honesty" [p. 4] with patients), and beneficence and nonmaleficence (through its focus on empathy and avoidance of any behavior that blames or shames a patient; Jobes, 2016). Similarly, the interventions recommended by Joiner et al. (2009) that focus on patient self-determination and involve patients in a team approach are anchored by the overarching ethical principles of respect for patient autonomy, beneficence, and nonmaleficence, even if the authors had not framed their innovations in terms of principle-based ethics.

Ethical principles can also help psychotherapists make decisions when the benefits and risks of options are not clear. Sometimes ethical principles will collide so that psychotherapists will not be able to fulfill one moral principle without violating another. Fortunately, principle-based ethics provides a decision-making format to guide psychotherapists in those situations. Good ethical decisions are made when psychotherapists stop, think, and reflect carefully before they engage in any action that appears to violate an overarching ethical principle.

Psychotherapists can act with more confidence when they can identify overarching ethical principles to justify their behavior. Nonetheless, how psychotherapists implement these principles depends partially on their personality and contextual influences. For example, psychotherapists ordinarily respect patient autonomy. However, one could imagine that some psychotherapists may temporarily allow their fear of a patient suicide to override their normal ethical inclinations and lead them to emphasize beneficence (protecting the life of a patient) so much that they inadvertently become paternalistic or overbearing toward a patient. Ironically some paternalistic actions based on misguided notions of beneficence may increase the risk of a suicide. This illustrates the importance of self-awareness. As noted in Cramer et al.'s (2013) list of competencies, part of being an effective psychotherapist involves the ability to monitor one's feelings and reflect on one's behavior (self-reflection is discussed in more detail in Chapter 5).

Should Psychotherapists Intervene?

Some graduate students may ask, with complete sincerity, whether they have the ethical obligation or right to try to persuade suicidal individuals to live. They may claim that beneficence (promoting the well-being of the patients) may sometimes conflict with respect for patient autonomy. The obligation of psychotherapists to ensure the life and safety of their patients may appear to run counter to the rights of patients to make the important decision about whether they will live. The inquiring graduate student may claim that, in some cases, psychotherapists should give priority to respect for patient autonomy over beneficence, and they should respect or even support, the wishes of patients who say that they want to die. This perspective has many limitations to it, although many believe that there is a limited window for rational suicide under narrow conditions.[5] A response requires understanding the nature of suicide and a bioethical perspective on health care.

Suicide is an atypical act that flies against the natural evolutionary tendency toward self-preservation. All suicidal patients who enter the offices of a psychotherapist have some part of them that wants to live. If not, why would they be there? If they were completely convinced beyond any doubt that suicide was the best solution, why would they bother to stop by to see their psychotherapists? Patients can always kill themselves if they want to. They can leave the treatment room, look up lethal doses of drugs on the Internet, go to a drugstore and buy over-the-counter medication, make a lethal milkshake, and drink it. Except for very limited circumstances (e.g., when a highly suicidal patient has revealed sufficient information to justify an involuntary civil commitment to a psychiatric hospital), patients can get up and leave any time they want to. And if patients really want to die, they certainly would not have told their psychotherapists of their intention and given psychotherapists the option of initiating an involuntary hospitalization. One might say that these patients are "trumping their own autonomy" (M. Recendez, personal communication, July 19, 2018). Therefore, if patients are exercising their free will to stay in the office with their psychotherapists, then psychotherapists can assume that some part of them wants to live.

Also, suicidal behavior almost always occurs in the context of a mental illness and intense emotions that inhibit rational thought.[6] Most patients who have attempted suicide expressed relief that they did not die, and the suicidal thoughts usually dissipate or at least substantially diminish once the acute suicidal episode begins to lift. More than 90% of persons who attempted suicide will eventually die from causes other than suicide, suggesting that the suicidal crises do not represent a well-thought-out or long-term goal on their part (M. Miller & Hemenway, 2008). Even if we assume the hypothetical that the patient "really wants to die," according to principle-based ethics, one may temporarily override patient autonomy when it conflicts with another overarching ethical principle (examples are given in Chapter 3).

How Should Psychotherapists Intervene?

Although the principle of respect for patient autonomy can be misapplied when considering whether psychotherapists can intervene with suicidal patients,

---

[5]Rational suicide is a complex topic beyond the scope of this book. Most psychotherapists know little about this area of practice. If they encounter a patient with a painful and terminal disease who expresses a will to die that appears rational, I recommend that the psychotherapists seek consultation.

[6]Controversy exists considering the relative role of mental illness and suicide. This issue is discussed in detail in Chapter 3.

it is often underappreciated when considering how to manage and intervene with suicidal patients. That is, patients should control as much of their treatment as is clinically feasible. Decisions about suicide assessments, management, and interventions should involve the patients as much as possible. In addition, empowered collaboration (active involvement of the patient in treatment) is one of the essential quality enhancement (risk management strategies) discussed in Chapter 5.

Furthermore, the importance of patient collaboration finds support in self-determination theory (SDT; Ryan & Deci, 2008). SDT has identified autonomy, competence, and relatedness as key factors in leading a fulfilling life. According to SDT, these are fundamental and intrinsic motivators of human behavior. That is, people will work to seek autonomy, strive for competence, or look to affiliate with other persons, without any extrinsic motivation. According to SDT, people have a natural tendency toward psychological growth, but these drives can be thwarted by especially harsh environments that lead to frustration and defensiveness. Patients may feel frustrated if their autonomy, competency, and affiliation needs are not met (Ryan & Deci, 2008). Conversely, patients will feel more invested in treatment if it addresses autonomy, competence, and affiliation needs.

Because of the emphasis on patient autonomy, psychotherapists should seldom override patient decisions in terms of hospitalization, when to disclose patient information without their consent (break confidentiality), how to implement means safety plans, ways to involve family members, topics of psychotherapy, and other issues. But in rare circumstances it could be justified to give a higher priority to beneficence (promoting the well-being of the patient) over that of respecting patient autonomy. Chapter 3 goes through the decision-making process involved when those situations arise.

Some psychotherapists tend to become paternalistic and adopt a low threshold for overriding respect for patient autonomy out of a fear that the patient will die from suicide unless they do so. They may be influenced by a *righting reflex*, which is "the desire to fix what seems wrong with people and to set them promptly on a better course, relying in particular on directing" (W. R. Miller & Rollnick, 2013, p. 6).

However, those who work effectively with suicidal patients know that some healthy part of them wants to live. For example, Joiner et al. (2009) identified the "ultimate self-determination by clients" combined with "a sense of togetherness" and "openness about all aspects of treatment" (p. 146) as key ingredients for the effective treatment of suicidal patients. Psychotherapists can promote this respect by ensuring that they understand the perspectives of the patient, offer them choices, and give them rationales for the recommendations made (Joiner et al., 2009). More information on respecting patient autonomy is provided in Chapters 3 and 5.

2

Screening and Assessment

The first job of psychotherapists is to identify patients at risk for suicide and, if the risk of suicide is present, to conduct a more thorough evaluation. The ways that the screening and assessment processes play out in real life are illustrated in the following vignette, a situation with a patient named Mary.

An Initial Evaluation

A psychotherapist is having her first appointment with a new patient, Mary, a 22-year-old college student about whom she has limited information. All she knows about the patient comes from a brief phone call in which she learned that the patient has insurance coverage (the psychologist is in network) and the general presenting problem is "sadness following a romantic break-up." The patient has completed a background form and is bringing that into the intake session with her today. Mary is well dressed, attractive, and spoke optimistically about her plans when she expects to graduate from college. The initial impression is that Mary has an adjustment disorder with a depressed mood and would only need brief supportive psychotherapy.

A lot of information needs to be covered in the initial session, which, for this psychotherapist, typically lasts 90 minutes. Psychotherapists need to give out the Privacy Notice, go over office policies, get a grasp of the problems that the patient considers important, create a diagnostic impression, and start treatment. Given the demographics and the appearance of this patient, one could easily feel tempted to skip asking any questions about suicidal thoughts. After all, suicide rates are lower for women and especially women with a college education. A lesser trained psychotherapist might have assumed that

http://dx.doi.org/10.1037/0000145-003
Suicide Prevention: An Ethically and Scientifically Informed Approach, by S. J. Knapp

she was not suicidal because she had spoken so optimistically about college and had other positive aspects in her life. But this psychotherapist is well trained and understands the importance of screening for suicide with every patient. As it turns out, Mary has suicidal thoughts. She has no past attempts, but she has a plan how she would do it. The thoughts are infrequent, but they are upsetting and hard for her to interrupt. Further interviewing reveals that she feels socially isolated, does not sleep well, and recently started to cut herself, and her conversation was peppered with negative self-references.

After screening for suicidal thoughts, the next step for this psychotherapist is to assess the risk of suicide. This chapter walks readers through the steps necessary for psychotherapists to screen and assess patients for suicide risk.

DEFINING SCREENING AND ASSESSMENT

Screening and assessing are overlapping but distinct activities. The goal of screening is to identify patients who have suicidal thoughts. The primary goals of assessment are to estimate the risk that the patient will die from suicide and to gather information that will inform suicide management and treatment strategies. Other goals of assessment are to (a) label or describe the patient's presenting problem, (b) establish a baseline of patient functioning that psychotherapists can use to measure progress, and (c) build a trusting and productive relationship. To conduct a good assessment, psychotherapists must demonstrate the relevant competencies identified by Cramer, Johnson, McLaughlin, Rausch, and Conroy (2013), which are to elicit information on current suicidal plans, acquire information that will help inform collaboratively made management and treatment plans, and develop an empathic and collaborative relationship with their patients.

The assessment of suicidal patients is inherently difficult. Suicides involve psychological, social, and biological dimensions that interact in complex ways. No single test, checklist, or set of questions can lead to an objective score that will definitively identify those who will attempt suicide. Ideally, one should be able to estimate the risk of suicide on the basis of some objective behavioral or physiological marker. However, that is not the case at least so far. Ultimately, risk estimates depend highly on the self-report of patients, which is an inherently flawed source of data.

In addition, unexpected events could confound the best estimate. Although population-wide predictions can identify the number of persons at risk to die from suicide, individual estimates require an understanding of an individual's history and current life situation. Finally, the risk of a suicide can sometimes change rapidly, depending on external and internal factors (J. C. Fowler, 2012). However, the lack of precision in predicting suicide does not mean that clinicians have nothing to assist them. A body of literature based on research and professional experience can help professionals in this task.

Here is an overview of the assessment process. This chapter describes each of these steps in more detail. After patients have been screened and identified as having some suicidal risk, psychotherapists should interview patients and follow three steps:

- Obtain more detailed information about current suicidal thoughts, past suicide attempts, or current suicide plans (if any).

- Identify the warning signs. Gather information about the feelings, thoughts, and behaviors that occur when patients enter a suicidal crisis state.

- Look for themes related to suicide. Accrue details about the patient's life experiences, life change and chronic stressors, social relationships, physical health, mental illness and psychological health, and religion and values.

Psychotherapists could also add a fourth step of using a brief symptom inventory.

As it would apply to Mary, the patient in the vignette at the beginning of this chapter, the psychotherapist would need to follow the three steps delineated previously. First, the psychotherapist would need to understand more about Mary's suicidal thoughts and whether she has had past suicide attempts or has plans for future suicide attempts. Second, the psychotherapist would need to identify warning signs, or the behaviors, feelings, motivations, thoughts, and reactions that would indicate that she was at risk for a suicide attempt. Third, the psychotherapist would need to gather more information about her life history and life circumstances. Finally, the psychotherapist has the option of using a brief symptom inventory to supplement the diagnostic impression, to monitor progress in treatment over time, or because there is a concern that she is a *false denier*, or a person with suicidal thoughts or behaviors who denies them.

The interpersonal theory (IPT) of suicide and other idea-to-action theories can guide psychotherapists on the themes to look for during these interviews. The psychotherapist working with Mary can look for themes of perceived burdensomeness; thwarted belongingness; acquired capability; hopelessness; defeat; entrapment; and other feelings, thoughts, or behaviors. Special attention will be paid to the circumstances that could cause Mary to move from suicidal ideation to a suicide attempt. Information on how to synthesize the data to estimate suicide risk and create informed management and treatment plans are covered in Chapter 3. Exhibit 2.1 shows the sequence of the steps from screening to treatment.

Throughout the assessment, psychotherapists should conduct the interviews collaboratively and respectfully, and convey caring for the patients and an interest in their well-being. The goal is to try to understand the patient's situation from the standpoint of the patient. After the assessment has ended, patients should feel as if they had the chance to tell their stories. Relationship building is so important that it begins the discussion on screening and assessment.

EXHIBIT 2.1

Steps From Screening to Invention

Chapter 2
  Screen for risk of suicide

  Assess patients

   Step 1: Ideation, attempts, and plans (feelings, thoughts, circumstances associated
      with suicidal ideation, past attempts, or future plans)

   Step 2: Warning signs, especially informed by research on suicide crisis states, such as
      the acute suicide affective disorder

   Step 3: Life circumstances and history: look at the patient's history, life stressors
      or changes, health, social relationships, mental illnesses, and value systems
      guided by the themes found in the ideation-to-action theories of suicide

   Step 4: (optional): Using brief symptom inventories

Chapter 3
  Assess risk of suicide

  Develop safety and other suicide management plans

Chapter 4
  Treatment of conditions leading to suicidal behavior

THE RELATIONSHIP IN THE SCREENING AND ASSESSMENT PROCESS

Developing a good treatment relationship is one of the goals of the assessment and one of the core competencies in working with suicidal patients as
identified by Cramer et al. (2013). How psychotherapists ask about suicide
can be as important as what they ask. The process of interviewing can be as
important as the information obtained. A good relationship increases the likelihood that psychotherapists will get accurate information and therefore will
be more likely to make good decisions.

   In addition, successful suicide management and treatment plans require
a good treatment relationship. It is easy to lose sight of the relationship
when trying to cover many issues concerning the immediate risk of suicide.
Inexperienced clinicians may focus too much on the mechanics of assessment and under appreciate the importance of developing a good relationship.
Many psychotherapists are understandably anxious when treating suicidal
patients, but they should not let their anxiety disrupt their efforts to build
a productive relationship. The optimal attitude is to display a stance of
"curiosity, concern, and calm acceptance" (J. C. Fowler, 2012, p. 87).

   One of the primary goals in the initial meeting is to get the suicidal patient
to come back. Nonetheless, data on the failure to seek treatment showed
that only half of the persons with suicidal ideation in the past year sought treatment (I. H. Stanley, Hom, & Joiner, 2015), and those who failed to get treatment were more likely to be Hispanic or Black, or male. Extrapolations from
the data suggest that many men or persons who are Hispanic or Black enter

treatment with more ambivalence. This points to the importance of working with men who may perceive that discussions of personal problems are a sign of weakness. It may point to the importance of working with Hispanic or Black patients who may have a greater distrust of health care professionals or who have more difficulty connecting with a White or non-Hispanic psychotherapist. Sometimes it can be indicated to say directly to patients, "Am I understanding you correctly?" "Have I gotten this correct?" or "Tell me if I understand you correctly." If they sense that their patients feel ambivalence about continuing in treatment, psychotherapists can say, "I want you to come back next week," or ask them, "Do you feel ambivalent about coming back for another appointment?" or "Do you think you will come back for the next appointment?" and then ask them why they gave their response.

As discussed earlier in this chapter, patients who express suicidal thoughts are in great emotional distress, and they may feel relief if they can talk about their feelings without shame. The stigma and shame associated with mental illness and suicidality are common impediments to seeking or staying with treatment (Alonzo, Moravec, & Kaufman, 2017; J. Han, Batterham, Calear, & Randall, 2018). Shame tends to impede therapeutic progress and contributes to suicidality through self-punishment and concealment. The nonjudgmental behavior of the psychotherapist during the assessment will reduce the shame and expedite patient recovery. Ideally, patients will eventually think of their suicidal thoughts with the same nonjudgmental attitude that they would think of a broken leg or a bout of the flu (Ellis & Newman, 1996).

The interviewer should be respectful, nonjudgmental, and caring. "It is essential that the suicidal patient actually *feel* well understood" (Jobes, 2012, p. 641; italics in original). Often it is appropriate to say, "Thank you for sharing those thoughts with me" when patients first reveal their suicidal ideation. Psychotherapists should attempt to validate patients' feelings and emotional pain. This does not mean endorsing the idea of suicide but allowing patients to feel that their suffering has been understood and accepted (Schechter & Goldblatt, 2011). Ideally, at the end of the session, patients will feel that they had a chance to tell their stories and that their psychotherapists cared about them (Meichenbaum, 2005).

This nonjudgmental and caring attitude facilitates disclosure among patients and helps them to sort out their thoughts and feelings. Often patients experience many painful emotions and disturbing thoughts that seemingly appear without provocation and are hard to understand. Good interviewing, over time, will help patients find patterns or coherence to these feelings and thoughts.

A good relationship also increases the willingness of patients to adhere to the treatment program ("conforms to the directives from a clinician"; Alonzo et al., 2017, p. 158). More important, a good relationship will help patients do more than just adhere to directives, but also to engage in treatment that Alonzo et al. (2017) defined as occurring when "a person is involved in a process through which he incorporates practical wisdom and advice in accordance with his needs, preferences, and capabilities in order to improve mental health outcomes" (p. 158). The vignette that follows describes how important a good treatment relationship will be.

A Motivated Patient

I had a patient with whom I worked hard to help him accept a voluntary psychiatric hospitalization. I spent a lot of time listening to him and trying to understand his story. While in the hospital, he made substantial progress. Before he transferred to an outpatient substance abuse program, he said, "You took the time to listen to me. you helped me when I could not help myself, and now I am going to help myself *and others.*"

It is hard to overemphasize the importance of a caring relationship. Many patients reported that they refrained from attempting suicide because they knew that their psychotherapist cared about them.

SCREENING FOR SUICIDE

Psychotherapists should screen all mental health patients over the age of 12 for suicidal risks using both a written and verbal question. There may be some exceptions, however. Psychologists do not need to screen clients who are receiving psychological services unrelated to health care, such as career counseling or life coaching. Psychotherapists working with medical patients should screen all of them with a written question and, if there is a suspicion of mental illness, include a verbal question as well. These recommendations attempt to balance the need to identify patients with a risk of suicide with the need to avoid mandate creep, or a tendency to mandate more and more screening procedures with less and less likelihood of promoting patient care.

Settings Involved Only in the Treatment of Mental Illness

Psychotherapists should routinely assess all new mental health patients over the age of 12 for thoughts of suicide. Many people, especially African Americans, will not volunteer information about suicidal thoughts unless they are asked directly (Morrison & Downey, 2000). Psychotherapists will be more likely to identify suicidal patients if they include both a written question on suicide as well as asking the patient directly about suicide. Regardless of the patient's response to the written question about suicide, psychotherapists should ask about suicide again during the first interview or as soon as feasible. Appendix A includes a sample patient information form that patients can receive and complete before their first treatment appointment. This sample form includes a third question about suicide taken from the Patient Health Questionnaire—9 (PHQ–9).[1] Psychotherapists should feel free to modify this form, including

---

[1]The Patient Health Questionnaire—9 or PHQ–9 may be found at http://www.phqscreeners.com/sites/g/files/g10016261/f/201412/PHQ-9_English.pdf. No permission is required to reproduce, translate, display or distribute.

the wording of the question about suicide. Experienced psychotherapists have given examples where asking a patient about suicide might have been contraindicated, so the general rule of asking every patient may have some exceptions.

Various authorities have emphasized the importance of asking about suicidal thoughts with patients receiving mental health services (e.g., *The Guidelines for the Psychiatric Evaluation of Adults* [J. J. Silverman et al., 2015] and recommendations of the Joint Commission, 2016).[2] Unfortunately, 30% or more of psychotherapists do not routinely ask patients about suicidal behavior (Hom, Stanley, Gutierrez, & Joiner, 2017; Roush et al., 2018).

Settings Not Involved in the Delivery of Health Care

Psychologists and other professionals do not need to routinely assess for suicide when delivering services unrelated to the assessment or treatment of mental illness. Such activities could include educational testing (except when social or emotional disturbance was a focus on the evaluation), testing for job performance, career counseling, or life or executive coaching. The rate of suicide among these clients is probably not higher than that of the population in general. Of course, psychologists can ask the clients about suicide if they show behaviors or express ideas that raise the suspicion that they may have a risk of suicide. However, there is no reason to routinely screen for suicide with such clients.

Settings Involved in Both Physical and Mental Health Care

Many psychotherapists work in settings that serve medical patients, although they may be called health psychologists or behavioral health psychologists in such settings. The decision to screen medical patients is influenced by institutional and regulatory concerns and by clinical need.

Institutional or Agency Practitioners

Some psychotherapists work for institutions that have policies on suicide screening influenced by the recommendations from the Joint Commission or incentives from Medicare's Merit-Based Incentive Payment Systems (MIPS) program, the federal quality incentive program. The Joint Commission's (2016) *Sentinel Alert* recommends that its facilities "screen all patients for suicide ideation using a brief, standardized, evidence-based screening tool" (p. 3) and then recommends several options including the PHQ–9. There is also the option of modifying the Patient Health Questionnaire—2 (PHQ–2) by adding a question about suicide. The PHQ–2 serves the same screening function as the PHQ–9, except that it is only two items.

---

[2]The Joint Commission is a nonprofit voluntary accrediting association for hospitals and other health care organizations.

In addition, large institutions may have practical reasons for using the PHQ–9. Institutions or agencies that participate in MIPS can gain bonus payments or avoid payment penalties according to the frequency with which they perform and report certain activities called *measures*. One measure (134—screening for depression) permits professionals to use either the Beck Depression Inventory (BDI)[3] (Beck, Steer, & Brown, 1996) or the PHQ–9. Another measure (411—depression in remission) requires professionals to use the PHQ–9. For these agencies, this practical consideration appears to override other considerations in the choice of screening instruments. It does not appear practical to use additional screening instruments for suicide if they are already using the PHQ–9 or BDI to fulfill MIPS standards. Although MIPS only applies to Medicare patients, many facilities find it easier to have one standardized screening instrument for all adults. Fortunately, the PHQ–9 has value in assessing suicide. Those who identify suicide risk on the PHQ–9 are far more likely to attempt suicide than those who do not identify such risk (G. E. Simon et al., 2013). The BDI similarly helps identify the risk for suicide (Runeson et al., 2017).

Solo or Small Group Practitioners

Many psychotherapists who treat patients with serious medical concerns do not work for large institutions who follow Joint Commission recommendations or who are exempt from MIPS because they see a low volume of Medicare patients. Some of these psychologists conduct traditional psychotherapy, but others provide more targeted interventions for patients with no psychopathology. These psychotherapists who do not have to comply with a Joint Commission or Medicare policy would have more flexibility in deciding how to screen for suicide.

This book recommends asking all medical patients about suicide at least once in a written question and following up with a verbal question if the patient has a mental disorder or has a high risk of developing a mental disorder. Medical conditions and mental disorders are linked. About 68% of adults with mental disorders have medical conditions, 29% of adults with medical conditions have mental disorders, and 17% of adults have comorbid mental and medical disorders (Druss & Walker, 2011). A medical disorder can place a patient at risk to develop a mental disorder or exacerbate an existing one. For example, a patient with diabetes complications may become depressed because she has restricted mobility and becomes socially isolated. Also, a mental disorder can place a patient at risk for developing a medical condition or exacerbating an existing one. For example, a patient with diabetes might get worse because the depression keeps him from following through with the

---

[3]The Beck Depression Inventory is a brief instrument used to measure depression. The copyright is held by Pearson Assessments.

medical regimen.[4] Finally, some medical and mental disorders have common risk factors. The example of diabetes applies here as well because both diabetes and depression are more common among patients who report a history of adverse childhood events or who have a lower socioeconomic status.

A comorbid mental disorder is more common with patients who have heart disease, cancer, dementia, diabetes, or traumatic brain injury. A recent diagnosis of a serious illness increases the risk of suicide. Other patients of concern include postpartum women, those who have chronic pain or extreme functional limitations, and those with poor sleep quality including insomnia and nightmares. Other disorders that are statistically linked to an increased risk of suicide in some studies include patients with asthma, epilepsy, osteoporosis, or skin disorders such as eczema or psoriasis (e.g., Erlangsen, Stenager, & Conwell, 2015; Fässberg et al., 2016; Kavalidou, Smith, & O'Connor, 2017; R. T. Webb et al., 2012).

In evaluating the decision concerning screening, psychotherapists need to balance the benefits of asking about suicide with the burden it places in terms of time and documentation requirements. On the one hand, one could argue against routine screenings for all medical patients because most of these patients do not need psychological services, and many of those who receive psychological services receive short-term and focused interventions that are unrelated or tangentially related to mental health. Psychologists in integrated care settings may encounter patients with a very low risk of suicide such as a mother who is having problems toilet training her child or a patient who is learning relaxation to control Raynaud's disease. These will be billed under the health and behavior codes, indicating a medical condition as the focus of treatment. Of course, psychologists can decide to ask any patient about suicide if circumstances warrant. On the other hand, one could argue for requiring such screenings for all medical patients because many patients who have died from suicide had seen a health care professional in the month before they died and often that health care professional had either failed to ask or failed to detect suicidal intent (Ribeiro et al., 2017).

This book recommends a balanced approach consistent with the Joint Commission (2016) recommendation to screen all medical patients for suicidal thoughts with a written question or a very brief screening instrument. If the psychologists believe these patients have a mental illness or show risk factors for a mental illness, they can supplement the written question(s) with a verbal question. As with patients with mental health problems, there may be situations where the psychologist could give a clinical reason not to ask about suicide. In screening patients, psychologists could consider the PHQ–9 (or the PHQ–2 modified by including the PHQ–9 question about suicide) or simply

---

[4]In this and in other short examples in this book, the assignment of the gender to the hypothetical patients is arbitrary and has no clinical significance.

adding their own question about suicide, such as "Have you ever had thoughts of killing yourself?"

ASSESSMENT STEP 1: ASKING ABOUT SUICIDE

As soon as a patient states that they have had thoughts of suicide, the assessment process beings. The next steps are to gather information on the nature of and circumstances surrounding the suicidal thoughts, any past suicide attempts, and any plans for future suicide attempts.

Asking About Suicidal Thoughts

The screening process categorizes patients as either having a risk of suicide or not having a risk of suicide. The schema works well for most patients. However, psychotherapists may be unable to confidently categorize other patients because they give conflicting information in their self-reports or show risk factors inconsistent with what one would expect given the patient's self-report of their suicidal risk. It is appropriate to give special attention to these patients.

The first step would be to look at the patient's responses to the written question or questions about suicide. Written questions will identify some suicidal patients who would not be identified by interviewer questions alone (Louzon, Bossarte, McCarthy, & Katz, 2016). Also, interviewer questions will identify some patients who would not be identified by the written question alone. Of course, there may be some initial overidentification. For example, Hom, Joiner, and Bernert (2016) found that about 40% of undergraduates who reported having a suicide attempt in a printed survey did not report a suicide attempt in a follow-up interview. Perhaps they took an expanded definition of a suicide attempt or were too quick in responding. Nonetheless, the benefits of having both a written and a verbal question appear to outweigh the downside.

Part of the problem with written questions may rest in their wording. For example, the relevant question on the PHQ–9 asks, "Have you had thoughts that you would be better off dead or of hurting yourself in some way for at least several days in the last two weeks?" So, this question asks about both active and passive suicidal thoughts ("You would be better off dead"), includes nonsuicidal self-injury (NSSI; "hurting yourself"), adopts a threshold of having the thoughts for "at least several days," and restricts the time frame to "the last two weeks" (Berman & Silverman, 2017). This is not to denigrate the usefulness of using this question, only to note that this question, like other written questions, has some limitations. Regardless of the patient's response to the written form, psychotherapists should follow up with a verbal question on suicide as soon as feasible.

Of course, some patients may not develop a risk of suicide until after treatment has already started. The patients may have accurately enough denied suicidal ideation during the initial interview. But sometimes harsh intervening events can precipitate suicidal thoughts in a patient who did not have them at the start of treatment. If suicidal thoughts emerge during treatment, psychotherapists should elicit the same information about suicide as found with new patients.

The Initial Question About Suicidal Ideation

This section presents questions to ask patients about suicidal thoughts and explains why asking these questions is important. Psychotherapists should not assume that patients will reveal suicidal thoughts on their own. Some may be reluctant to reveal such thoughts because of shame. For other patients, suicidal thoughts might not be their major concern at the time they entered treatment. Data from the Center for Collegiate Mental Health (2018) are instructive here. Although 9.5% of students seeking counseling identified suicidality as a concern, only 1.5% identified suicidality as their primary concern. This suggests that patients might come in and identify their primary issue as depression, anxiety, relationship problems, and so on, even though suicidal thoughts may have been lurking in the background.

It is recommended that psychotherapists ask their patients if they ever had suicidal thoughts (e.g., "Have you ever had thoughts of suicide?"), followed up, if appropriate, with a question about current thoughts (e.g., "Have you had thoughts of suicide in the past 2 weeks?" "Do you currently have thoughts of suicide?").

Psychotherapists should modify the exact wording to suit their own style, but they should avoid using negative wording such as "You're not going to kill yourself, are you?" (Berman & Silverman, 2017). Negative phrasing tacitly encourages patients to deny suicidal thoughts (Quinnett, 2018). Psychotherapists should also avoid euphemisms ("Do you feel like you will do harm to yourself?"). Harming oneself through an NSSI is an important clinical symptom, but the goal here is to discern the extent of the thought of suicide, not thoughts of NSSIs. When patients indicate suicidal thoughts on the screening instrument, psychotherapists can ask them about their suicidal thoughts early in the interview because it allows psychotherapists to spend the rest of therapeutic time discussing those thoughts, if necessary.

When patients do not indicate suicidal thoughts on the screening instrument, psychotherapists can ask them about the suicidal thoughts later in the interview. Some patients are slow to open up because of embarrassment or anxiety. For such patients, psychotherapists may delay asking the question about suicide until they have spent more time with their patients to develop better rapport. Bryan and Rudd (2006) recommended asking the patients about their life in general and, after a discussion on that broad topic, move into symptoms, then to thoughts of wanting to die, and finally to the questions on suicide. They believe that this sequence will allow time for psychotherapists to build rapport with their patients and to normalize any feelings of suicide by placing them in context.

Cultural factors may be relevant here. Takahashi (1997), for example, recommended approaching the topic of suicide with Japanese patients indirectly by asking about stressors, sense of personal worth, and visions for the future. Many Asian patients will deny suicidal thoughts because they consider such thoughts to be shameful but will acknowledge being very fatigued and without the energy to complete daily tasks (J. Chu, Khoury, et al., 2017). Similarly, patients from Muslim cultures are very reluctant to admit to suicidal thoughts given the gravity of the sin of suicide in Islam. It is appropriate, however, to ask them about thoughts of death.

Asking about suicide does not increase the likelihood that it will happen (K. M. Harris & Goh, 2017). In fact, just talking about it might reduce suicidal risks (Dazzi, Gribble, Wessely, & Fear, 2014). The idea that a psychotherapist who asks about suicide will implant the idea of suicide in the head of a patient is about as reasonable as the idea that a neurologist who asks about migraine headaches will implant migraine headaches into the head of a patient (Joiner, 2010).

If the patients deny any current suicidal thoughts, do not report suicidal thoughts in their answers to the initial printed questions given to them, and have no other high-risk factors for suicide, then psychotherapists can discontinue questions about suicide and proceed with the regular intake. Usually "no" means "no" and pursuing the issue unnecessarily will only divert psychotherapists from the real presenting problems of their patients.

If patients showed a discrepancy between their verbal and written responses to questions about suicide, then it is appropriate to ask them the reason for the discrepancy. "Can you help me understand why you gave different responses to these questions?" Sometimes the reasons for the discrepancy are benign, such as the patient read the question too quickly and responded incorrectly. Other patients may have idiosyncratic reasons for their responses. Some may respond "no" to the question about suicidal thoughts because they are so good at suppressing the suicidal thoughts that they believe the thoughts don't really count or that they only have suicidal thoughts infrequently or only under certain circumstances. Nonetheless, Podlogar et al. (2016) found that those few who denied suicidal behavior on a written screening instrument but disclosed it at a later interview showed higher risk factors for suicide than those who acknowledged suicidal behavior on a written screening instrument.

Following Up With High-Risk False Deniers

Risk is not always obvious, and some who deny suicidal thoughts have them. About three fourths of patients who died from suicide denied suicidal intent at their last appointment with a health care professional (Berman, 2018). It is possible that some of the patients did not have suicidal thoughts at their last appointment with a health care professional. But it is likely that many did.

There is no definitive way to identify false deniers. Berman (2018) found that admitters were similar to deniers. Suicidal decedents who denied suicidal ideation at their last health care appointment differed from suicidal decedents who acknowledged suicidal ideation at their last health care appointment on four out of 34 variables. But these variables did not fit into any easily identifiable theme, suggesting the differences might have been random fluctuations.

Nock and others (e.g., Nock, Park, et al., 2010) have done some promising work using implicit association tests to identify those who have suicidal thoughts, and this might be used with some patients who are false deniers. Suicidologists are watching this research carefully to determine if the positive results will be replicated or applied to a wider range of patients than have been found in the initial studies. In the present, however, the data on implicit tests do not justify its routine use in suicide assessments.

The optimal strategy may be to take a second look at patients who deny suicidal ideation but have high risk factors for suicide. Those high-risk deniers may have a high degree of psychological distress; have experienced a recent major loss or setback in romance, finances, or health; or have few social supports. Psychotherapists may ask these patients again after they have taken a suicide assessment instrument; talk to them about passive ideas of death; identify suicidal imagery; or take time to develop a relationship that is more conducive to an honest response.

This further discussion should not be done in an adversarial manner that assumes willful deceit on the part of the patient. Instead, psychotherapists should take a calm and collaborative approach with the goal of trying to explore the patient's experiences from the standpoint of the patient.

Psychotherapists can rephrase the question, such as asking, "Have you ever had a fleeting thought that you would kill yourself?" "Did you ever in the past have thoughts of killing yourself?" "Do you think that you will ever develop suicidal thoughts in the future?" "Do you ever have mental images of killing yourself?" The new phrasing might tap a different source of data than the question "Do you currently have thoughts of killing yourself," where patients would respond only to current thoughts.

Some patients may "think" about suicide in the form of mental images and not words. Consequently, it may be indicated to ask if they have mental pictures of themselves dying from suicide or dying in general. They may picture themselves in a coffin or undergoing the process of dying. Although these pictures may not involve words in the literal sense, they have the psychological impact equivalent to suicidal ideation.

Some patients may feel annoyed after being asked about suicide a second time. Psychotherapists can be honest about their motives. They might say, for example, "I guess I must come across as overprotective or overconcerned. Maybe I am, I just want to be certain that you are safe."

Passive Thoughts of Death

Some patients deny an intent to kill themselves but express a preference for dying. Although individuals with passive death thoughts (sometimes called passive suicidal ideation, death ideation, or morbid ruminations) may not represent as high a risk for suicide as those with suicidal ideation, their death thoughts need to be taken seriously. Psychotherapists can ask them, "Have you ever felt that life is not worth living?" or "Do you ever wish that you could go to sleep and never wake up?" According to the IPT, patients with passive thoughts of death have the desire to die but not the acquired capability for suicide. Other patients may not allow themselves the option of killing themselves because their religion forbids it, but they nonetheless wish for death.

Nevertheless, these patients are a special concern for several reasons. First, such thoughts represent great emotional distress. Second, these patients may not engage in the self-care behaviors necessary to ensure adequate health. The desire to die may lead them to miss medical appointments, fail to comply with medical regimens, eat poorly, fail to exercise, or otherwise neglect their health.

Furthermore, patients with passive thoughts of suicide may place themselves in situations where the risk of an accidental death increases. People with mental disorders die from accidents at a rate higher than the population in general, and some of the risk factors for accidental death are similar to those for suicide (Crump, Sundquist, Winkleby, & Sundquist, 2013). Most accidents are just that: unfortunate events that occurred because of unforeseen circumstances or common human error. Nonetheless, some of these deaths may be due to confusion, poor judgment, or a reckless disregard for one's well-being.

The distinction between accidental and deliberate death is not always clear. For example, persons who die from an accidental overdose of opioids share many of the same characteristics of those who die from an intentional opioid overdose. Both are more likely to have a history of chronic pain, lack stable resources and consistent family support (Yarborough et al., 2016), abuse three or more substances, and have a history of depression (Bohnert, Roeder, & Ilgen, 2011). Perhaps some cases classified as overdoses from drugs are really suicides that are misclassified. Or perhaps the dichotomy of overdoses into accidental and deliberate may not capture the complex motives involved. A diminished value on the worth of one's life or a willingness to take unreasonable risks with one's safety could motivate an overdose even if it was not explicitly suicidal.

Finally, patients with passive suicidal ideation can move into an active stage of suicide if they, over the course of time, develop the acquired capability for suicide (i.e., habituate themselves to suffering and lose their fear of death) or begin to feel entrapment or that they are in a situation that is too terrible to bear.

Helping False Deniers Open Up

It may help to understand why patients would withhold crucial information from their psychotherapists. Of course, concealment might not be a dichotomous variable. Some patients may, for example, disclose suicidal thoughts, but minimize their severity or frequency, or admit suicidal thoughts but withhold their thoughts on suicide plans, and so on.

A review of the reasons why people do not seek mental health treatment might suggest the reasons why those in treatment fail to disclose feelings openly. Many adults do not seek mental health treatment because they feel embarrassed by these thoughts and because of self-stigma ("one's own stigmatizing attitudes about help-seeking"; I. H. Stanley, Hom, & Joiner, 2018, p. 34). They may also fear being perceived as weak, fear the loss of privacy, or fear being hospitalized or forced to take medications. Others have failed to seek treatment because they believed that their suicidal symptoms were normal or not severe enough to warrant treatment, or that treatment would not be effective (Carrara & Ventura, 2018; Czyz, Horwitz, Eisenberg, Kramer, & King, 2013; D'Agata & Holden, 2018; Hom, Stanley, & Joiner, 2015; Hom, Stanley, Podlogar, & Joiner, 2017). A patient may have more than one reason to conceal, and the different reasons may overlap.

Of course, psychotherapists will not know at the start of the interview if their patients are false deniers or why they are denying. Subsequently, the only recommendation is for psychotherapists to use their judgement in discerning the likelihood of false denial, and likely reason for denial, and to choose their intervention accordingly. Suggestions are offered next on how to address some of these issues. A list of reasons why patients may deny or minimize suicidal thoughts and suggested responses is given in Table 2.1.

Self-Stigma. Those who have internalized the social stigma associated with suicidal behavior may feel angry at themselves because they failed to live up to their standards of conduct. Shame is a powerful motivator of behavior and usually in a bad way. It leads to self-deception, deception of others, and demoralizing self-disgust. Not only do these patients have suicidal symptoms, they also feel shame from having these symptoms and experience the burden of concealing these symptoms from others. Self-stigma is also associated with poorer adherence to treatment, demoralization, lack of self-esteem, and increased hopelessness (Carrara & Ventura, 2018).

TABLE 2.1. Possible Reasons for Concealment and Responses

Reason	Therapeutic response
Self-stigma/shame or fear of being seen as weak	Seeking treatment takes courage and shows character and strength; nonjudgmental, accepting attitude
Prefer self-management	Treatment involves self-management
Fear of hospitalization or punitive measures	Preference for voluntary and respectful treatment
Minimizing symptoms (lack of perceived need or sense that they are not bad off)	Keep them talking about their experiences and feelings
Belief that treatment will not work	Reference experience and outcome data

Insights from psychoeducational programs addressing self-stigma may be helpful (I. H. Stanley, Hom, & Joiner, 2018). Psychotherapists can explain that patients who reveal their vulnerabilities and disclose suicidal thoughts are showing positive traits such as willpower, resourcefulness, self-determination (taking control over their lives), or strength by investing in their health. Instead of being a weakness, the ability to disclose shortcomings and challenges, and to seek to improve one's well-being, represents psychological strength and courage.

Fear of Being Perceived as Weak. Other patients or prospective patients may believe that engaging in psychotherapy makes them weak, vulnerable, or defective in some way. A certain amount of positive self-presentation is normal. Problems occur, however, when patients do not want to admit to any shortcomings or imperfections. This concealment may lead patients to feel distant, isolated, and unconnected to others.

Patients are more likely to disclose their thoughts if they think that their psychotherapists will be nonjudgmental, offer emotional support, and take their concerns seriously (Hom, Stanley, Podlogar, & Joiner, 2017). Psychotherapists can help reduce the fears of being judged by normalizing suicidal thoughts by how they phrase questions. For example, they might say, "Many people who feel depressed have thoughts of suicide. Do you have such thoughts?" (paraphrased from Shea, 2011). Or if patients have been through many stressful experiences or are having severe emotional distress, psychotherapists might note, "Many depressed (or stressed, or anxious) persons think of suicide, are you having such thoughts as well?" Psychotherapists can also note that such standards can be a substantial burden and lead to unnecessarily harsh self-criticism, and that patients should feel free to be less critical of themselves.

As noted previously, some patients may acknowledge some suicidal thoughts but greatly minimize their frequency, duration, and intensity. Or they may acknowledge suicidal thoughts but fail to disclose their suicidal plans or past attempts. Consider the experience of this psychologist.

A Patient Opens Up

A patient had been in treatment for several weeks when she told her psychotherapist that she had been "lying to her" about the intensity and duration of her suicidal thoughts and the fact that she had a well-developed plan about how she would kill herself. Although the psychotherapist was surprised by this disclosure, it represented an important milestone in treatment wherein the patient now felt confident and comfortable enough to share important information that heretofore she had felt the need to withhold.

Apparently, the psychotherapist was doing something right in terms of creating conditions in treatment that made the patient feel safe. She thanked the patient for her honesty and acknowledged that it took courage for her to share these important facts about herself.

Preference for Self-Management. Some patients or prospective patients may prefer to "handle things on my own" without the need for outside help. This attitude is not entirely problematic if it is qualified appropriately. Self-reliance can be positive if it leads them to seek out useful information and initiate productive change. It becomes problematic if they reject services that are likely to help them. For these patients, psychotherapists can respond on two levels. First, they can reference self-reliance in their description of the treatment protocol. Psychotherapists can point out that treatment requires collaborative efforts with the goal of getting patients to manage their own lives more effectively. Psychotherapy ultimately supports self-directed life management; it does not undercut it. They can state, "My way of doing psychotherapy is for you to manage your own life. Psychotherapy will only work if you are invested in the process. I can't make you get better; only you can do that."

Fear of Punitive Responses. Patients with active suicidal ideation may deny any suicidal thoughts because they fear that their psychotherapists will send them to a hospital against their will, tell their family about their suicidal thoughts without their consent, or take other steps that deprive them of autonomy or compromise their privacy. Psychotherapists can assure patients about the high importance that they place on patient autonomy and confidentiality. They can point out that treatment is most effective when patients are collaboratively involved in treatment.

The discussion of protections of confidentiality might occur during the discussions of the Notice of Privacy required by the Health Insurance Portability and Accountability Act of 1996 (HIPAA) Privacy Rule in which psychotherapists describe the exceptions to confidentiality. I suspect that most patients pay minimal attention to this review, but patients with suicidal ideation may attend to the part where psychotherapists say that they have the option of disclosing information without the patient's consent (breaking confidentiality) if the patient presents an imminent danger to self or others. Psychotherapists who suspect that a patient is withholding information can explain how they interpret and implement the exceptions to confidentiality. Psychotherapists can explain that thoughts of suicide seldom require them to disclose patient information without their consent or result in a psychiatric hospitalization and almost never lead to an involuntary psychiatric hospitalization (Bongar & Sullivan, 2013).

Minimizing the Symptoms. Some patients or prospective patients may believe that thoughts of suicide are normal. Their beliefs may have developed through their family history where prevalent pathology has become normalized. Or these beliefs may be reinforced by those in their immediate social network who expect to have a hard life. For them, "life's a bitch, then you die."

The appropriate response may be to encourage them to discuss their experiences and feelings. Often discussions about their life issues demonstrate that the events or experiences are more salient or disruptive then they were first willing to acknowledge. Psychotherapists can also talk about their inherent worth as a person deserving of positive emotions or how these symptoms can impede them in their quest for legitimate self-goals, such as becoming an effective teacher (nurse, business person, etc.), a loving parent, a good Christian, and so on. The following vignette describes a patient who greatly minimized her problems.

A Highly Disturbed Family

One patient was referred by her physician for "stress management." She came reluctantly and described herself as having great mental health except for some temporary stressors at work. She proudly proclaimed that her family life was wonderful, her husband was very supportive, her children were doing well, and so on. I started her on progressive muscle relaxation, but over the weeks it gradually leaked out that her family life was chaotic. Her husband was having an affair, the children were struggling in their personal lives, and she had a suicide attempt several years ago for which she received no medical attention and never reported to anyone.

Belief That Treatment Will Not Work. Often self-negation reflects the help-lessness or pessimism inherent in persons who are suicidal. They do not have faith in the available treatments. However, psychotherapists can instill hope by directly addressing the outcome data dealing with their treatments, including reductions in painful symptoms, increases in global functioning, and greater integration into social groups.

Certain themes run through all the psychotherapeutic responses. Psychotherapists should come across as nonjudgmental, caring, and transparent. Nonetheless, on its face, concealment appears to be driven by some of the same factors (e.g., hopelessness, mistrust, self-disgust, and shame) that drive suicidal behavior.

More Questions on Suicidal Ideation

When patients report that they have thoughts of suicide, psychotherapists should ask more specific questions about suicidal behavior, including the nature of their ideation, past suicide attempts, and suicide plans. The first task of psychotherapists is to determine if the patient presents an immediate risk of suicide. The discussions may also gather information to inform management and treatment plans, to establish a baseline to evaluate progress in treatment, and to build or deepen the treatment alliance.

It is not sufficient for psychotherapists to learn a list of steps to follow when they assess suicidal patients. Instead, highly effective psychotherapists will understand why these recommendations were made and feel confident to ignore, modify, or add to a specific recommendation on the basis of patient or contextual factors. They will be more effective in making these changes if they know why the recommendations were made in the first place. As a result, the following discussion of what to do includes a discussion of why to do it.

Psychotherapists will want to learn more about their patient's suicidal thoughts. It is often best to start with open-ended questions, such as "Tell me about these thoughts of suicide that you are having" or with other questions that allow patients to add details that they think are important. The goal of an open-ended question is to allow patients to tell their stories in their own words. Psychotherapists should listen with the goal of trying to understand the patient. Sometimes their narratives may reveal unusual or illogical reasoning. But the goal here is to understand the patient, not to argue (Michel, 2011). Arguing with or criticizing causes patients to be defensive; listening sensitively helps patients to disclose their feelings. Good psychotherapists will generally listen more than they talk.

Psychotherapists can ask forced-choice questions later, if necessary. Some of those might be, "How often do you have suicidal thoughts?" "How long do these thoughts usually last?" "How long did the thoughts continue the last time you had them?" "Do thoughts of suicide upset you or give you a sense of relief?" "If they upset you, how would you rate the intensity of the thoughts or the degree that they upset you?" "How would you rate the unpleasantness of the thoughts on a scale of 1 to 10?"

Some patients report feeling relief at having suicidal thoughts, however. The reasons for this are unclear, but perhaps the suicidal thoughts give them an option that their emotional pain will end. For such patients it may be worthwhile to ask about the emotional distress immediately before they had the suicidal thoughts. These patients may be feeling a sense of entrapment and see suicide as the only way out of their suffering. Paradoxically, for some patients, suicidal thoughts may be reinforcing (Kleiman et al., 2018).

It is important to learn more about the suicidal ideation. Rogers and Joiner (2018a) found that high levels of suicidal ideation were more positively related to suicide risk factors than low levels of suicidal ideation. Responses about the frequency, duration, and intensity of the thoughts can tell a lot about the degree of distress and suicidal risk. Thoughts that are more frequent, have a longer duration, or have greater intensity suggest a greater risk of suicide. The frequency, duration, and intensity are often highly correlated, but not always. For example, a patient may think about suicide many times a day (high frequency), but this would be less of a concern if the thoughts were fleeting (short duration) and were not particularly intrusive or upsetting (low intensity). On the other hand, a patient may think about suicide only a few times a day (low frequency), but this would be a matter of more concern if the patients could not get the suicide thoughts out of their mind (long duration) or if the thoughts were very upsetting (high intensity).

Psychotherapists should document patients' responses to these questions. As noted previously, one of the goals of an assessment is to develop a baseline by which to measure progress. Psychotherapists can use changes in the frequency, duration, and intensity as a benchmark to measure patient progress (Rudd, 2012). Monitoring patient progress and documentation is discussed in more detail in Chapter 5.

Asking About Past Suicide Attempts

Psychotherapists can ask their patients with suicidal thoughts if they have ever attempted suicide or if they have ever taken steps to kill themselves. The single best predictor of a suicide is a recent suicide attempt (even then most people who die from suicide do not have a previous suicide attempt). The risk of suicide increases when the attempt was more recent. But, attempts more than 20 years ago do not increase the risk of another attempt (C. Chu et al., 2015). Multiple attempters tend to have more psychopathology and subsequent suicide attempts. This makes sense according to the IPT because individuals can increase their capacity for self-harm through repeated exposure to self-violence.

Psychotherapists can ask, "Did you ever attempt suicide with some intent to kill yourself?" This should capture some situations in which patients might have been sufficiently ambivalent about their attempt that they would otherwise not classify it as an attempt. This phrasing is adapted from Rogers and Joiner (2018b).

Or psychotherapists can ask, "Did you ever take steps to kill yourself?" Sometimes patients will take an idiosyncratic interpretation of the phrase "suicide attempt." One patient denied that she attempted suicide by jumping out of the window, saying that she expected the angels in heaven to lift her to the ground safely. One patient placed a loaded gun to his head and then changed his mind at the last minute; because he did not pull the trigger he did not report this as a suicide attempt. Another patient, who shot himself in the head and survived, reported the event as accidental. He was sufficiently ambivalent about shooting himself at the time that he interpreted the self-inflicted wound as accidental. These patients might be more willing to disclose what happened if the questions asked were about "steps" to kill themselves as opposed to just asking about a suicide attempt.

Some psychotherapists do not learn of a patient's past suicide attempts until they review the records of previous psychotherapists that documented attempts that the patient did not mention. When asked about these past events, the patient might say, "It happened so long ago, I did not think it mattered," or "I was not really trying to kill myself that time," or give other reasons for the nondisclosure. Some patients fail to tell their current psychotherapists about a past attempt because they feel shame over it.

When asking about the details of the attempt, it is often best to start with open-ended questions such as "Tell me about that time," "What do you remember about that time?" or some other question that allows patients the chance to add details that are important to them. Then psychotherapists can ask forced-choice questions later, if necessary. However, the goal is to allow patients to tell a narrative of the attempt and how it fits into their overall life history. Patients are the experts of their own experiences (Michel, 2011). Contrary to popular belief, most people who attempt suicide do not leave suicide notes. About one third of suicide decedents left notes (Stone et al., 2018).

Rudd (2012) suggested asking patients about the precipitants, motivations, outcomes, and reactions to past attempts. Precipitant questions tap the details about the stressors that prompted the attempt. Motivation questions tap the reasons and seriousness of the attempt. Outcome questions tap the results of the attempt, such as whether the patient suffered physical damage or had to get medical treatment. Reaction questions tap how patients feel about surviving the attempt.

If a patient has had multiple past attempts, psychotherapists can ask about the worst (most serious) suicide attempt. Patients can choose which one they consider to be the worst, but it is usually the one in which they came the closest to dying. Worst-point suicide planning or behavior is associated with future suicide attempts (Joiner et al., 2003).

Precipitants

Psychotherapists can ask patients if a specific event or stressor appeared to precipitate the attempt. "What happened in your life at the time to lead you to this suicide attempt?" Often such attempts occur shortly after a significant social loss, a financial setback, or a decline in health. Many may feel entrapped or humiliated as would be predicted by the integrated motivational–volitional (IMV) theory of suicide. Precipitants could include emotional states as well as objective external events. The details on the psychological state of the patient could help psychotherapists understand the suicidal crisis state or external circumstances that led to the past attempt, with the expectation that similar suicidal states or events could precede future attempts.

Motivations

Psychotherapists can ask patients why they made the attempt (e.g., "What were your reasons for trying to take your life?"). Emergency room patients gave four common reasons for why they attempted to kill themselves: reducing distress (e.g., "to stop bad feelings," "to get away or escape"), communication (e.g., "to communicate to others how desperate [I am]"), perceived better alternative for living (e.g., "to die," "to be with people you love"), and self-loathing (e.g., "to punish yourself," "to stop feeling self-hatred or shame"; S. S. O'Connor, Comtois, Atkins, & Kerbrat, 2017, p. 50). One of these factors, communication, does not necessarily need a suicide to fulfill its goal. The other factors involve ending negative feelings, the opportunity to be with deceased loved ones, and self-punishment.

The strength of the motivation to die can sometimes, but not always, be inferred from the suicidal mode of the patients before the suicide attempt. Previous attempts that used especially lethal means predicted future suicide attempts better than previous attempts with less lethal means (Liotta, Mento, & Settineri, 2015).

But patients may not accurately understand what constitutes lethal behavior. A patient may have taken a dozen pills that might appear to be an attempt designed primarily to elicit reactions from persons in her environment.

But an apparently half-hearted attempt might have been done with a clear intent to die. Subjective reports of intent do not always correspond well to the intent that an objective observer would infer given the lethality of the means used.

Outcomes

Psychotherapists can ask patients about the medical severity of the attempt or the extent to which medical care was required. The degree of medical severity may reflect the patient's access to or knowledge about the means of suicide. Furthermore, it could be useful to learn whether the patient took steps to avoid being rescued.

Reactions

Psychotherapists can ask patients how they felt about surviving that attempt. "How did you feel about surviving the attempt?" The attitude of the patients toward the attempt is important. Some patients will regret that they made the attempt and vow not to do it again. Others will regret that they survived the attempt and vow "I will do it right the next time." Those who regretted surviving expressed a greater intent to die (Kleespies et al., 2011) and had an increased risk of future suicide attempts (Henriques, Wenzel, Brown, & Beck, 2005).

The reactions of others to the attempt are relevant to the assessment. On the one hand, it is a good prognostic sign if others responded with appropriate concern because this suggests that the patients had a supportive social network that may help keep them alive. On the other hand, it is a poor prognostic sign if others responded with indifference or anger or if the patient did not tell anyone because this suggests the lack of a supportive social network. Shame at the attempt may also drive nondisclosure. Suicidal patients may intuitively sense what research has found: Many people view those who attempted suicide as weak, selfish, cowardly, or immoral (Corrigan, Sheehan, Al-Khouja, & Stigma of Suicide Research Team, 2017).

The Role of Suicide Contagion and Clusters

If the patients have past attempts (or even if they have just expressed suicidal ideation), then it is indicated to ask them if they have any friends or family members who have talked about suicide, attempted suicide, or died from suicide. The evidence for suicide contagions is mixed, but a review by Sinyor et al. (2018) suggested that media reports can have an influence on suicidal behavior. The evidence is stronger for the presence of suicide clusters; suicide risk appears to increase when suicidal persons know each other.

The social network approach of Christakis and Fowler (2009) may be helpful here. Christakis and Fowler presented the *three-degree rule*, which holds that social influence can be felt up to three degrees of separation. For example, the likelihood that a person is happy is 15% higher if he or she has one degree of separation with a happy person (i.e., they have a mutual friend who is happy), but this drops to 10% at two degrees of separation (i.e., they have a friend of a friend who is happy), and 6% at three degrees of separation (i.e., they have a friend of a friend of a friend who is happy). After three degrees of separation the relationship becomes nil. The degrees of separation data do not necessarily indicate causation (does your happiness influence the happiness of your friends, or vice versa?), and the magnitude of the relationship even with one degree of separation (15%) indicates that happiness involves multiple factors, of which the social network is only one. Nonetheless, Christakis and Fowler argue that social networks influence many dimensions of life including health (such as sexually transmitted infections or obesity), suicidal risks, and other behaviors.

This would suggest that those who had a person in their social network who died from suicide would be at an increased risk to die from suicide themselves. Some evidence supports this interpretation. For example, Hom, Stanley, Gutierrez, and Joiner (2017) found that military service members and veterans who lost a friend to suicide had an elevated risk for suicidal behavior themselves.

Consequently, it seems appropriate to ask patients about friends or friends of friends who have attempted or died from suicides. It may be profitable to ask them what feelings emerged when they learned of these attempts. If the patient had a family member who died from suicide, then the risk of suicide is even more elevated because suicides are statistically more likely to occur in families in which suicides have already occurred. Part of the increase might be due to a biologically shared temperament or a shared stressful environment that makes individuals more vulnerable to suicide. Also, their exposure to suicidal behavior could reduce their fear of death or make suicidal behavior appear more normative.

Suicide clusters occur especially among adolescents. Knowing someone who attempted suicide increases the suicidal thoughts of adolescents (Abrutyn & Mueller, 2014). The reasons for the connection are not entirely clear. Perhaps knowing someone who died from suicide makes it a more normative or socially acceptable response to problems. Or perhaps there is no causation involved, only the "birds-of-a-feather" phenomenon whereby individuals who have certain personality traits tend to develop friendships with each other (Youyou, Stillwell, Schwartz, & Kosinski, 2017). Multiple suicides, two or more persons deciding to die by suicide together, are rare, but they do occur and account for .03% of all suicides, and about 2% of all suicides appear to be precipitated by the suicide of a loved one (Stone et al., 2018).

Asking About Suicide Plans

Psychotherapists should ask suicidal patients if they have suicide plans. Suicide planning can be considered a dangerous subtype of suicidal ideation (Bryan, Garland, & Rudd, 2016). Having a plan increases the risk of a suicide, and those who report suicidal plans are more likely to use lethal means when they attempt suicide. Understanding suicidal plans is so important that Cramer et al. (2013) identified it as one of the core competencies in treating suicidal patients.

If patients state that they have plans for a suicide attempt, then it is often best to start with an open-ended question such as "Tell me about the plan." Psychotherapists can ask forced-choice questions later if necessary. Psychotherapists will want to learn the details of such plans, including how the patients intend to do it, where they would attempt it, when they would attempt it, whether they have plans to circumvent efforts at rescue, and what preparations have been made for the attempt. Patients who reveal more detail in planning are at a higher risk to attempt suicide. A patient who says that she intends to take an overdose of medication is worrisome, but a patient who says that she intends to take a specific number of a specific medication or combinations of medications based on her reviews of the lethality of these drugs is even more worrisome. A patient who says that he intends to shoot himself is worrisome, but a patient who says that he intends to shoot himself and has ready access to a gun is more worrisome. It is still even more worrisome if the patient has experience using guns, so that the process of loading and firing the gun involves automatic processes that do not require him to stop and think through the steps involved.

It is also indicated to ask patients when and where they plan to kill themselves and why they choose this time and location. For example, a high-risk patient might say that he will do it late at night in the garage and that he chose that time and location because interruptions would be less likely.

Psychotherapists can ask patients, "Do you have access to the means to kill yourself?" "Do you have access to a gun?" "Do you know how to get the pills needed for an overdose?" or "How would you get to that high bridge where a jump would be lethal?" Psychotherapists can ask patients if they have rehearsed their suicide. For example, some patients who intend to shoot themselves may place a loaded gun to their heads or place an unloaded gun to their heads and pull the trigger. Some patients who intend to jump from a high place will go up to that high place and mentally rehearse jumping.

If patients reveal a plan to attempt suicide, it may help to ask them if they have secondary or tertiary plans. "Have you considered other ways to kill yourself?" This information is important. Chapter 3 discusses the process of means safety (also called means restriction) and the steps that individuals can take to remove access to the means of suicide. For means safety efforts to be effective, psychotherapists need to know all the means of suicide that the patients have considered.

Also, patients can discuss any external or internal triggers to these thoughts, and their feelings, while they plan the event. Sometimes it can help to ask patients if they have any images or mental pictures associated with their planned suicide attempt. Psychotherapists can also ask about feelings that arise when the patients hold that image in mind. As with past suicide attempts, the emotions and behaviors that accompany thinking about suicidal plans may help identify the warning signs that could foreshadow future suicide attempts. Sometimes patients who plan to kill themselves will prepare for their deaths by making out or revising their wills or by giving away precious or personal objects to loved ones.

Estimating Risk

Psychotherapists can then ask patients, "On a scale of 1 to 5, what is the likelihood that you feel that you will definitely kill yourself?" (1 being *definitely no* and 5 being *definitely yes*; paraphrased from Weissberg, 2011). Their response to this last question is especially important. Czyz, Horwitz, and King (2016) found that youth who predicted that they would eventually die from suicide were more likely to attempt suicide in the future; Roaldset and Bjørkly (2010) found that hospitalized women who reported a high likelihood that they would attempt suicide after discharge were more likely to do so; and Peterson, Skeem, and Manchak (2011) found that hospitalized patients' perception of their risk of self-harm predicted actual self-harm 8 weeks later. The rating question can be followed by an open-ended question such as "What led you to give yourself that score?"

Analyzing the Information

If the patients reveal a very short duration, low frequency, and low intensity of suicidal ideation, and low suicide intent (they rated their risk of dying from suicide as a 1), had no suicide attempts or attempts more than 20 years ago, have no current plans, and otherwise show a low risk of suicide, then psychotherapists can discontinue the further assessment of immediate suicidal risk and focus on other aspects of their intake interview.

If the patients reveal longer duration, more frequency, and higher intensity of suicidal ideation, and high suicidal intent (they rated the likelihood that they will die from suicide as a 2 or higher), had recent past suicide attempts, have current plans, show a very high level of subjective distress, or otherwise show a risk of suicide, then psychotherapists can ask them more questions about their thoughts about suicide, how acceptable it is to them, how they would feel about dying in general, whether they know anyone who has died from suicide or attempted suicide, whether they have thoughts of dying by other means (e.g., from an accident), or other questions to determine the strength of their will to live. Passive suicidal thoughts, such as "I wish I were dead" or "I would like to go to sleep and not wake up," are also cause for concern.

Often the patient's self-reported estimate of the likelihood that they will attempt suicide is consistent with what one would expect given the totality of the stressors and protective factors in their lives. At times, however, the patient's self-report may not correspond to an objective determination of their risk (Bryan & Rudd, 2006).

It would be prudent for psychotherapists to address any apparent discrepancy. "Ordinarily I would feel reassured that you believe that you will not attempt to kill yourself, but you have attempted to kill yourself in the past. Are you being overly optimistic about avoiding a future suicide attempt?" Or, "How bad does it have to be for you to kill yourself?" "How much more can you take, before you will kill yourself?"

The Trajectory of Suicidal Thoughts, Plans, and Attempts

The assumed trajectory is for patients to go from suicidal ideation to suicidal plans and then to suicide attempts. Having a suicide plan substantially increases the risk of a suicide. Those who have plans are more likely to use more lethal means when they attempt suicide. Having previous suicide attempts or having current suicide plans increases the risks of a suicide. Suicide attempts with highly lethal means predict future suicide attempts better than suicide attempts without highly lethal means (Liotta et al., 2015). Good treatment will try to stop the movement from ideation to planning or attempts.

However, this sequence of suicidal ideation to suicidal plan to suicide attempt does not always appear to occur. Kessler, Borges, and Walters (1999) found that 34% of respondents went from suicidal ideation to a suicide plan, and that 72% of those suicide ideators with a reported suicidal plan went on to an attempt. However, 28% of respondents with suicidal ideation went directly to a suicide attempt without reporting the intermediary step of developing a plan. Liotta et al. (2015) found that about 10% of those with suicidal ideation went directly to a suicide attempt without reporting the intermediary step of developing a plan. So, one could estimate that between 10% and 28% of those with suicidal ideation will go directly to a suicide attempt without reporting a plan. Most move from suicidal ideation to suicidal plan to suicide attempt (Pathway 1). But some appear to move directly from suicidal ideation to suicide attempt (Pathway 2). In other words, most attempted suicides occurred among those who entered the suicide state after revealing a suicide plan, but some attempted suicides occurred among those who entered the suicide state without revealing a suicide plan.

Pathway 2 attempts to raise questions. Do the apparently unplanned attempts in Pathway 2 occur among persons who have troubles controlling their impulses, or who had their normal inhibitions reduced because they consumed alcohol or other drugs? Do Pathway 2 attempts occur among patients who quickly and impulsively develop a plan to die from suicide, often within minutes before their attempt?

The assumption that Pathway 2 always represents impulsivity has several problems, including the fact that individuals who attempt suicide in the absence of a known plan show only a small elevation in trait impulsivity (Anestis, Joiner, Hanson, & Gutierrez, 2014). Also, some patients cannot identify their own thinking patterns at the time of the attempt, and despite efforts on the part of their psychotherapists to clarify their patients' experiences, they simply state that it just happened or words to that effect (Rimkeviciene, O'Gorman, & De Leo, 2016).

Furthermore, the role of alcohol consumption in Pathway 2 suicide attempts is unclear. It is true that those who had been drinking moved more quickly from suicidal ideation to a suicide attempt than nondrinkers (Bryan, Garland, & Rudd, 2016). So, it is possible that alcohol or other drugs reduced the inhibition against suicide for some patients, but most patients in Pathway 2 had not taken alcohol or other drugs at the time of their attempt (Rimkeviciene et al., 2016).

Finally, it is possible that some involved in Pathway 2 attempts had dormant or incomplete plans. Perhaps they had plans for suicide in the past but had taken these plans off the shelf for the time being (Joiner, 2010), and their psychotherapists had not learned about them. Or perhaps some patients had incomplete plans. They may not have reported a suicidal plan because, in their minds, they had only identified the method, but not the time or place. Or perhaps they had identified the general method of suicide (e.g., "taking pills") but had not yet identified the specific type of pills or quantity.

The practical implication is that conscientious and detailed screenings can identify some persons at risk to die from suicide who would not be detected by less-detailed screenings. More precision in the interviewing, including information on secondary or tertiary plans and the psychological state that occurred during past attempts or while thinking about or planning future attempts, will lead to more effective suicide management and intervention plans.

ASSESSMENT STEP 2: IDENTIFYING WARNING SIGNS

An important goal of asking about ideation, past attempts, and plans is to try to understand how the patients enter the suicidal crisis state. The psychological states or behaviors that precede or accompany suicidal attempts reveal *warning signs*. The term warning signs was originally developed to help laypersons identify common signs or symptoms of suicidal behavior, akin to the way that they could identify the warning signs of a heart attack. So, teachers could be alert to the possibility of a suicide if students were, for example, reporting that they felt anxious, were not sleeping well, were seeking revenge, or showing other symptoms. However, the traditional notion of warning signs of suicide ran into problems in that the varying lists of warning signs became so long that they were essentially meaningless and led to an unacceptable level of false positives.

It would be more appropriate, however, to use the term warning signs in a different sense to help patients or psychotherapists to identify patient-specific signs, symptoms, or experiences that could precede a suicidal crisis (Tucker, Crowley, Davidson, & Gutierrez, 2015). By understanding the psychological experiences associated in the past with suicidal ideation or attempts, patients and psychotherapists will be better able to anticipate what may happen in the future. Although the experience of every patient is unique, practitioners can be guided as to which emotions or behaviors to look for by considering research on the suicidal crisis states.

Warning Signs and Suicidal Crisis States

Researchers and clinicians have long recognized the presence of acute states of disturbance that occur before a suicidal crisis. Suicidal patients may feel agitated or experience physical or mental activity characterized by pacing, handwringing, unease, unrest, or a sense of wanting to crawl out of one's skin (Ribeiro et al., 2013). Some patients say it is hard to distract themselves from the continuing internal monologue of fear, anxiety, and self-hate. They often report that they attempted suicide to end the seemingly unbearable emotional pain (S. S. O'Connor et al., 2017).

Selby, Anestis, and Joiner (2008) used the term *emotional cascade* to describe a process of going into a state of emotional arousal. Events that disrupt an important social relationship or a represent a substantial failure at work may set off a cascade, especially if the individual has a high baseline of dysphoria. Events that seemed quite minor on the surface can also set off a cascade if they trigger feelings of self-disgust or worthlessness.

Suicide Crisis States

Psychotherapists can identify the symptoms to look for in suicide crisis states by looking at the descriptions of the acute suicidal affective disturbance (ASAD; Rogers, Chiurliza, et al., 2017; Tucker, Michaels, Rogers, Wingate, & Joiner, 2016), the suicidal crisis syndrome (SCS; Galynker, 2018), or the *direct drivers* identified in the Collaborative Assessment and Management of Suicide (CAMS) intervention (Jobes, 2016), which are "psychological forces idiosyncratic to the patient . . . that may propel the patient into acute suicidal states" (p. 93).

Although none refer to their suicidal crisis states as suicidal modes, their descriptions of these states could align with or overlap with the concept of a suicidal mode in that they describe the behaviors, thoughts, and feelings that precede or accompany ruminations about suicide or a suicide attempt.

Some may question the importance of looking at these intense emotional states by pointing out that some suicidal persons appear to have a sense of calm about them before they die. Perhaps some of them do have such a sense of calm. However, some of the reports of apparent calm before a suicide attempt may be misinterpreted or missed by an outside observer. Other patients with a commitment to die may have reasons to minimize or deny their suicidal motivation and may not reveal the symptoms usually found in a suicidal crisis (Galynker, 2018).

The ASAD involves a series of physical and psychological symptoms that appear to aggravate each other. The ASAD is marked by either or both "social alienation (e.g., severe social withdrawal, disgust with others, perception that one is a liability on others)" or "self-alienation (e.g., views that one's selfhood is a burden, self-disgust)" (I. H. Stanley, Rufino, Rogers, Ellis, & Joiner, 2016, p. 98). The terms *social alienation* and *self-alienation* overlap considerably with the concepts of thwarted belongingness and perceived burdensomeness found in the IPT. Also, this state is characterized by at least two of the following: agitation, insomnia, nightmares, or irritability. Of course, a patient might have other unpleasant symptoms in addition to those identified in the ASAD, or there may be an atypical presentation of symptoms.

According to Tucker, Michaels, et al. (2016), patients can reach this acute state rapidly. Sometimes patients will enter the suicidal crisis several hours before they attempt suicide, but other patients will enter the suicidal crisis state in less than half an hour before they attempt suicide. The likelihood of an attempt increases with the severity of the arousal.

The ASAD items were derived from clinical experience, descriptors of the near-term factors of those who died from suicide, and from contemporary theories of suicide, such as the IPT. Rogers, Chiurliza, et al. (2017) were careful to note the limitations of their work and the need for longitudinal studies, and studies with more diverse populations, including those who seek treatment and those who do not seek treatment. Also, they noted the need to compare the ASAD with the SCS.

Galynker's (2018) suicide crisis state differs from the ASAD in several ways, but there is much overlap. According to Galynker, the SCS is a state of cognitive and behavioral dysregulation characterized by frantic hopelessness (a feeling of entrapment and hopelessness), ruminative flooding (automatic negative thoughts), and strange somatic symptoms experienced in the context of extreme anxiety or panic. These factors form a negative feedback loop where physical symptoms aggravate psychological symptoms and vice versa. Unlike the ASAD, the SCS hypothesizes that the onset of the suicidal crisis can be more gradual or fluctuating.

An important difference is the emphasis that Galynker (2018) gave to entrapment ("an urgency to escape or avoid an unbearable life situation when escape is perceived as impossible" [p. 150]) and desperation ("mental anguish so intense that it requires immediate relief, and any relief in the future appears irrelevant" [p. 150]). In this sense Galynker's SCS is similar to what one would expect from the IMV theory. Both entrapment and desperation overlap with the concept of hopelessness that is implicit in the IPT. But entrapment does not necessarily require a motivational state to escape (Siddaway, Taylor, Wood, & Schulz, 2015), and desperation refers to an immediate state compared with hopelessness that refers to a more long-standing attitude (Galynker, 2018).

Finally, Jobes (2016) described suicidal behavior as coming from direct drivers. Suicidal behavior is accompanied by psychological pain, self-rated stress, agitation, hopelessness, and self-hate. Jobes also considers the role of sleep problems, shame, impulsivity, and hopelessness.

At first glance it appears that clinicians are forced to choose between three competing systems for identifying suicidal crises. However, these systems are not entirely in opposition to each other.

First, none of the research teams alleges that the common symptoms in the suicide crisis state are entirely comprehensive. So, for example, a psychotherapist working using the ASAD may encounter a patient with one of the symptoms uniquely identified by the SCS such as panic dissociation ("the somatic experience of unfamiliar sensations felt all over the body" [Galynker, 2018, p. 158]). Although this is not listed as one of the symptoms in the ASAD, clinicians working with the ASAD model can certainly accept that some of their patients may have panic dissociation.

Second, the actual symptoms listed overlap considerably, even when the terminology differs. For example, both the ASAD and the SCS explicitly identify insomnia as a factor in this acute suicidal state, and Jobes (2016) recognized that insomnia often occurs with suicidal thoughts. Both the ASAD and CAMS identify the importance of hopelessness, although Galynker (2018) used the term *desperation*, which he described as a more acute manifestation of hopelessness.

Also, the ASAD includes self-disgust. Galynker (2018) did not identify self-disgust per se but noted the role of self-disgust when patients "ruminate about their own failures" (p. 165) or actions that caused them guilt. Jobes (2016) used the term *self-hate*, which appears to overlap with self-disgust. Tucker, Michaels, et al. (2016) and Jobes (2016) referred to agitation, but Galynker's description of "frantic anxiety" appears to overlap with agitation.

Finally, a main difference among the ASAD, CAMS, and SCS appears to be that the SCS describes cognitive processes, such as rigid thinking, rumination, or the failure to suppress thoughts, and not just the content of the thoughts. However, Jobes (2016) and researchers from the Joiner laboratory have also written about the role of cognitive processes; it is just not included as one of the identifying features in the ASAD, even though Rogers and Joiner (2018b) found a relationship between a lifetime of past suicide attempts and rumination focusing on suicidal themes. Global rumination is associated with suicidal ideation and suicide attempts (Rogers & Joiner, 2017), although suicidal specific rumination (focusing on suicidal thoughts or plans) may be more useful in predicting a suicide.

Galynker (2018) identified the rigid cognitive processes in the suicidal state as ruminative, circular, and inflexible. Although Galynker did not identify cognitive absolutism specifically in his description, it appears that this could be a component of this rigidity, and this would be consistent with cognitive therapy, which sees perfectionism, seeing things in black-and-white terms, and the failure to look at grays as vulnerabilities for depression and suicide (Wenzel, Brown, & Beck, 2009). Recent research by Al-Mosaiwi and Johnstone (2018) found that absolutist thinking was common in Internet forums that focused on suicidal ideation.

In discussing processes, Galynker (2018) also noted the role of rumination or "repetitive thoughts focused on one's own distress" (p. 165). Although Galynker used the term broadly to refer to rumination about one's symptoms, or one's life failures, Rogers and Joiner (2018b) noted that suicide-specific ruminations predicted a lifetime suicide attempt better than other variables. Galynker also introduced the term *ruminative flooding*, which differs from ordinary rumination in that it is perceived as uncontrollable and may result in somatic symptoms such as headaches.

One form of rumination, *brooding* ("dwelling on the consequences of a depressed mood"; Law & Tucker, 2018, p. 68), appears more closely linked to suicidal thoughts than the other form of rumination, *reflection* ("reflecting upon reasons for a depressed mood as a means of problem solving"; Law & Tucker, 2018, p. 68). Rumination may contribute to suicidal thoughts through activating overarousal in the form of agitation or nightmares (Rogers, Schneider, et al., 2017).

Interviewing Patients About Their Suicidal Crisis State

It can also help for patients to describe their pain. It is often best to start with open-ended questions ("Tell me how you feel") and supplement with more specific questions if necessary: "Is it more depression or anxiety?" "Often anxious people feel queasy in their stomachs. Do you have those sensations?" "How well do you sleep at night?" and so on. Depending on the patient, it may be indicated to ask about any psychotic experiences that they may have had.

Some patients have a limited awareness of their physiological reactions and their own internal states. They may be less aware of when they are hungry, angry, distressed, or in pain. If patients have trouble identifying or describing their feelings, psychotherapists can at least acknowledge their pain and strive to understand their experiences. Some men have difficulty expressing or acknowledging emotions except anger. Consequently, it may help to ask them about their *perceptions*, what they *thought* about something, or how they *reacted*.

Psychotherapists can usually discern the emotional pain in the tone of the voice of the patient, their posture, or other behavioral indices. It often helps patients to rate the intensity of their pain on a scale of 1 to 10, with 10 being the highest (Jobes, 2016, included a rating of 1 to 5). Questions that psychotherapists could ask patients include "How would you describe the emotional pain you feel on a scale of 1 to 10 with 10 being the highest amount of pain?"

When it comes to identifying the specific feelings and behaviors associated with the suicidal crisis state, psychotherapists can incorporate information obtained during discussions of the patient's suicidal ideation, past attempts, or suicidal plans. Often patients can identify the emotions they experienced when they have suicidal thoughts or plans. In addition, psychotherapists can ask patients to describe their experiences or psychological state right before a suicide attempt. They may ask patients to pretend that they are watching a slow-motion movie where they can describe the events and experiences in detail.

Psychotherapists should be especially alert to experiences and emotions as described by the ASAD, SCS, or CAMS. Using a "big tent" approach, I suggest looking first for any symptoms identified as most important by these theories or that occur across all theories. These would be entrapment, perceived burdensomeness, thwarted belongingness, insomnia, agitation, and hopelessness, which are described next. Then psychotherapists can look for other symptoms that appear in some but not all of the descriptions of suicidal crisis states, which include self-hatred, shame, social withdrawal, and impulsivity. Exhibit 2.2 lists these warning signs.

Of course, these symptoms can interact in complex ways. For example, shame may have a bidirectional relationship with anger (Cassiello-Robbins, Wilner, Peters, Bentley, & Sauer-Zavala, 2019), wherein patients who feel shame may cover up that emotion with anger or patients with anger problems may feel shame over their behavior.

Often the descriptions involve definitions or nuances in how the symptom is described. These seemingly minor points can have meaningful clinical implications if they help psychotherapists become more precise about what they are looking for. For example, looking for global traits of impulsivity might not help psychotherapists understand patients very well. But a form of impulsivity, such as negative urgency, may be an important factor for some patients.

Entrapment and Hopelessness

Psychotherapists should look for entrapment, defeat, and hopelessness, which are interconnected constructs. *Entrapment* is defined "as urgency to escape or avoid an unbearable life situation when escape is perceived as impossible"

EXHIBIT 2.2

Warning Signs From Suicidal Crisis States

Most salient warning signs
  Sense of entrapment, defeat, or humiliation
  Self-alienation—includes self-hatred/self-disgust
  Social alienation—social withdrawal, perceived burdensomeness
  Agitation or frantic anxiety
  Hopelessness or desperation
  Insomnia

Other warning signs
  Irritability
  Impulsivity
  Nightmares
  Anhedonia
  Dissociative panic
  Depressive turmoil
  Fear of dying
  Cognitive rigidity, cannot process information well
  Rumination, especially brooding (dwelling on consequences of one's mood) or
    ruminative flooding: uncontrollable and associated with physical symptoms

---

(Galynker, 2018, p. 150). Entrapment and defeat are postulated to be major determinants of suicidal behavior according to the IMV theory, although some researchers view them both as interacting dimensions of a higher order construct, involuntary subordination (A. W. Griffiths, Wood, & Tai, 2018). Hopelessness is an implicit component of the IPT and a component of entrapment. The difference is that hopelessness does not necessarily involve the motive to escape and does not necessarily involve the sense of diminished status. An important element of entrapment is that it may involve either external circumstances that block goals or internal states imposed by the patient's thoughts, interpretations, or feelings. R. C. O'Connor and Portzky (2018) allowed for the possibility that the importance of entrapment may vary according to the patient's gender, stage of life, or culture.

Irritability

Researchers have defined irritability differently (Toohey & DiGiuseppe, 2017). However, many consider it as having a low threshold for anger, or a tendency to react aggressively when provoked. It may also indicate a tendency to overreact to a perceived offense (Orri, Perret, Turecki, & Geoffroy, 2018). For purposes of suicide assessment, it may be indicated to look at irritability in both the frequency of anger or the proportionality of the anger to the perceived offense.

In one study on the ASAD, it was measured with a clinical anger scale (Rogers, Chiurliza, et al., 2017). Anger toward others appears related to thwarted belongingness and perceived burdensomeness (K. A. Hawkins et al., 2014). Anger may be related to social isolation if the angry person avoids contact with others. Psychotherapists can ordinarily identify excessive anger through the discussions of life events, social relationships, or other topics.

Irritability or anger may be important to explore with men who have intimacy problems. They may have difficulty expressing tender emotions such as love or hurt because they are perceived as feminine emotions. However, anger is socially acceptable in the cultural stereotype of masculine emotions. Because homicide and suicide are statistically linked, it is prudent to ask suicidal patients if they have thoughts of harming others. Tucker, Michaels, et al. (2016) identified irritability as part of the suicidal crisis state. Galynker (2018) noted that heightened irritability was a component of the agitation in the suicidal crisis state.

Self-Hatred or Self-Disgust

Self-hatred or self-disgust appear to be the affective dimension of intense self-criticism without the possibility of redemption through positive change. Some of the items in the self-hatred scale are as follows: "I hate myself," "I am a failure," "I am ashamed of myself," "I feel disgusted when I think of myself" (Turnell, Fassnacht, Batterham, Calear, & Kyrios, 2019, p. 782). Self-hatred or self-disgust can lead to perceived burdensomeness to the extent that others would be better off if one were dead. Self-disgust may arise because individuals lack the ability to forgive themselves or to show self-compassion. Tucker, Michaels, et al. (2016) identified the importance of self-disgust, and Galynker (2018) noted that self-disgust was often present in the ruminations of patients. Jobes considered self-hate a concept sometimes seen as identical to self-disgust and an important factor to assess.

Shame

Guilt and shame are overlapping but distinct emotions. In common parlance, they are often used as synonyms for each other, and both involve a violation of a social norm. But they are not identical. According to Tangney, Miller, Flicker, and Barlow (1996), guilt involves remorse over a behavior and a prosocial desire to repair a relationship or make restitution. A person feeling guilt is likely to problem solve ways to rectify the situation.

On the other hand, shame involves feelings of "worthlessness, inferiority and incompetence, and often leads to a desire to escape and withdraw socially" (Bastin, Harrison, Davey, Moll, & Whittle, 2016, p. 456). Whereas guilt may lead to productive results, shame is likely to lead to unproductive self-recrimination. Guilt encourages problem-solving; shame encourages rumination. Guilt can lead to better behavior; shame discourages such behavior because the shamed person assumes that they will always be defective. Guilt allows the individual an option of reuniting or reconciling with the offended person. Shame offers no such option and is more likely to lead to social isolation.

Psychotherapists may identify shame in self-criticism that is disproportionate to the offense. Shame can be detected through discussions of life events or social relationships. Neither Tucker, Michaels, et al. (2016) nor Galynker (2018) identified shame as part of the suicidal mode, but shame is linked to suicide in other studies (e.g., Dodson & Beck, 2017) and may motivate social withdrawal. Also, Jobes (2016) considered shame a unique risk factor that can lead to such an intolerable state that it could prompt a suicide attempt.

Agitation

Agitation is a "time limited state of both psychological and behavioral over arousal often characterized by restless and/or repetitive behaviors coupled with expressions of emotional turmoil and/or mental anguish or unrest" (Ribeiro et al., 2015, p. 26). It differs from anxiety in that anxiety tends to be future oriented, whereas agitation focuses on immediate physical or psychological unrest. Items on the Brief Agitation Scale give a good sense of the feeling of agitation. The three items deal with wanting to crawl out of one's skin, feeling emotional turmoil in one's gut, and feeling so stirred up that one wants to scream (Ribeiro, Bender, Selby, Hames, & Joiner, 2011). The heightened energy associated with agitation provides the impetus for a suicidal person to follow through with their impulses (Ribeiro et al., 2015). Tucker, Michaels, et al. (2016), Galynker (2018), and Jobes (2016) identified agitation as an important dimension to assess.

Social Withdrawal

Social withdrawal involves avoiding social situations and relationships because they are no longer rewarding. Individuals may fail to disclose personal behaviors or struggles out of shame or a fear of being humiliated or a lack of trust in others (Dodson & Beck, 2017). Tucker, Michaels, et al. (2016) identified social withdrawal as part of their suicidal mode. Jobes (2016) highlighted the role of relationship loss, relationship stress, and the perception of being a burden on others, although he did not identify social withdrawal as an immediate warning sign of a suicide attempt.

Insomnia and Nightmares

It is always indicated to ask suicidal patients about their sleep habits. Asking about total sleep time might be the most prudent way to start because it is linked to suicidal behavior (Michaels, Balthrop, Nadorff, & Joiner, 2017). If patients report that they consistently receive less than 7 hours of sleep a night, psychotherapists can follow up with additional questions concerning trouble falling asleep, early morning wakening, or nightmares.

Nightmares are "vivid, disturbing or frightening dreams that awaken the individual" (Nadorff, Lambdin, & Germain, 2014, p. 225). Bad dreams are distinguished from nightmares in that they do not lead to awakening. However, many researchers lump nightmares and bad dreams together. Nightmares may contribute to insomnia in that patients will awaken from nightmares or wish to stay awake to avoid having more nightmares.

Self-reported sleep disturbance is related to suicidal ideation. EEG sleep patterns of patients with suicidal ideation tend to differ from those without suicidal ideation. For example, they tend to have shorter periods with delta waves (indicating the deepest level of sleep; Dolsen et al., 2017).

Sleep problems (trouble falling asleep, trouble staying asleep, or having nightmares) can take their toll on a patient. "Exhaustion and complete tiredness seemed to take control of daily life" (Bonnewyn et al., 2014, p. 617). Trouble sleeping predicts suicidal behavior even when depressive symptoms are controlled for (Bernert, Turvey, Conwell, & Joiner, 2014). The level of insomnia appears to predict increases in suicidal ideation and not the other way around (Zuromski, Cero, & Witte, 2017). Insomnia likely contributes to suicide because poor sleep leads to fatigue, cognitive rigidity, or other difficulties in thinking through problems.

Tucker, Michaels, et al. (2016) identified insomnia and nightmares as related to the suicidal crisis state. Jobes (2016) identified the importance of insomnia and nightmares, whereas Galynker (2018) identified only insomnia as related to the suicidal crisis state.

Impulsivity

Impulsivity refers to "actions that are unduly hasty, risky, and ultimately dangerous to the individual" (Chamberlain, Redden, & Grant, 2017, p. 11). It could be a major factor in moving a person from suicidal ideation to suicidal threat according to the IMV theory of suicide. However, impulsivity may have several dimensions or causes. It can be caused by a lack of premeditation, an inability to follow through with tasks, a desire for sensation seeking, or *negative urgency* ("the tendency to act rashly when experiencing negative affect"; Valderrama, Miranda, & Jeglic, 2016, p. 16). Some hypothesize that impulsivity may account for suicide attempts that occur in the absence of a self-reported suicide plan (called Pathway 2 suicides). However, the evidence in support of this perspective is mixed. Nock, Hwang, Sampson, and Kessler (2010) found that suicide risk increased in persons with impulsive disorders, although this was primarily due to an increased risk among those with conduct disorders or intermittent explosive disorders. Also, Chamberlain et al.'s review (2017) found mixed results when looking at impulsivity and suicidal behavior, which may be due to different ways of defining and measuring impulsivity.

Impulsivity was not identified as a risk factor for entering the suicidal mode by either Tucker, Michaels, et al. (2016) or Galynker, although Jobes (2016) considered it in his risk-assessment protocol. Jobes suggested asking patients to rate their own impulsivity and its relationship to a potential suicidal attempt.

ASSESSMENT STEP 3: THE TOPICS AND THEMES APPROACH

Questions about suicidal ideation, plans, past attempts, and the suicidal mode are only the start of the assessment. Unless the risk of suicide is low, it is recommended that psychotherapists inquire in more depth about vulnerability and protective factors related to suicide risk. The background information can also provide context for the patient's responses to questions about suicide.

Psychotherapists obtain additional information through an intake interview. The content and documentation required for the intake interview comes from multiple sources. Psychologists need to be aware of the record-keeping guidelines of the American Psychological Association (2007), and psychotherapists need to be aware of the regulations of their state, provincial, or territorial licensing board. In addition, most commercial insurers follow the standards of the National Committee on Quality Assurance, but many insurers also have unique requirements, so that it is not possible to give one document that meets the standards for all legal entities or commercial insurers. Fortunately, the requirements of these different sources overlap considerably.

Appendix A contains a patient information form that gathers much of the information needed for an intake interview. Psychotherapists should feel free to modify the form as they see fit. Psychotherapists can give the information form to patients before their first meeting. They could also post the form on their website for patients to download and complete, or they could have patients arrive for their sessions a few minutes early and complete the form in the waiting room. Psychotherapists should feel free to modify the form as they wish.

Of course, psychotherapists are seldom able to acquire all the necessary information they need to make the best decisions in the first session. For some patients with a high risk of suicide, it may be necessary to move quickly into suicide management strategies and defer getting more detailed information. If psychotherapists focus too much on getting a comprehensive evaluation and ignore the distress of their patients in the first session, then they may have done an adequate risk assessment, but they are left with patients who do not feel valued or heard and are less likely to return for a second session. Nonetheless, psychotherapists should try to get the intake information as soon as feasible.

When conducting an intake interview with a suicidal patient, this book takes a topics and themes approach. *Topics* refer to the content areas that psychotherapists should cover as part of the usual intake, and *themes* refer to the common motifs related to suicide found in each of the topics. The six topics are (a) patient background; (b) life changes or stressors; (c) social relationships; (d) physical health; (e) religion and values; and (f) mental illness and psychological health, including a mental health diagnosis, emotional pain, and psychological resilience. Table 2.2 presents the topics and salient issues related to suicide prevention.

TABLE 2.2. Topics and Themes Related to Suicide Risk

Topic	Themes
History	Acquired capacity: exposure to suffering or violence as victims, perpetrators, or witnesses including child abuse, trauma, or serious physical illnesses
	Desire to die: relationship to family and others, attachment to others, integration in a community
Events	Acquired capacity: events including exposure to violence or harm
	Desire to die: anything that decreases social field, or results in a loss including loss of self-esteem (humiliation)
Health	Acquired capacity: perception of poor health, especially chronic pain or anticipation of death
	Desire to die: chronic pain, or decline in activities of daily living, or anything that leads persons to believe that they are a burden to others
	Possibility of defeat, entrapment, and hopelessness
Social networks	Acquired capacity: exposure to suicides in social network, being in an abusive relationship, being aggressive toward others
	Desire to die: alienation or social losses
	Possibility of defeat and humiliation
Religion (values)	Desire to die: look for life-protecting or life-promoting factors
Emotional pain	Acquired capacity: Is diagnosis linked to exposure to violence or suffering?
	Desire to die: Is diagnosis linked to intense unpleasant emotions or faulty thinking processes?
	Possibility of defeat, humiliation, or entrapment

The themes identified help determine the risk of a suicide attempt or of entering a suicidal crisis state. The themes are derived from the ideation-to-action theories of suicide and include acquired capacity, the desire to die (perceived burdensomeness, thwarted belongingness, and so on), protective factors, and the emotions and behaviors that characterize the patient's suicidal crisis state.

The six topics overlap considerably. For example, questions about physical limitation may lead to information about a recent life event (such as a major disease) that may impact the patient's ability to maintain social relationships or may evoke certain religious attitudes about suffering or divine retribution. Or, questions about social relationships may lead to information about intimate partner violence, emotional distress, physical pain, and a diagnosable *International Classification of Diseases, Tenth Revision* (ICD–10) disorder.

The topics and themes approach helps psychotherapists gain a fuller picture of their patients and how their suicidal thoughts make sense in the totality of their lives. Psychotherapists can preface these questions with statements such as "I want to understand more about you," and they should maintain the same caring attitude that they showed when asking the initial questions about suicidal thoughts.

Of course, the template presented here only represents a general guide for information gathering. Psychotherapists may modify their inquiries depending on the unique circumstances and characteristics of their patients. For example, when treating military veterans, police officers, correctional officers, or firefighters, it may be appropriate to ask for more detail about their exposure to violence or other life endangering situations. Or when treating older adults, it may be appropriate to ask more detail about their physical health, the loss of loved ones, and any decline in their social contacts. Appendix B contains a review of common items found in the intake interviews with an emphasis on suicide-related topics.

Protective Factors

A thorough assessment also requires consideration of the protective factors, or variables that are "associated with a decreased risk of morbidity or mortality" (Kleespies, 2014, p. 98). The commonly identified protective factors are strong social connections, psychological resilience, and religious beliefs or personal values that disapprove of suicide. On the surface, protective factors may appear only to represent the absence of risk factors. For example, the protective factor of belonging to a strong social group may appear to be the lack of thwarted belongingness, and having life-affirming religious beliefs may appear to represent the opposite of hopelessness and self-disgust.

Protective factors are more than the absence of risk factors. Social connections, psychological resilience, and religious or spiritual beliefs are multifaceted (Rutter, Freedenthal, & Osman, 2008). It would be possible for an individual to feel socially rejected in some domains of life, but still have life-saving social connections in other domains. Child-rearing obligations, for example, appear especially important as a reason for living (Bakhiyi, Calati, Guillaume, & Courtet, 2016), even though caregivers may feel socially rejected in other areas of their lives.

Psychological resilience may be more than just the absence of psychopathology. According to the *dual-factor* (or *two continua*) model of mental well-being, "the absence of mental illness is not the presence of mental health" (Keyes, 2007, p. 95). Good mental health and psychopathology might not be opposite ends of one single continuum, but rather separate dimensions that often, but not always, correlate with each other. For example, Teismann, Brailovskaia, et al. (2018) found that psychiatric inpatients with suicidal ideation were less likely to engage in suicide attempts over time if they also scored high on positive mental health.

The protective factors of social connectedness, psychological resilience, and religion may overlap. For example, psychologically resilient individuals may know how to elicit support from friends in their social field when they are distressed, and religion may confer psychological resilience through optimism. Also, friends and social contacts can help individuals reduce their distress by suggesting more productive ways for them to view their problems, and participation in a religion may provide opportunities to find social support or give a way to find meaning through offering supports to others.

Although protective factors reduce risk, no protective factor is an absolute veto on suicidal risk. For example, patients might say that they would not attempt suicide because they have strongly held religious beliefs against it. However, while under stress or under the throes of strong negative emotions, life-protecting beliefs may lose their salience and effectiveness.

Avoid Focusing on Tangential Risk Factors

Psychotherapists need to avoid going into areas that are less directly related to suicide, unless they can identify clinical reasons for doing so. Hundreds of variables could be linked to suicidality (May & Klonsky, 2016). Many of these factors contribute very little additional predictive power or tap overlapping concepts, especially when conducted with samples with a low risk of suicide (Witte, Holm-Denoma, Zuromski, Gauthier, & Ruscio, 2017). A psychotherapist could spend countless hours accumulating all sorts of information that may slightly improve the estimated risk of harm but, in the meantime, lose time that could best be spent helping the patients manage their suicidal risk.

In addition, many variables are confounded. For example, suicides tend to be higher in rural states as opposed to urban states (Western and Northwestern states have the highest suicide rates; Rossen, Hedegaard, Khan, & Warner, 2018). But rural living itself might not be responsible for the increased risk of suicide. Rural living might increase the risk of social isolation, but it is social isolation, not rural living, that increases the risk of suicide. Or rural living might mean a reduced access to health care, but it is the lack of access to health care, and not rural living, that increases the risk of suicide.

Topic One: Patient Background

The essential points that psychotherapists should remember about demographics and personal history are that

- demographic factors such as age, race, or gender can be used to estimate the risk of a suicide in the long run;

- psychotherapists should not overvalue the role of these factors—they only indicate the likelihood that an individual has been exposed to the life experiences or circumstances that influence the risk of suicide; and

- psychotherapists should be especially alert for elements of the patient's history that indicate exposure to violence and suffering either as a perpetrator, victim, or witness.

Consider this situation:

Is This Patient at High Risk?

When working in rural Pennsylvania, I had an intake with an older White male who was a retired coal miner referred by his family physician for depression following the recent death of his brother. He walked with a cane and had apparent discomfort moving around.

Without knowing anything more about the patient, I knew that, demographically, he was at a high risk for suicide given his age, gender, race, occupation, and likely access to weapons.

Fortunately, this patient has a positive disposition, although he was currently experiencing a complicated bereavement. He had a loving family, liked to read, and had no thoughts of suicide.

Consider this other situation:

Is This Patient at Low Risk?

When working at a university counseling center I had an intake with an African American student who was referred by her resident assistant for difficulties in adjusting to college. She was attractive and had a high grade point average. She did not have a steady boyfriend but had options of interest to her.

Without knowing anything more about the patient, I knew that, demographically, she was at a low risk for suicide given her age, gender, race, performance in school, and sexual orientation. Unfortunately, she found adjusting to college very difficult and had recently had thoughts of suicide. These stories illustrate the facts that every patient is different and demographics do not mean destiny.

The information about the patient's background is often called a static or fixed factor. Static factors such as age, race, and personal history do not change. Gender and sexual orientation are generally static, although they sometimes do change. Static factors contrast with other factors that are dynamic or changing.

As stated in Chapter 1, men die more often from suicide than women, although women attempt suicide more often than men. Race and ethnicity are also static factors. Older White or Native American men are at a higher risk of suicide, although rates of suicide among African Americans may be underreported (see the discussion in Chapter 1). Hispanics tend to have rates of suicide higher than non-Hispanic White Americans, but there is diversity within diversity. Some Hispanic groups, such as Puerto Ricans, have high rates of suicide, whereas other Hispanic groups have much lower rates. Asian Americans have low rates of suicide, although there is diversity among the specific nationalities. A patient's current socioeconomic status (SES) is a static factor. Educational level is often used as a proxy variable to determine SES, and those with high school educations have rates of suicide twice as high as those with college educations (Phillips & Hempstead, 2017). But the usefulness of looking at SES alone is open to debate because it is often confounded with other risk factors such as financial strain, unemployment, mental illness, social isolation, or disability.

Sexual minority youth have an increased risk of suicide (Silva, Chu, Monahan, & Joiner, 2015; Stone et al., 2014), but there is some evidence that the risk is highest with individuals with bisexual orientations (Pompili, Girardi, Tatarelli, & Tatarelli, 2006). Similar patterns occur for sexual minority adults (Hottes, Bogaert, Rhodes, Brennan, & Gesink, 2016). Persons who are transgender or gender nonconforming have rates of suicide higher than the population in general, especially if they have experienced rejection, discrimination, or victimization (Testa et al., 2017). The factor most likely associated with the higher risk of sexual minorities is rejection by an important social group, such as their families of origin.

Age, gender, race, SES, sexual orientation, and other demographic factors do not inherently predispose a person to suicide. Rather, these factors increase the likelihood that the individual will be exposed to the experiences that increase risk. For example, Americans who live in Native American communities (Indian reservations) have higher rates of suicide because they have a disproportionate number of risk factors, such as unemployment, exposure to trauma, substance abuse, lack of access to health care services, and other life circumstances that increase the likelihood that they will experience hopelessness, social isolation, or other factors more directly related to suicidal risk (Gray & McCullagh, 2014). And older adults have higher rates of suicide because they are more likely to have serious health problems and social isolation than younger people.

Some occupations have higher rates of suicide than other occupations, but this is often because the members of that occupation have had life experiences that increase the risk of suicide. Physicians have elevated rates of suicide. There is no reason to believe that persons inclined to suicide become physicians. However, physicians are exposed to many situations that increase the likelihood of suicide. According to Wible (2017), suicides often occur among physicians who have developed on-the-job posttraumatic stress disorder (PTSD), have lost patients through death, feel dehumanized, have lost personal connections to patients through the practice of assembly-line medicine, or who otherwise have developed psychopathology created or aggravated by on-the-job stress.

Farm workers, including ranchers, farm owners, and farm hands, die from suicide at a rate higher than any other occupation. They often have social isolation, less access to health care, and easier access to weapons, and many are experiencing a very substantial decline in income with the likelihood of foreclosure ever looming (Weingarten, 2017).

Of course, these static factors only address general trends as reflected by the vignettes at the start of this section. Older White or Native American men, physicians, and farmers do not always die from suicide, and some well-educated young Black women do. Nothing about a person's demography inherently makes them suicidal. But nothing in a person's demography makes them immune from suicide either.

Certain historical factors, such as a stressful childhood, are related to suicide. Psychotherapists can ask general questions such as "Tell me about your childhood" "What was your family life like?" "Did you like school?" "Did your parents do a good job with you?" or "Did you have any particularly difficult experiences growing up?" It is best to start with open-ended questions and move to forced-choice questions later if needed.

This background information can help psychotherapists to better understand their patients. Psychotherapists may learn, for example, that their patients were victims of abuse, received little positive attention from their parents, had family or residential instability, or lived in precarious conditions where the necessities of life could not be ensured. A higher amount of adverse childhood experiences is associated with a younger age for having the first suicide attempt (Choi, DiNitto, Marti, & Segal, 2017). Often children raised in these environments may adopt strategies that help them to adapt in these environments, such as developing a mistrust of others or having a heightened reactivity to stress, but which do not help them to adapt to environments later in life (Ellis, Bianchi, Griskevicius, & Frankenhuis, 2017).

Psychotherapists should ask patients if they have been exposed to physical suffering or violence in their lives, either as victims, perpetrators, or witnesses. The reason for these questions is that the acquired capability for death or fearlessness of death often develops because of habituation to violence or injury and an increase in pain tolerance, although evidence also suggests that the acquired capability for death may have a genetic component (A. R. Smith et al., 2012). Also, it is possible that some individuals with genetically influenced impulsivity or adventurousness may expose themselves to more dangerous situations.

Nonetheless, the history of the patient becomes an important predictor of suicide for those who have been a recent victim of a military sexual assault (e.g., Soberay et al., 2016), were a college student with a history of sexual assault (e.g., Chang et al., 2015), had a history of childhood abuse (e.g., Harford, Yi, & Grant, 2014; Mortier et al., 2017), lived in a family where there was domestic violence (e.g., Fuller-Thomson, Baird, Dhrodia, & Brennenstuhl, 2016), were a survivor of domestic violence (e.g., Dufort, Stenbacka, & Gumpert, 2015; McLaughlin, O'Carroll, & O'Connor, 2012), or were victims of human trafficking (Borschmann et al., 2017). Although all adults who experienced child abuse had an increased risk of dying from suicide, those who experienced violent child abuse had rates of suicide attempts higher than those who experienced nonviolent child abuse (Sachs-Ericsson, Stanley, Sheffler, Selby, & Joiner, 2017).

Topic Two: Life Changes and Chronic Stressors

The essential points that psychotherapists should remember about life changes and chronic stressors are that

- the risk of suicide increases after a negative life change, especially the loss of a social relationship, and

- other losses increase the risk of suicide if they involve defeat or humiliation, or lead to a sense of entrapment.

The interview should ask about recent life changes and ongoing stressors. Patients may spontaneously bring up recent stressful events or chronic stressors, sometimes called daily hassles. If patients do not spontaneously bring up such events, it is useful for psychotherapists to directly ask them "Have you had any recent stressors or major changes in your life?" or "Are there any things in your daily life that you find particularly stressful or upsetting?" followed by other open-ended questions such as "Tell me about it?" or "How do you feel about these changes?" After asking these open-ended questions, psychotherapists can ask for more specific information if needed, such as "Has this change been positive or negative?" "Was it anticipated?" or "How are you adjusting to it?"

Relationship losses are the most common precipitants of a suicide attempt (see more information in the section on Social Relationships). Other common precipitant events are legal problems (Overholser, Braden, & Dieter, 2012), job loss, or financial difficulties (Coope et al., 2015). These losses may increase the risk of suicide because of their link to perceived burdensomeness as would be predicted by the IPT theory or to defeat, humiliation, or entrapment as would be predicted by the IMV theory. Some men who are socialized into identifying their worth with their ability to provide for their families may lose self-esteem and perceive themselves as a burden following the loss of their breadwinner role. In addition, patients may have chronic stressors, such as an unpleasant job, a disruptive marriage, problems with neighbors, or other daily hassles that degrade the quality of their lives.

The sample patient information form (Appendix A) includes a question about the patient's arrest history. A recent arrest or incarceration, especially if it involves humiliation, increases the risk of suicide. Nearly one third of suicide victims had court involvement, twice the rate of controls (Cook & Davis, 2012). Prisoners in county jails have a high rate of suicide. Prisoners in long-term

TABLE 2.3. Common Precipitants of Suicide

Relationship problems[a]	42%
Physical health problem	22%
Job/financial problem	16%
Legal problems	13%

Note. Data from Stone et al. (2018).
[a]Relationship problems include family arguments, intimate partner problems, death of a loved one, and being a victim or perpetrator of interpersonal violence.

prisons have lower rates of suicide in part because they are monitored closely, but also because they have already passed through the crisis phase that commonly occurs immediately on incarceration. Shame following an arrest may be especially difficult for patients from honor cultures, where status in the community or saving face is particularly important. The known precipitants of suicide and their percentages are found in Table 2.3.

If patients recently immigrated to the United States or belong to a group that has been traditionally marginalized, it may be profitable to ask them about minority stress. "Do you feel free to interact in society without discrimination or mistreatment?" "Have you been subjected to racial, ethnic, or religious slurs or microaggressions?" Cultural strain can increase social isolation, especially for patients who recently immigrated to the United States. For example, adult children of immigrant families may feel conflicts between their parent's wishes for them to keep family traditions and their own wish to integrate more into the mainstream of American society (Bhugra, 2013).

Topic Three: Social Relationships

The essential points that psychotherapists should remember about social relationships are that

- social relationships, such as marriage, typically promote well-being and protect against suicide;

- losses or conflicts in social relationships are related to perceived burdensomeness and thwarted belongingness;

- family conflicts may be an especially important precipitant of suicide among non-White Americans;

- psychotherapists should evaluate the role of social media in the lives of their patients; and

- psychotherapists should be alert for any social contagion influences on suicide.

Psychotherapists can ask patients about their social lives including family, friends, social groups, and colleagues at work. Social isolation is related to an increased risk of suicide (Calati et al., 2019). This occurs whether looking at objective indices of loneliness (such as being unmarried or living alone) or subjective reports of loneliness. The finding is consistent across cultures.

Some of the questions that psychotherapists could ask would be open-ended, such as "Tell me about your friends," or "Tell me about your family." After these open-ended questions, psychotherapists may wish to ask more direct questions, such as "Do you go out together often with friends or families?" "Do you find these contacts meaningful?" "Do you ever feel lonely?" "Do you feel close to people?" "Do you have close friends?" "Do you feel close to your family?" "What do you like most about your friends?" "Are you involved in any social groups?" "Do you belong to a church?" "Are you involved in any community or religious groups that do charitable work?" "Tell me about those activities." "How would you rate your relationships with your co-workers?" "Do you like your work?" The interview can look at the overall social network of the patient, their attachment style, marital relationships, and use of social media.

Social support is "the belief that one is cared about and has available assistance" (Bell et al., 2018, p. 88). It can be fulfilled through family, friends, or larger social groups. Social connectedness is a well-identified protective factor. Social support could mean (a) instrumental support such as the sharing of resources with others; (b) informational support, such as advice on how to access certain resources; or (c) affectional support, such as expressions of caring or reassurance. Even knowing that others are available to provide support can reduce stress.

Marital advantage refers to the health and well-being advantages of being married. Married people tend to report greater happiness than unmarried people. However, the quality of the marriage is important as well. People who are in long-term unhappy marriages have lower self-esteem and less life satisfaction and happiness than divorced persons (D. N. Hawkins & Booth, 2005).

If patients are married or in long-term relationships, it is useful to ask about the quality of their relationship. "How well do you and your husband/boyfriend [wife/girlfriend] get along?" "Does your husband/boyfriend [wife/girlfriend] know how distressed you are?" "How would they feel if they learned how distressed you are?" Sometimes marital quality can degrade when couples face serious external stressors, so information on recent stressors may sometimes clarify the reasons for martial conflict.

Nonmarried individuals, especially nonmarried men, have a greater risk of suicide than those who are married (Kyung-Sook, SangSoo, Sangjin, & Young-Jeon, 2018). The breakup of a marriage or long-term relationship can be very difficult. After a breakup many people become depressed, especially if they planned to get married or if they were living together (Rhoades, Kamp Dush, Atkins, Stanley, & Markman, 2011). Although some may feel a boost in happiness after a divorce, it is stressful for most people (H. S. Friedman & Martin, 2011), and it may also mean a change in social circles and residence, and a decrease in discretionary income.

Compared with controls, individuals who died from suicide were more likely to have interpersonal conflicts before their deaths (Overholser et al., 2012). These may include relationship problems with spouses or romantic partners. Some of the features associated with poor quality relationships include betrayals (affairs), partner violence, coldness, lack of emotional support, or unproductive quarreling. Separations or threats of separations can also precipitate suicidal ideation. Of course, the relationship between separation and low marital quality is complex because sometimes a preexisting mental disorder may cause or exacerbate both marital problems and suicidal ideation (Kazan, Calear, & Batterham, 2016).

The quality of social relationship may, for many patients, represent difficulties in establishing and maintaining good relationships. In addition, several studies have found a link between adult attachment styles and risk of suicide (Lizardi et al., 2011). Attachment theory holds that patients develop patterns of relating to significant others during early childhood. Parents who are responsive and concerned about their children are likely to have children who have secure attachment or a basic trust in others and an ability to develop close relationships. These models for relating to others persist into adulthood, although the models may change through experience and self-reflection, so that a child with insecure attachment (relatively little trust or confidence in others) may develop secure attachment as an adult. Lizardi et al. (2011) found that attachment problems were linked to past suicide attempts, and attachment-focused therapies with adolescents tend to reduce suicidal behavior (Ewing, Diamond, & Levy, 2015).

Psychotherapists should pay attention to themes of perceived burdensomeness, thwarted belongingness, and hopelessness that may arise in these conversations about social connections. It is one thing for a patient to say that he had an argument with his sister. It is another thing for a patient to say that he had an argument with his sister and that the rift will never be repaired. It is one thing for a patient to say that she has lost a job and is temporarily unemployed. It is another thing for a patient to say that she has lost a job and is not looking for another one because the employment opportunities for her are so bleak and she will always be a burden on others.

On the other hand, some patients in great emotional pain will often adamantly refuse to consider suicide because their friends or family members need them. As would be predicted by the three-step theory of suicide, the social connectedness of these patients inhibits suicidal behavior, despite whatever pain the patients feel. Those who have identical twins, are mothers, or are pregnant have lower rates of suicide, although an unwanted pregnancy may increase the risk of suicide in some women. Within the United States, those who attend religious services report higher levels of well-being than those who do not attend religious services. The reasons for this correlation are not clear, but one reason may be the social connections created or maintained by attendance at religious organizations.

The social connection does not necessarily have to be with humans; it could also occur with nonhuman companions. The following vignette illustrates this point.

The Protective Role of Nonhuman Companions

I have known patients who were so committed to their pets that they would never attempt suicide. They knew, accurately enough, that the quality of life for the pets would be seriously compromised if they were to die and the welfare of their animal companions were put in the hands of relatives, neighbors, or SPCA officials. In one case I took a great sigh of relief when I learned that a patient with chronic suicidal thoughts had just acquired a new dog (her old pet had died a year before). I knew her relationships to her dogs was very strong, and I could not imagine her doing anything that would hurt them.

Cultural Factors

Cultural variables need to be considered. Shame or disgrace and family discord were especially strong predictors of suicide among Asian Americans, and family conflict was related to suicidal behavior among Latinx (J. P. Chu, Goldblum, Floyd, & Bongar, 2010). Other cultural factors to consider include minority stress, cultural sanctions against suicide (discussed in Chapter 2), and idioms of distress (discussed later in the section on Mental Illness and Psychological Health; J. P. Chu, Hoeflein, et al., 2017).

Shame may also be important in honor cultures, or cultures where one's self-worth is determined by reputation and efforts must be sustained to ward off threats to one's honor. Suicide rates tend to be higher in honor cultures, perhaps because of the difficulties in always protecting one's honor (Crowder & Kemmelmeier, 2018).

African Americans who experience microaggressions have an increased risk of suicide, perhaps reflecting the social isolation or marginalization that are related to microaggressions (Hollingsworth et al., 2017). Ruminations about historical losses are associated with an increased risk of suicidal ideation among Native Americans (Tucker, Wingate, O'Keefe, Hollingsworth, & Cole, 2016). This finding makes intuitive sense. One would expect those who have had difficult lives and exposure to many adverse events would look for explanations, including the historical losses created by American policies toward Native Americans.

Social Media

With all patients, and especially younger patients, it is helpful to ask about their social media presence because that could be a major part of their social lives. It may help to start with open-ended questions such as "Tell me about your social media presence." Then if necessary psychotherapists could follow up with more specific questions such as "How much time do you spend on social media?" "Do you find it rewarding?" "Does it help you feel more connected with others?" Twenge, Joiner, Rogers, and Martin (2018) found that adolescents who spent the most screen time on social media had poorer mental health and more suicidal thoughts than adolescents who spent less screen time on social media and more time in other activities such as in-person social interactions, sports, reading, or attending religious services. It is unclear if the increased screen time or lack of other social activities accounted for this finding. Nonetheless, it is worth evaluating social media in the total context of the patient's life.

Clark, Algoe, and Green (2018) found conflicting data on the relationship of social media to psychological well-being for adults. They concluded that "social network sites benefit their users when they are used to make meaningful social connections and harm their users through pitfalls such as isolation and social comparison when they are not" (p. 32). For some patients, Facebook and other media may help them to keep up-to-date with relatives or friends who live at a distance. For other patients, social media may be associated with a lack of meaningful personal relationships.

Topic Four: Physical Health

The essential points that psychotherapists should remember about physical health and suicide are that

- poor physical health predicts suicide, especially if there is chronic pain or a decline in activities of daily living;

- insomnia has an especially strong link to suicide; and

- some of the cognitive processes found in some chronic pain patients, such as catastrophizing, are similar to the cognitive processes found in patients who have suicidal thoughts.

Psychotherapists should ask patients about their physical health. They can ask open-ended questions such as "How is your health?" When reviewing the patient's medical condition, psychotherapists can ask patients to tell them more about that condition and how it impacts their daily life, such as restricting their activities of daily living, causing them chronic pain, keeping them from meeting up with friends, or leading them to experience workplace discrimination (Khazem, 2018). The patient information form (Appendix A) contains a question about current medications including prescription, over-the-counter, and alternative drugs or herbs. Psychotherapists can use the patient responses on the patient information form as a basis for discussing medications. "What are you taking this medication for?" "How is that working for you?"

Self-reported health may predict suicidality more than actual health. Some patients will report their health as good, even though they have numerous chronic illnesses and functional limitations. Other patients will report their health as poor, even though their conditions are minor.

Physical and mental health are intertwined. A medical condition can place a person at risk for developing or exacerbating a mental disorder, especially depression, and can also increase the risk of suicide. It is not possible, however, to identify precise correlations between specific medical conditions and suicidality. This is due to methodological issues, including differences in the populations studied (e.g., Western or non-Western populations; older adults or population in general); the way that diseases are classified; or whether the index is suicide, suicidal ideation, or suicide attempts.

Nonetheless, cancer, diabetes, neurological disorder (e.g., epilepsy), osteoporosis, pulmonary disorders (e.g., asthma), skin disorders (e.g., eczema, psoriasis), and visual and hearing disorders appear to increase the risk of suicide (Erlangsen et al., 2015; Fässberg et al., 2016; Kavalidou et al., 2017; Khazem, 2018; Kye & Park, 2017; R. T. Webb et al., 2012). The polytrauma triad of PTSD, traumatic brain injury, and chronic pain increases the risk of suicide (Blakey et al., 2018).

It may be indicated to ask patients with chronic or severe illnesses about their activities of daily living. Patients often feel depressed if they cannot drive or otherwise leave their houses because of physical limitations or because they depend on others for mobility. Even simple tasks such as taking a shower on one's own or opening a can of olives can be frustrating and discouraging. That may help explain, for example, why osteoporosis increases the risk of suicide.

Chronic pain is associated with an increased risk of suicide, but the exact nature of the relationship is unclear, especially because many chronic pain patients have risk factors for suicidal thoughts (e.g., being female, isolated, having a comorbid substance misuse disorder; Campbell et al., 2016). Also, some of the personality traits or behaviors that contribute to suicide, such as catastrophic thinking or depressed mood, exacerbate pain-related distress, and some of the personality traits or behaviors that reduce the risk of suicide such as having a positive affect also mitigate pain related distress.

Pain and sleep problems appear to have a bidirectional influence, with changes in sleep problems predicting changes in pain and, to a lesser extent, changes in pain predicting sleep patterns (Koffel et al., 2016). This is especially relevant given the influence that sleep problems have on suicidal behavior (see discussion of sleep disturbance and suicide later in this chapter). The sample patient information sheet (Appendix A) includes a question about the patient's quality of sleep.

Some patients will attempt to control chronic pain through opioids, although opioids seldom reduce chronic pain. Nonetheless, some patients are so afraid of the chronic pain that they become deeply committed to and invested in continuing to take opioids. The long-term use of opioids increases the risk of opioid addiction among patients who have a background of substance abuse. Also, some patients may develop depression from long-term opioid use.

Sometimes the news of a serious medical condition, such as dementia among younger adults, can precipitate suicidal thoughts. Of course, the issue for the patient is perceived burdensomeness; patients often misconstrue the extent to which they are a burden.

If any patient reports significant health problems, it is indicated to communicate with the health professionals treating the patients. It is useful for psychotherapists to have a clearer understanding of the physical limits of their patients. As noted in Chapter 4, sometimes health care professionals are unaware of the psychological impact that disabilities are having on their patients.

In some rare occasions, patients may have suicidal thoughts secondary to a physical illness or as a side effect of a medication. I once promptly hospitalized a new patient following a serious suicide attempt. While in the hospital, this patient was diagnosed with a tumor, which was successfully removed, and the mental health symptoms quickly dissipated. Shea (2011) reported evaluating a man with strong suicidal thoughts. During the interview, he learned that the man was on a medication that sometimes had suicidal thoughts as a side effect. When the medication was removed, his suicidal thoughts lifted. These events do not commonly occur. But it is prudent to ask for a review of medications including nonprescription drugs or herbal supplements for all patients regardless of whether or not they present with suicidal thoughts.

Topic Five: Religion and Values

The essential points that psychotherapists should remember about religion and values are that

- values, including religious and spiritual values, can often reduce suicide risk; and

- suicidal patients often go on "values autopilot," where they fail to connect their values to their lives.

Religion is a major force in the lives of many people. One of the questions on the sample patient information form (see Appendix A) asks patients if they would like treatment to incorporate their religious or spiritual beliefs. If patients respond "yes," psychotherapists can ask them about their religion. If patients respond "no," psychotherapists can ask them about their value system. Some patients do not want to talk about religion, perhaps because they believe it is irrelevant or perhaps they fear that their psychotherapists will denigrate or criticize their belief system.

If patients are willing to talk about it, then psychotherapists can say, "Tell me how your religious traditions make you stronger" or "What is helpful in your religious tradition?" Or they could ask, "What gives you strength during these stressful times?" "Who do you rely on for support while you are going through all these struggles?" or use similar phrasing.

Even if patients decline to talk about religion, psychotherapists can nonetheless ask about values, what is important to them, or what kind of person they would like to be. Often patients will state that they value being a good parent, a caring spouse, or a conscientious employee. Unfortunately, because of their emotional distress, many patients feel divorced from their values and are living in a state of values autopilot, wherein they fail to connect their values to their daily lives.

Religious beliefs are a subset of a broader category that has been called *global meaning systems* (C. L. Park, Currier, Harris, & Slattery, 2017) or *centers of meaning* (Silberman, 2005). Nonreligious persons may have strongly considered values that form the bedrock in their lives. Psychotherapists can help patients identify their values. Whether patients express this in terms of religion, spirituality, or values is less important than the salience the beliefs have for them. Some patients may be in "values autopilot" and have difficulty identifying their values. The following vignette illustrates this point.

A Patient Identifies Meaning

A nurse who was depressed and suicidal denied having any values. Despite her depression, she always went to work and took her work seriously. The psychotherapist pointed out that she must value the well-being of others highly given that she worked conscientiously as a nurse despite her subjective distress.

The data on the relationship between religion and suicide are mixed. Most studies find that religion is associated with a reduced risk of suicide, although some studies found it unrelated to suicide risk and a few studies finding that it increased suicide risk (Gearing & Alonzo, 2018). One of the reasons for the inconsistent finding is that religion is a complex and multidimensional phenomenon that could involve both internal and external factors, and different dimensions of religion could impact different dimensions of the social and psychological lives of patients. Part of the protective nature of religion may be that it involves participation with a social group (e.g., attending communal worship services or participating in church functions together), encourages healthy lifestyles (e.g., discouraging smoking or excess alcohol consumption), or offers instrumental support in the form of concrete or material resources (e.g., bringing meals to those who are temporarily disabled, providing transportation to doctor's appointments). Also, many people find that being of service to others reduces their own sense of isolation.

In addition to its instrumental support, religion often advocates for life-protecting beliefs ("I have an obligation to follow the commandment not to kill myself") and life-promoting beliefs ("I have an obligation to live my life fully and contribute to others"). A *life-protecting belief* is a negative commandment: Do not kill oneself. A *life-promoting belief* is a positive commandment: Improve my life and the lives of others. A life-promoting belief typically involves hope, a sense of self-worth (e.g., one is made in the image of God), and social obligations to others, including an obligation to be a good family member, congregant, or citizen. Life-promoting beliefs encourage coping strategies that religiosity provides (e.g., solace in the face of stressful events). It is preferable for patients to express life-promoting beliefs, but life-protecting beliefs may temporarily inhibit patients from attempting suicide. Patients who had high moral objections to suicide were less likely to attempt suicide than patients with low moral objections to suicide (Lizardi et al., 2008).

Topic Six: Mental Illness and Psychological Health

The essential points that psychotherapists need to remember about mental illness and psychological health are that

- although suicide is a transdiagnostic symptom, it is more common among patients with some diagnoses;

- traditional notions of mental illness may not capture all the suffering that suicidal individuals experience;

- regardless of the specific diagnosis, psychotherapists should look for experiences that increase their desire to die or their acquired capability for suicide; and

- psychological resilience can reduce the risk of suicide.

Psychotherapists have been trained to link treatment procedures to the diagnoses of their patients. This makes some sense for the treatment of suicidal patients, but two caveats need to be made. First, suicidal behavior occurs across a wide range of diagnoses. Second, the current diagnostic system might not capture all the emotional suffering of patients, and for purpose of suicide prevention, psychotherapists need to supplement their knowledge of the ICD–10 with knowledge of the life circumstances and cultural experiences of their patients.

It is often stated that about 90% of patients who die from suicide have a mental disorder (e.g., Liotta et al., 2015). Studies that obtained that estimate often looked through the medical records of patients who died from suicide and determined if the patients had a diagnosis or had the symptoms recorded in the medical record sufficient to warrant a diagnosis.

J. Chu, Chi, Chen, and Leino (2014) stated that this 90% figure is too high, at least as it applies to Asian Americans. They claimed that physical illness, functional limitations, shame at being a burden on other family members, family conflict, or acculturation stress may create suicidal thoughts even in the absence of a mental disorder. Only 67% of their sample of suicidal Asian Americans had psychiatric disorders. They opined that psychotherapists should look at sociocultural factors in addition to diagnosed mental illness to treat mental illnesses among Asian Americans.

On the other hand, Joiner, Buchman-Schmitt, and Chu (2017) claimed that this 90% figure is too low, and that many suicide decedents have undiagnosed mental illnesses or subclinical features of mental illnesses. The differences between these findings may be more apparent than real. It may be profitable to look back and see how mental illness is defined. According to one common definition, mental illness is "on-going patterns of thoughts, feelings, and actions that are deviant, distressful, and/or dysfunctional" (Myers, 2008, p. 594). If family problems, interpersonal conflicts, feelings of burdensomeness, and acculturation stress cause great emotional turmoil, perhaps they should be included in the definition of mental illness, even if the patients do not fit into current diagnostic formulae developed for predominately Western populations.

This interpretation of what should constitute a mental illness does not detract from the important implications of the work of J. Chu et al. (2014): Psychotherapists should recognize that suicides frequently have precipitants in Asian Americans that differ in strength and valence from those found in the majority population, and a greater sensitivity to these cultural differences will help improve suicide detection. Good psychotherapists are sensitive to the idioms of distress found in different cultures.

Cultural factors can also influence the interpretation of suicidal behavior. J. Chu, Khoury, et al. (2017) found that Caucasian Americans were more likely to endorse mental health or medical reasons for their suicidal behavior, whereas Latinx and Asian Americans were more likely to identify interpersonal conflicts as the reason for their suicidal behavior.

The mental disorder, or its cultural or subclinical variant, may create or facilitate a cognitive predisposition to consider suicide. In addition, the mental disorder may be precipitated by or coexist with external stressors, such as recent job loss, disruptions in social relationships, or physical illness or disability.

Although suicidal behavior can occur in a wide range of diagnoses, some diagnoses present a higher risk of suicide than others. Kessler et al. (1999) found that manic disorders (bipolar) represented the greatest risk of a suicide attempt, followed by depression and substance abuse. Other researchers have included anorexia and PTSD as especially high-risk diagnoses for suicide (Nock, Hwang, Sampson, & Kessler, 2010). Psychotic processes are cause for special concern. Patients with acute psychotic features present as especially high risk to attempt suicide. Referrals for medication are always indicated, and hospitalizations may sometimes be required.

Patients with comorbid mental health diagnoses may have a higher risk of a suicide attempt probably because they increase the likelihood that the individual has more of the features associated with suicidal behavior, according to the ideation-to-action theories of suicide. For example, as it applies to the acquired capability for self-injury, anorexia, substance abuse (especially the use of injected drugs), trauma, NSSI, and aggressive behaviors may be related to higher risks of suicide regardless of the specific diagnoses because they increase acquired capability in that they involve experiences that may habituate an individual toward suffering and pain and decrease their fear of death. Or, they involve a sense of humiliation, defeat, or entrapment.

Hopelessness or entrapment are common features associated with suicide. But psychotherapists should not assume that having plans for the future means an absence of hopelessness. In their review of psychological factors, psychologists should not give too much weight to the presence of future plans or the appearance of the patient. Patients can have plans for the future and still be highly suicidal. They may report that they intend to take such-and-such a trip, have ideas for business expansion, or are working on an important project, and still present a high risk of suicide. Joiner (2010) provided anecdotal information about decedents who had made plans or had talked about plans before, and sometimes even hours before, they died from suicide. Furthermore, R. C. O'Connor, Smyth, and Williams (2015) found that positive future thinking was associated with a subsequent suicide attempt. The reason for this counterintuitive finding is not clear. Perhaps the respondents had unrealistic goals or perhaps they felt acute disappointment if their goals were not met.

Grooming should not be overvalued either. It is true that grooming may have clinical implications. In addition, persons who are in an immediate state of preparing for suicide will often slow down their blink rate (Joiner et al., 2016), which probably reflects a degree of commitment to act within minutes. Nonetheless, physical appearance alone is a poor prognosticator of suicidal status. Other than blink rates, no data on physical appearance differentiates suicidal patients from nonsuicidal patients. Suicidal patients can often present well, be poised, and appear well dressed and immaculately groomed.

The following section reviews several of the mental health conditions most commonly linked with suicide: depression, substance abuse, anorexia, and serious personality disorders. Then it reviews specific transdiagnostic factors such as aggression, trauma, and NSSI. It ends with a review of suicide among older adults, including those with dementia.

Depression

Major depressive or bipolar disorders are associated with suicide in the common mind. It is likely that the social isolation associated with depression or that the disruptions in interpersonal relationships caused by bipolar disorder may lead to the thwarted belongingness, perceived burdensomeness, or entrapment that are associated with suicide according to the ideation-to-action theories of suicide. Unipolar depression also increases risks of suicide, most probably through the social alienation, self-disgust, and hopelessness that often accompanies depression. Expressions of fatigue or lack of energy may be equivalents for sadness and loneliness in some cultures.

In addition, bipolar disorder is believed to be heavily influenced by genetic factors, and it is possible that the genetic predisposition to bipolar disorder may account for the clustering of suicides in some families, although the data on this is currently unclear (McGuffin et al., 2010).

Misuse of Alcohol

Alcohol misuse is related to suicide in two ways. First, those who have chronic problems with alcohol have an increased risk to die from suicide, especially if the alcohol misuse is comorbid with other mental disorders (Conner, Bagge, Goldston, & Ilgen, 2014). About 27% of suicide decedents had alcohol in their bloodstream at the time of their deaths, but not all of those were intoxicated (Anestis, Joiner, Hanson, & Gutierrez, 2014). When intoxication precedes a suicide attempt, it is not known if the alcohol increased suicidal thoughts, if the alcohol removed inhibitions against self-harm, or if the alcohol influenced different persons differently (Conner et al., 2014). Nonetheless, it is helpful to ask suicidal patients about their use of alcohol or other drugs, even if it is not part of the presenting problem. Alcohol appears to facilitate suicide attempts more than other drugs (Bryan, Garland, & Rudd, 2016).

Misuse of Opioids and Other Drugs

Drug overdoses are now the leading cause of accidental death within the United States. The number of drug overdoses in the United States has tripled since 1999, and of the 52,000 drug overdoses in 2015, 63% involved opioids, with sharp increases in fentanyl- and heroin-related deaths (Rudd, Seth, David, & Scholl, 2016). Overdoses from heroin increased fivefold from 2001 to 2013 and increased threefold from 2010 to 2014.

Opioid, cocaine, and polysubstance addictions are also associated with increased risks of suicide (Yuodelis-Flores & Ries, 2015). Bogdanowicz et al. (2016) found that more than one fourth of patients being treating for opioid misuse disorders had a previous suicide attempt. In addition, prolonged opioid use can cause depression among some patients who had no history of depression. The relationship between substance misuse and suicide becomes more complex when considering that many of the sequalae of substance misuse, such as legal difficulties, loss of employment, or disruptions in relationships, are also risk factors for suicide.

Patients who abuse opioids or other drugs are more likely to die from suicide if they have a comorbid mental illness such as depression (Ortíz-Gómez, López-Canul, & Arankowsky-Sandoval, 2014) or if they inject drugs (Artenie et al., 2015). According to the IPT, repeated self-injections may habituate drug users to pain and reduce their natural inhibition against self-harm (Joiner, 2005).

It is often hard to distinguish between an accidental or intentional death, and many overdoses listed as accidental may have been intentional (Bogdanowicz et al., 2016). The factors commonly used to distinguish intentional from unintentional deaths are a history of past suicide attempts, the statements of the patients immediately before the overdose, and the likelihood of mis-calculation of drug effects. Accidental overdoses often occur among those who have recently been through withdrawal or have otherwise reduced their intake of drugs over time and lost the tolerance their bodies once had to high levels of drugs. When they take the level of drugs that they previously needed to get high, they may unintentionally take a level that kills them. Nonetheless, this methodology for distinguishing between intentional and accidental overdoses has limits to it, and Rockett et al. (2014) argued that suicides from drug overdoses are substantially underrepresented in official statistics.

The distinction between deliberate and accidental deaths may be too arbitrary. The word *accident* implies that the event was random and unpredictable. Perhaps many drug deaths listed as accidental were not random or unpredictable but reflected indifference or disregard for personal safety. Patients might say something to the effect of, "I did not care whether I lived or died at the time I took those drugs."

The ability to distinguish between accidental and intentional drug deaths are further complicated because both usually involved more than one drug, such as alcohol, marijuana, heroin, or other illegal drugs, or other prescription medications, especially benzodiazepines (Yarborough et al., 2016). Also, those who had overdoses of opioids listed as accidental often shared characteristics with suicidal patients: chronic pain, the lack of stable resources and consistent family support (Yarborough et al., 2016), the abuse of three or more substances, and a history of depression (Bohnert, Roeder, & Ilgen, 2011). One implication is that psychotherapists should get details about past overdoses, even if patients labeled them as accidental. Even if labeled accidental, past overdoses at least raise the possibility of an indifference toward living.

Anorexia

Patients with anorexia have rates of suicide that are significantly higher than the rates of suicide for patients with most other mental disorders. Aside from the medical complications caused by anorexia, suicide is the most common cause of death for those who have anorexia (Brausch & Perkins, 2018). One theory is that the poor health caused by anorexia makes the individuals less able to withstand the physical trauma caused by a suicide attempt. However, this claim lacks strong evidence. Anorexic women who die from suicide often use violent means that would likely kill anyone (Joiner, 2010).

Another theory is that anorexia is a form of passive suicide or slow death by self-starvation. However, this claim also lacks strong evidence. Only a small percentage of patients with anorexia die from suicide. Furthermore, the goal of restricted eating is not death but a change in physical appearance (Joiner, 2010).

According to the IPT, patients with anorexia gradually lose their inhibition against pain and death because of their continued experiences with self-starvation (Joiner, 2005). However, the data on this are mixed, and the research is complicated by the fact that NSSIs often co-occur with anorexia and other eating disorders (Brausch & Perkins, 2018). Also, as would be predicted by the IPT, A. R. Smith, Zuromski, and Dodd (2018) suggested that suicidal patients with eating disorders have low belongingness and perceived burdensomeness. It appears that patients with eating disorders may have strained social relationships because of the demanding nature of their disorder that makes relationships hard, which may explain the link to suicide through thwarted belongingness or perceived burdensomeness (Goldstein & Gvion, 2019).

Serious Personality Disorders

Some suicidal patients have serious personality disorders (e.g., borderline personality disorder [BPD]). They often have histories of childhood traumas, self-mutilation, or repeated suicide attempts that, according to the IPT, increase their acquired capability for suicide because it habituates them to the fear of dying. They often cannot control their distress. In addition, they may have life stressors, emotional pain, feelings of hopelessness, and a lack of connections with others, or they may also have comorbid diagnoses of eating disorders, substance abuse, major depression, or a pattern of NSSI that will further increase the risk of suicide.

Some psychotherapists believe that the suicide attempts by patients with BPDs are designed to elicit reactions from those in their immediate social circle or to gain special attention or privileges. Because the assumed goal is to alter or manipulate the behavior of others, they are called *manipulative attempts*. Those threats of suicide may come across as selfish, insensitive, and representing a sense of entitlement. If so, then it appears that a history of a previous suicide attempt should not generate the same degree of concern with a patient with BPD as it would with a patient without BPD.

But the issue is more complex. First patients who show the symptoms of BPD do sometimes die from suicide, even if it had been assumed that they were only trying to solicit responses from others. In a follow-up study that lasted 26 years, Paris and Zweig-Frank (2001) found that 10% of patients with BPD died from suicide.

Second, clinicians should not always assume that patients are telling the truth when they say that they did not intend to die from the attempt. Some patients who survive a suicide attempt will minimize the strength of or even outright deny their wish to die. Also, patients themselves may not always fully understand the reasons for their attempts. Furthermore, suicidal attempts can have more than one motive. A desire to influence the environment, to communicate one's distress, or to solicit support from others may be combined with a sincere desire to die.

In addition, psychotherapists should take all threats seriously, even if not always literally. It is dangerous to assume that if the patients were seriously suicidal, they would have died by suicide long ago, or that if they were serious about suicide, they would "stop talking about it and just do it" (Jobes, Rudd, Overholser, & Joiner, 2008). It is more productive to assume that the threats were the patient's effort to express the degree of their distress. Often threats of suicide with BPD patients are linked to negative emotions arising out of interpersonal conflicts (Wedig, Frankenburg, Bradford Reich, Fitzmaurice, & Zanarini, 2013). Although the emotional suffering of the patients might not always lead to a suicide attempt, the suffering is very real.

Exposure to Trauma and PTSD

Traumas could include any threat to the safety or life of a person or assaults or threats that cause substantial pain or fear of harm. Witnessing a trauma can, for some persons, be as upsetting as experiencing a trauma directly. Whether an individual develops PTSD after a trauma depends on the severity of the trauma, the psychological resources of the individual, and many contextual factors. PTSD creates fear and high vigilance and high emotional arousal, but also feelings of danger, lack of trust in others, and other distressing thoughts. Some may even experience moral distress or guilt and shame over actions or lack of actions that occurred at the time of the trauma.

Exposure to trauma is a risk factor for suicide. One trauma increases the risk of suicide, and multiple traumas increase the risk even more. The risk of a suicide attempt with PTSD patients increases if they also abuse alcohol (Rojas, Bujarski, Babson, Dutton, & Feldner, 2014) or if they are especially sensitive to anxiety (I. H. Stanley, Hom, Spencer-Thomas, & Joiner, 2017). The presence of PTSD predicted suicide risk better than exposure to trauma itself (LeBouthillier, McMillan, Thibodeau, & Asmundson, 2015). The arousal and reactivity associated with PTSD may be the factors most closely associated with suicide risk (Brown, Contractor, & Benhamou, 2018).

The reasons for the connection between PTSD, trauma, and suicide are not clear. Perhaps the pain from traumas reduces the inhibition against self-violence and increases the acquired capability for self-harm as would be predicted by the IPT (Bryan, Grove, & Kimbrel, 2017). Perhaps the symptoms such as poor mood, depression, or poor temper control disrupt social relationships and increase social isolation (Poindexter et al., 2015). Perhaps the trauma leads to psychological distress that patients perceive as unbearable and create a sense of entrapment as would be predicted by the IMV theory. Or perhaps all three factors could be involved and interact in complex ways.

Nonsuicidal Self-Injury

NSSI refers to cutting, burning, hitting, or other self-inflicted pain in the absence of any suicidal intent. Skin cutting is the most common form of NSSI. It is commonly found in patients with BPD, but it occurs across other disorders as well, and it also occurs in some individuals with no psychiatric diagnosis. Perhaps as many as one in five university students will engage in a NSSI (Willoughby, Heffer, & Hamza, 2015).

Many patients self-injure because it reduces distressing emotions such as anger, fear, anxiety, or tension. Other patients seek to punish themselves or elicit attention from others. Motivations for NSSI can change between episodes or even within episodes (Kapur, Cooper, O'Connor, & Hawton, 2013). Acts of self-harm may temporarily reduce negative emotions, but they do not teach individuals how to circumvent or manage strong emotions. Acts of self-harm may sometimes elicit an immediate response from others in the short run, but they seldom improve social relationships or feelings of closeness with others in the long run.

NSSI differs from suicide in that the patients do not intend to die. NSSI typically involves less severe medical damage than a suicide attempt and occurs more frequently. Whereas most suicidal people will "only" attempt suicide a few times in their lives, a nonsuicidal self-injurious patient might have dozens or even hundreds of acts of self-inflicted harm. In addition, adolescents or young adults are more likely to engage in NSSI than middle-aged or older adults.

Nonetheless, NSSI and suicide ideation often co-occur. Also, many patients with NSSI will express passive suicidal thoughts (e.g., "I don't care if I live or not"). The risk of suicide increases if the patient has had multiple episodes of harm, uses different methods of self-harm, has inflicted more serious medical damage, reports a decrease in the amount of pain from self-harm, and has a higher level of overall psychopathology (Ward-Ciesielski, Schumacher, & Bagge, 2016). NSSIs increase the risk that a person with suicidal ideation will develop a plan and the risk that a person with a suicidal plan will make a suicide attempt (Kiekens et al., 2018).

The IPT claims that suicidal behavior is more likely to occur when individuals become habituated to pain, such as may occur from NSSI. A review of self-injury studies found that those who engage in NSSI will show an increase in pain tolerance (Kirtley, O'Carroll, & O'Connor, 2016). In the case of NSSI, the repeated exposures to pain may lead to a decrease in fear about death or the pain and injury associated with suicide (Joiner, Ribeiro, & Silva, 2012). Willoughby et al. (2015) found support for this in their prospective study wherein repeated incidents of self-harm reduced the patient's fear of death and perceptions of pain. Consequently, NSSIs may represent a stepping stone or a progression of self-harm that goes from nonlethal self-harm to suicide attempts (Bryan, Bryan, May, & Klonsky, 2015).

Aggression

Suicide is related to aggression regardless of the diagnosis of the patient. For example, in a sample of men court ordered for treatment for intimate partner battering, 22% had suicidal ideation (Wolford-Clevenger et al., 2015). Also, soldiers who have externalizing disorders have a greater risk of suicidal behavior (M. J. Friedman, 2014). Except for antisocial personality disorder, the presence of an aggression-related mental disorder increased the risk of a suicide (McCloskey & Ammerman, 2018). Violence toward others, being a victim of violence, and violence to self are highly correlated (Monahan, Vesselinov, Robbins, & Appelbaum, 2017), and 1.6% of suicides are murder/suicides (Stone et al., 2018).

Persons who act violently often have comorbid substance abuse and impulsivity problems (Murrie & Kelley, 2017). They may also show some of the same absolutist and catastrophizing thinking patterns that occur among suicidal persons.

Thus, it is prudent to consider acts of violence or victimization when estimating suicide risk, and it is appropriate to ask persons with strong suicidal thoughts whether they have acted violently or are at risk to do so. The link makes sense from the standpoint of the IPT where repeated exposure to violence gradually reduces an individual's fear of death or harm.

Dementias and Other Considerations With Older Adults

Older adults have rates of suicide that exceed that of the population in general. The rates of suicide are especially high among the oldest old (those who are 80 years old or older). However, nothing about being an older adult necessarily leads a person to become suicidal. Instead, older adults are more likely to have life circumstances or experiences that predispose them to suicide. For example, poor physical health is associated with an increased risk of suicide. Cheung, Merry, and Sundram (2015) found that one-third of older adults who left suicide notes gave poor physical health as the reason for their suicide and almost three fourths had underlying medical conditions. These physical problems may involve a loss of autonomy, physical pain, or a perception that they are a burden to others. Other self-reported reasons for suicide attempts among older adults include psychological pain, family conflicts, and a lack of meaning in life (Van Orden et al., 2015).

Suicides are more likely to occur when individuals have recently transitioned into a nursing home or have had a loved one transition to a nursing home. Otherwise, Mezuk, Rock, Lohman, and Choi (2014) could not find any consistent list of factors associated with suicide risk in nursing homes, other than the long-term predictors associated with suicide in general: depression, social isolation, loneliness, and functional decline. But larger facilities tended to have higher rates of resident suicides (Mezuk, Lohman, Leslie, & Powell, 2015).

Some older adults have passive wishes to die, although they might not necessarily express an intention to kill themselves. Often these adults have had recent losses, such as the loss of a loved one or the loss of independence and physical functioning. They may say, "I hope to die in my sleep," or "I am just waiting for God to take me." Indirect self-destructive behaviors include refusal to eat, or drink, or to cooperate with medical regimens. These statements and behaviors usually warrant clinical interventions designed to improve the quality of their lives and expand their social relationships. However, these statements, in and of themselves, would not warrant considering a patient to be suicidal.

Patients admitted to nursing homes must be screened for psychiatric conditions, including the possibility of suicidal thoughts or intent. This screening can identify residents who need to be monitored or receive mental health services.

Qin's (2011) review found mixed results when looking at the relationship of dementias and other forms of cognitive decline to suicide. Some studies have found an increased risk, whereas others have found a decreased risk. The analysis of this contradictory data requires considering the type of cognitive decline, how it is measured, preexisting risk factors, the living conditions of those who have dementia, and other factors.

Qin (2011) opined that dementia represented an increased risk for suicide, although the risk is far less than the risk created by other mental disorders. Furthermore, the increased risk is highest for younger adults with dementias. It is possible that a recent diagnosis of dementia may increase the desire to die from suicide, but individuals who progressed to more debilitating forms of dementia may lack the executive functions necessary for planning a suicide or may live in facilities or have caregivers who closely monitor them.

Psychological Strengths

Protective factors may include *psychological resilience* or "a set of skills or behaviors that help them [people] understand or manage a stressful event"

(C. L. Park et al., 2017, p. 186). Psychological resilience could include the ability to gain distance from one's problems, to have hope or a sense that one could change the future for the better, or the ability to distract oneself from intensely unpleasant emotions.

The evidence on the role of psychological resilience on protecting patients from suicide come from several studies wherein hardiness (commitment, control, and accepting life as a challenge; Abdollahi, Abu Talib, Yaacob, & Ismail, 2015), ability to face adversity (Min, Lee, & Chae, 2015), a sense of purpose and control (Pietrzak et al., 2010), gratitude (N. B. Smith et al., 2016), ability to tolerate distress (I. H. Stanley, Boffa, et al., 2018), and positive mental health (Teismann, Forkmann, et al., 2018) all appear to be negatively associated with suicidal ideation, although not all researchers found such connections (e.g., Liu, Fairweather-Schmidt, Burns, Roberts, & Anstey, 2016). Humor can be a sign of psychological resilience if it focuses on building relationships with others, but aggressive humor could alienate others and impair social relationships (Tucker et al., 2013).

It is suggested that psychotherapists look for psychological strengths unique to the patient in both their life overall and in response to suicidal thoughts. Psychotherapists can ask patients to identify their psychological strengths or to describe a recent challenge that they handled well and what about their behavior caused that event to turn out well. These may give psychotherapists some clues as to what strengths may reduce the likelihood of suicide in the long term and give suggestions for what strengths to use in the service of an effective treatment. Of course, psychological resources can sometimes be stressor specific and can vary across time and situations. I knew a woman who weathered health problems and unemployment with remarkable inner strength until her health returned and she could return to work. But years later she fell apart when her pet died.

In addition, psychotherapists can look for suicide-specific coping abilities. B. Stanley, Green, Ghahramanlou-Holloway, Brenner, and Brown (2017) referred to *suicide-related coping* as the "knowledge of and perceived self-efficacy in engaging in the use of internal coping strategies and external resources to manage suicidal thoughts with the goal of decreasing imminent risk and averting suicidal crises" (p. 190). These strategies or resources would include engaging in activities that reduce suicidal thoughts or being able to regulate one's emotions when suicidal urges appear.

ASSESSMENT STEP 4 (OPTIONAL): BRIEF SYMPTOM INVENTORIES

As noted earlier in this chapter, it is recommended that psychotherapists give every mental health patient at least one written question and one verbal question concerning suicide as part of a universal screening process. In addition, when patients express suicidal ideation, or have risk factors for suicide, psychotherapists can consider administering a brief suicide symptom test.

These tests will supplement, but not replace, the ordinary suicide evaluation process.

Psychotherapists might use brief tests to identify patients who appear to be false deniers. Results from the brief tests may confirm the clinical impressions of the psychotherapists. Or they may reveal that the patients have more (or less) suicidal risk than the psychotherapists had thought from the interviewing alone.

Also, psychotherapists may use brief tests to monitor suicidal ideation or measure treatment progress. Repeated administration of screening instruments does not appear to have an iatrogenic effect (Hom et al., 2018). However, very brief screening instruments that rely on historical data would not be appropriate to evaluate progress over time because historical data is less sensitive to change.

No suicide instrument predicts suicide with a high degree of both sensitivity (how well do they identify those at risk) and specificity (how well do they rule out those not at risk). Runeson et al. (2017) reviewed suicide assessment instruments and found "no scientific support for the use of suicide risk instruments for predicting suicidal acts" (p. 9). The author is not challenging this conclusion but noted that the goal here is limited to using tests to supplement psychotherapists impressions, identify false deniers, or monitor progress. Consequently, psychotherapists should never use a test alone to estimate the risk of suicide, but the results can be one component in an overall assessment. The tests that follow are not the only ones that could be used. Psychotherapists may use other instruments with which they have greater familiarity, or that are used regularly at their facility (e.g., if they are required as part of the facilities participation in MIPS), or that have more research with specific populations.

Psychotherapists who use tests must ensure that they score and interpret them. In one study, only about 20% of patients who endorsed suicidal thoughts on the PHQ–9 had subsequent discussions with their physicians about their suicide (Quinnett, 2018). If the worst should happen and a patient died from suicide and the psychotherapists got sued, it would be difficult for the psychotherapists to explain why they thought that giving the test was important but did not score the test or document the results. Psychotherapists should explain to patients that they are using these tests to obtain a better understanding of them, because they care about them and their welfare, or that they are using them to measure progress over time.

The instruments reviewed here include the Beck Depression Inventory, the Beck Hopelessness Scale, and the Beck Scale for Suicide Ideation. They are selected because they are high on sensitivity and thus may be better at identifying false deniers than a test high on specificity.

The Beck Depression Inventory (Beck, Steer, & Brown, 1996) contains 21 items that measure emotional, physiological, and behavioral symptoms of depression on a scale of 0–3 with 12 being a cutoff suggesting suicidal risk (Troister, D'Agata, & Holden, 2015). It takes 10 minutes to complete. Although it was originally developed with samples with depression, it has been found to predict suicidal behavior with patients with a wider range of diagnoses.

The Beck Hopelessness Scale (Beck, 1993) contains 20 items that measure expectations of failure and thoughts about the future. It takes about 5 minutes to complete. It was originally designed to measure motivational, affective, and cognitive aspects of hopelessness, although subsequent research on such factors has been mixed (e.g., Iliceto & Fino, 2015). Nonetheless, a score of 6 or higher suggests a risk for suicide (Troister et al., 2015).

The Beck Scale for Suicidal Ideation (Beck, 1991) consists of 21 items that measure the duration and frequency of suicidal ideation, protective factors, and suicidal plans. It is an interview-administered scale that takes 5 to 10 minutes to complete. The patient has the option of responding to each item with either a 0, 1, or 2, reflecting the suicidal intensity. The scale starts with five screening items. If patients report any passive or active suicide thoughts to those items, then 14 more items are added to assess duration and frequency of suicidal thoughts, sense of control over those impulses, preparation for an attempt, and deterrents to a suicide attempt. The last two items ask about previous suicide attempts. A score higher than 0 raises concern.

Although assessment and interventions are presented in separate chapters, the processes overlap considerably. With some patients with a high risk of suicide, it may be necessary to move directly into safety planning even if the assessment is incomplete. With all patients the assessment will allow the development of a good relationship between the psychotherapists and patients and provide information that will help inform the interventions.

3

Interventions Part One

Including Managing Suicide Risk

Good psychotherapy saves lives. Although few outcome studies have looked at suicide attempts as an outcome measure, a meta-analysis by Calati and Courtet (2016) found that, compared with patients who received medication alone or only brief or supportive psychosocial interventions, "patients who received psychotherapy were less likely to attempt suicide during the follow-up" (p. 8).

However, good psychotherapy with suicidal patients should first focus on managing the immediate risk of suicide. The goal of suicide management is to keep patients alive until psychotherapy has a chance to work. Addressing the mental illnesses that predispose patients to attempt suicide is important, but this concern is subservient to the need to ensure the patients' immediate safety. Treating the mental illness alone will not reduce the short-term risk of suicide (McKeon, 2009). Meerwijk et al. (2016) found that patients were 1 to 5 times more likely to die from suicide or to attempt suicide during treatment if they received an indirect intervention only (one that focused on the mental illness and not suicidal behavior itself) compared with receiving a direct intervention (one that focused on suicidal behaviors). Similarly, Dueweke, Rojas, Anastasia, and Bridges (2017) found that patients had a lower frequency of suicidal and self-harm thoughts if they received direct interventions as opposed to indirect interventions.

This chapter reviews effective psychotherapy with suicidal patients and the first parts of the intervention, including establishing the appropriate level of service, covering the informed consent process, promoting a good treatment

http://dx.doi.org/10.1037/0000145-004
Suicide Prevention: An Ethically and Scientifically Informed Approach, by S. J. Knapp

relationship, and managing suicide risk. Chapter 4 furthers the discussion of treatment and considers ways to modify psychotherapy to make it more effective with suicidal patients. Chapter 5 covers quality enhancement strategies that can be embedded throughout the assessment, management, and treatment processes as needed.

LEVELS OF SERVICE

The first step in planning the intervention is to determine the level of service or whether the patient should be treated as an inpatient or an outpatient. Throughout the assessment, psychotherapists have been gathering information to form a judgment about the patient's risk for suicide. By identifying the factors related to suicide risk, psychotherapists can estimate the risk of suicide and develop suicide management strategies and interventions to reduce that risk. Cramer, Johnson, McLaughlin, Rausch, and Conroy (2013) identified the determination of risk as one of the core competencies needed when treating suicidal patients.

Often psychotherapists must make decisions in less-than-optimal circumstances. Sometimes they must decide about risk immediately with a patient in a session, without the time to think through the decision or consult with others. Often they learn of the suicidal behavior in the intake interview and have little information on the patient and no history of a relationship to draw on. The stress may be particularly unnerving for novice psychotherapists. At its worst it may leave psychotherapists unsure as to what to do and cause them to lean toward the most conservative and restrictive interventions, such as a hospitalization, without thinking through the alternatives carefully. Ideally, psychotherapists who have had training or experience in dealing with suicidal patients will have a framework to draw on and that will guide them in their decisions, even if they must act quickly in less-than-optimal circumstances.

Psychotherapists must be realistic about the database available to guide them in estimating the risk of suicide for their patients. Years of research have identified only a few variables that are consistently associated with an elevated risk of suicide across many settings (Franklin et al., 2017). The imprecision may occur because the predictors of suicidal ideation may not be the same as predictors of suicidal attempts; because predictors for one culture may differ from predictors for another culture; or because of the inherent complexity of suicide that involves the interaction of numerous social, biological, or personality factors. So, for example, two individuals might share the same trait of loneliness, but its impact will be influenced by the other situational factors and personality traits.

Although short-term estimates of suicide risk are imperfect, this does not mean that psychotherapists should lapse into nihilism. Limitations in the data do not mean that psychotherapists have no data to draw on. A format for determining the immediate degree of risk and appropriate level of care is presented in the next section. This levels of service procedure has limitations to it, which are described. Nonetheless, it helps psychotherapists to decide whether to treat the patients in the hospital or as outpatients.

The following section describes the factors used to determine these levels of service, the ways to use levels of service charts, and their limitations. But first it must describe the fluid vulnerability theory (FVT) that influences how the levels are created.

Fluid Vulnerability Theory

Psychotherapists can estimate the risk of suicide by relying on the FVT (Rudd, 2006), which can be used along with ideation-to-action theories of suicide. According to the FVT, suicide risk can be seen from two dimensions: acute and baseline. Baseline refers to chronic or stable dimensions, whereas the acute dimension changes more quickly over time. The baseline represents a set point around which the risk of suicide can fluctuate. A stressful life event would be likely to change patients' acute risk, but less likely to change their baseline risk. The patients' suicide risk can move up or down depending on stressors or circumstances. Data from ecologically momentary analysis can be interpreted in a manner consistent with what the FVT would predict. For example, in their study using ecologically momentary analysis, Kleiman and Nock (2018) found that "suicidal ideation fluctuated close to a baseline with episodic peaks representing suicidal crisis" (p. 35). Similarly, Rogers and Joiner (2019) found variations in suicidal thoughts or suicide-related thoughts that seemed to fluctuate around a set point.

Patients with a high baseline of risk are more likely to experience a suicidal crisis or attempt suicide. It is easier for them to go into a suicidal crisis and harder for them to return to baseline. Patients with a lower baseline of risk are less likely to experience a suicidal crisis or attempt suicide. It is harder for them to go into a suicidal crisis and easier for them to return to baseline.

So, patients with a high baseline would be more likely to go into a suicidal crisis after an argument with a paramour, and they would take longer to return to their baseline. But patients with a low baseline would be less likely to go into a suicidal crisis after a similar argument. It would take less time for them to return to their baseline (Rudd, 2006).

The triggering event for the suicidal crisis is often related to the vulnerabilities of the patient. For example, a patient who had a suicidal crisis triggered by an interpersonal conflict would be likely to have loneliness or interpersonal deficiencies as a major vulnerability, which makes their baseline of risk high (Bryan & Rudd, 2018).

The FVT can be aligned with the ideation-to-action theories of suicide, which emphasize looking at the acquired capability for harm and access to means that may increase the risk of a suicide attempt. Information from the patient's background may influence the estimate of the patient's capacity for suicide.

Determining Risk

The risk of suicide could be considered imminent (hospitalization should be considered), serious (outpatient treatment with close monitoring should be appropriate), or moderate or low (outpatient treatment with some monitoring should be appropriate). The levels represent a continuum based on the degree of external control needed to ensure safety. However, these are not fixed categories, but heuristics, and psychotherapists should feel free to place patients in-between adjacent categories such as moderate/serious or serious/imminent and so on. Table 3.1 summarizes these levels of service.

The three factors used to formulate the level of service are (a) determining the baseline of distress, (b) identifying the likelihood of having a suicidal crisis, and (c) assessing access to lethal means. The determination of risk is made by looking at the interaction of these factors.

Determining the Baseline of Distress

The baseline of risk can be determined by looking at the subjective distress of the patient, scores on any test, and the acquired capability of harm. Psychotherapists can look for themes of emotional turmoil, perceived burdensomeness, thwarted belongingness, lack of reasons for living, or other factors that suggest that the patient wants to die. Brief symptom rating scales, as discussed in Chapter 2, may also give an indication of distress. Distress can be reduced if patients have protective factors such as a strong social network or a belief system that disapproves of self-harm.

According to Joiner, Van Orden, Witte, and Rudd (2009), psychotherapists can assume that patients have a high level of acquired capability for suicide if they have had multiple suicide attempts or if least three of the following applies to them: they had attempted suicide at least once; had a suicide attempt aborted; had self-injected drugs; had engaged in nonsuicidal self-injury; had frequent exposure to human suffering; or were exposed to physical violence either as a victim, witness, or perpetrator. This could include exposure to

TABLE 3.1. Levels of Service According to Estimated Risk

Level	Treatment option	Criteria
Imminent	Consider hospitalization	Easy to move into suicidal crisis (high baseline, few protective factors and suicide coping strategies) and access to means
Serious	Outpatient with intense monitoring	Not as easy to move into suicidal crisis (lower baseline or more protective factors or suicide coping strategies), *or* no access to means even if acquired capability is high
Moderate	Outpatient with monitoring	Harder to move into suicidal crisis (lower baseline or more protective factors or suicide coping strategies) *or* no access to means (or no plans) and may have lower acquired capability
Low	Outpatient with minimal monitoring	Unlikely to move into suicidal crisis, *and* acquired capability and no access to means or perhaps no plan for suicide

human suffering, as would be found among health care personnel, first responders, or disaster relief workers.

Using the parlance of Collaborative Assessment and Management of Suicidality (CAMS; Jobes, 2016), one could say that the baseline of the patient was determined or influenced by *indirect drivers* of suicide, or the "issues, or problems, or concerns that make the patient vulnerable to his or her direct drivers, but do not themselves cause suicidal states" (Jobes, 2016, p. 109). For example, a patient with a high daily level of irritability, agitation, or insomnia-induced fatigue would have a high baseline of distress.

Identifying the Likelihood of Having a Suicidal Crisis

Acute factors may change the suicidal risk and lead a patient to enter a suicidal crisis. So, patients could have a suicidal crisis if they experience a sudden stressor such as a fight with a loved one, job loss, or so on. From the standpoint of CAMS, one could say that the acute crises would be precipitated by *direct drivers*, which are patient-specific factors that "may propel the patient into acute suicidal states" (Jobes, 2016, p. 93).

Psychotherapists can estimate the likelihood that the patients would experience an external stressor or have difficulty responding to chronic stressors. Stulz et al. (2018) found patients often identified more than one precipitant of their suicide attempt and, like Stone et al. (2018), found that interpersonal conflicts were the most common precipitants. Other common reasons were financial problems, work stress, a recent death, and physical illness. Of course, no psychotherapist can predict all the events that could happen to patients, although some events could be expected. For example, if a patient says that his marriage is in trouble, then it could be expected that he might have stressors related to marital discord. Psychotherapists may consider their patients' abilities to weather such stressors in the past and could use this information to assess how well they could respond to similar stressors in the future.

A major goal of the assessment is to identify the potential triggers for the suicidal crisis and the warning signs (the psychological and behavioral symptoms that accompany the suicidal crisis). Data from the acute suicidal affective disturbance (ASAD; Rogers, Chiurliza, et al., 2017), the suicide crisis syndrome (SCS; Galynker, 2018), the CAMS, or other studies of acute psychological pain may identify warning signs that precede or accompany the patient's suicidal crisis (see the review in Chapter 2).

Assessing Access to Lethal Means

The final feature to consider is whether the patients have access to the means to kill themselves. As noted in Chapter 2, psychotherapists should also ask patients if they have secondary or tertiary plans.

Applying the Levels of Service

Hospitalizations should be considered for patients in the imminent category of risk. Patients in the imminent risk category have (a) a high baseline of distress including noticeable acquired capability of harm, (b) a likelihood of a suicidal crisis, and (c) access to the means to kill themselves. For example, patients in the imminent state may present a high indication of distress as indicated by the questions on suicidal ideation, display a mental health diagnosis accompanied by much psychological pain, score high on an inventory measuring emotional distress, or rate their daily level of distress is high. Patients may have described a suicidal crisis in the past, have numerous ongoing stressors, and report few protective factors that would keep them from entering into or interrupting that suicidal crisis. The patients may have an acquired capability for suicide as indicated by past suicide attempts, repeated incidents of nonsuicidal self-injury, and having access to firearms.

Patients in the serious risk category can likely be treated as outpatients with close monitoring. Patients in the serious risk category are similar to patients in the imminent risk category except that they either (a) have a lower baseline of distress or have more protective factors that reduce the risk of having a suicidal crisis, (b) have the skills to interrupt a crisis, or (c) lack access to the means to kill themselves.

Patients in the moderate or low categories of risk can likely be treated as outpatients with some monitoring. Patients in the moderate risk category have a lower likelihood of experiencing a crisis because they have sufficient psychological resilience or resources to prevent themselves from going into a suicidal crisis, are better able to interrupt a suicidal crisis, or have a lower baseline of distress. They may not have the acquired capability for self-harm, but if they do, they have no access to the means to kill themselves. A patient in the low risk category has a low baseline and little likelihood of having a suicidal crisis, or has a reduced acquired capability to kill themselves and no access to means, or perhaps does not even have a suicidal plan.

Consider the patient, Miguel, who appeared in the vignette opening Chapter 1. A levels of service approach could be applied to him.

Levels of Service With Miguel

Miguel has a high baseline of distress as represented by subjective reports of discomfort. Further information would be needed on his history, but his background as a hunter and a past suicide attempt suggests that he has some acquired capability of suicide. The mental state he is feeling now with depression, agitation, and trouble sleeping is like the emotional state he was feeling 10 years ago when he had a previous suicidal attempt by taking an excess of over-the-counter medications. However, he said, "I was not married then, and did not have as much to live for." Those and other comments suggest that Miguel has social connections that give him a reason for living. He rated the likelihood that he would die from suicide as "1" on a 5-point scale with 1 representing the lowest level of risk.

Miguel has access to weapons but expressed a willingness to secure them safely. He also appeared willing to allow his wife to be involved in psychotherapy.

It appears that Miguel would fall into the serious risk category and could be treated as an outpatient with close monitoring. If he had refused to involve his wife or had refused to secure his weapons, he might have been moved into the imminent risk category. Also, the level of risk might have changed if the suicide attempt had been recent, as opposed to 10 years ago. One of the factors to look for is a sense of hopelessness or entrapment. This can often be gauged by the manifest statements of the patient, but it can also be shown through actions. Miguel's cooperation in involving his family and restricting access to lethal means suggests some degree of hopefulness on his part. According to the three-step theory, one could say that Miguel's pain and hopelessness is not able to overwhelm his connectedness to his family.

Consider the patient, Mary, who appeared in the vignette opening Chapter 2. A levels of service approach could also be applied to her.

Levels of Service With Mary

Mary has a high level of distress. She initially presented very well, but as the interview went on, it became clear that she was in substantial emotional distress. She is performing well in school, but doing so is difficult; is feeling a lot of emotional pain; is sleeping poorly; and is feeling socially isolated.

The fact that she is cutting herself suggests that she is at risk of habituating herself to pain and suffering. More information is needed on the length of time she has been cutting herself, the medical severity of the cuts, and their frequency. However, she has never had a previous suicide attempt and has no suicide plan. Mary rated the likelihood that she would die from suicide as a 2 on a 5-point scale, with 1 being the *lowest* level of risk and 5 being the *highest* level of risk. She says that she wants to live so that she can pursue a career in teaching and spoke positively of the relationships she formed during her student teaching experience.

A recent romantic breakup precipitated this deterioration in her emotional life. The psychotherapist wondered if another social reversal could prompt another crisis.

It appears that Mary would fall into the serious category, where outpatient treatment is appropriate with close monitoring. If she had not been cutting and had not reported such intense emotional pain, the psychotherapist might have placed her in the moderate-risk category. However, the cutting indicates the possibility of habituation to pain and suffering and an acquired capability for self-harm. If she had a previous suicide attempt, a plan, and access to lethal means that could not be restricted, the psychotherapist might have considered her in imminent risk. In addition, she reported a connection to her career as a teacher and could give good and credible reasons why she wanted to live.

Advantages and Limitations of the Levels of Risk Methodology

The advantage of the levels of service chart is that it requires clinicians to slow down, assess the information systematically, and reach a conclusion about risk that can be justified on the data presented. Psychotherapists who document this in the patient's record have proof that they have reviewed suicide-related information systematically. Charts of this type provide a shorthand for determining the level of care in the short term.

In the cases of Miguel and Mary, the charts helped the psychotherapist to decide the appropriate level of treatment after the first meeting, even though much important information was lacking. Levels of service charts, such as this, may give inexperienced mental health professionals a false sense of certainty because there are several caveats in using them. However, the effective psychotherapists know the limitations of these charts and will revise their assessment of risk as more information comes to light or the condition of the patient changes.

The risk and protective factors can tell us which individuals are likely to act on their inclinations in the long run. But the issue before psychotherapists is to estimate the risk of suicide within the near future. This and similar charts are theory driven, not data driven. There are no data that these classification systems accurately estimate the risk of suicide in the short term (M. M. Silverman, 2014). Most patients who fall into the serious or imminent risk category will not die from suicide (Carter et al., 2017), and some patients who fall in the low-risk category will die from suicide.

Second, the risk factors are always changing and could change suddenly. A job loss, disruption of a relationship, or a sudden decline in health could abruptly transform the risk assessment for a patient.

In addition, the methods of determining the baseline of distress or the acquired capability of harm are only heuristics. This formula describes some of the relevant factors as dichotomies, even though they are continuous. So, a psychotherapist may identify a patient as having the acquired capability for self-harm, even though acquired capability is best seen either as multifaceted or on a continuum, or as a trait that is activated only under limited circumstances. For example, it was somewhat of a judgment call to estimate the degree to which the patients Miguel and Mary in the vignettes had acquired the capability for self-harm. For example, patients who engage in extensive self-injury will use multiple means, have repeated incidents, and report a lower sensation of pain. This does not appear to be the case for Mary, but this part of her life needs to be monitored carefully. Effective psychotherapists are aware of this mismatch and thus use the level of risk model with this limitation in mind.

Also, the mere act of placing a patient into a discrete risk category commits psychotherapists to a position on the risk of suicide. A problem could occur if psychotherapists overvalue this placement and fail to see that it is only a heuristic concerning a patient at a point in time. All psychotherapists have a risk of *confirmation bias*, or a tendency to find evidence that supports their previous positions. There is a risk that psychotherapists may look for future information to justify the original estimate instead of seeing it as a hypothesis that needs to be continually challenged and revised as new data emerges or as the circumstances of the patient's life change.

Finally, no one can estimate the suicide risk of many patients with a high degree of certainty. According to Rose's theorem of public health (Khaw, 2008) as applied to suicide, more cases of suicide will occur in the larger population with fewer risk factors than will occur among the smaller population with more risk factors.[1] Consequently, practitioners need to attend both to the actuarial risk factors and to the unique life circumstances of each individual. As stated by Berman and Silverman (2014), "in our legal work, we have encountered too many cases of individuals who had died by suicide who were married with children, were religious leaders . . . were in treatment with a mental health professional, or had future plans" (p. 438).

Although it is most productive to focus on identifying individuals at a high risk for suicide on the basis of the available data, our ability to accurately estimate the risk of suicide is limited, and many individuals in the general population without the common risk factors will die from suicide. A substantial portion of individuals who died from suicide were already receiving some health care, including mental health care. Often the professionals were shocked by the death, claiming that they saw no warning signs for suicide. In some cases, it is possible that the treating professionals had not assessed the patient adequately. However, in many cases it is likely that the professionals had delivered adequate or excellent services but the knowledge of, opportunity to, and ability to detect suicidal inclinations is limited.

The imprecision in estimating the risk of suicide should not discourage psychotherapists from using levels of service charts. As noted previously, psychotherapists can use the charts to justify management or treatment decisions in the short run, but they should not overvalue them or give them more gravitas than they deserve. They represent a snapshot of the patient at one point in time but are no substitute for continuing to monitor and reevaluate the patient.

After the level of service has been established, psychotherapists can then proceed with providing the best suicide management and treatment that they can. The first part of interventions, informed consent and suicide management, is covered in the rest of this chapter.

---

[1]Rose's theorem may represent an overestimate as it applies to suicidal patients. Nonetheless, several studies show that many persons in low-risk categories die from suicide. According to Kessler, Borges, and Walters (1999), 9% of the population had three or more risk factors for a suicide attempt and accounted for 55% of all suicide attempts. The other 91% of the population accounted for the other 45% of attempts. The limitation of Kessler's research is that it relied on self-report data on attempts and therefore cannot include people who completed their suicides. Data from Mattisson, Bogren, Brådvik, and Horstmann (2015) also partially support this interpretation. In their longitudinal study of community residents with mood disorders, 25 males with depression (the high-risk group) died from suicide out of a pool of 195 subjects, whereas 43 other residents (a lower risk group) died from suicide over the same time period out of a pool of more than 3,500 residents. Although more suicidal decedents were from the low-risk group, they only had an approximate rate of 1:800 dying from suicide compared with suicidal decedents from the high-risk group who had an approximate rate of 1:8 dying from suicide. Finally, according to Large et al. (2016), almost half of the suicides reported occurred in those considered to be lower risk patients.

OVERVIEW OF EFFECTIVE INTERVENTIONS
FOR SUICIDAL PATIENTS

Treatments that have demonstrated effectiveness in reducing suicidal behavior are cognitive behavior therapy for depression (Ghahramanlou-Holloway, Neely, & Tucker, 2015; Rudd et al., 2015)[2] and dialectical behavior therapy for borderline personality disorder (Linehan et al., 2015). CAMS (Jobes, 2016) and B. Stanley and Brown's (2012) safety plans are effective interventions for managing suicidal risks, and they can be combined with other, more comprehensive interventions.

Other programs have reported success in reducing suicidal risk, although more research is needed to verify the results. These include psychodynamic interpersonal psychotherapy (Guthrie et al., 2001), an attempted suicide intervention prevention program (Gysin-Maillart, Schwab, Soravia, Megert, & Michel, 2016), and mentalization-based psychotherapy (Bateman & Fonagy, 2009, 2019). In addition, attachment-based family therapy appears to be a promising intervention for suicidal adolescents, and problem adaption therapy (PATH) and interpersonal therapy appear to help older adults (Calati, Courtet, & Lopez-Castroman, 2018). Finally, a multisite study in Japan found that assertive case management (case managers trained in suicide interventions actively reaching out to vulnerable individuals) reduced episodes of self-harm (Furuno et al., 2018).

This book urges psychotherapists to know the outcome literature on effective treatments but acknowledges that psychotherapists must decide which treatments to use on the basis of several factors such as the clinical presentation of the patients, including comorbidities, patient preferences, and their areas of competence. For example, psychotherapists who are skilled in psychodynamically informed psychotherapy and are getting good patient results with that treatment should not start cognitive behavior therapy with a patient unless they underwent the study and training necessary to be proficient in that modality. Even those psychotherapists who are skilled in both modalities might choose psychodynamically informed psychotherapy depending on the patients' preferences and their unique clinical presentation. Psychotherapists should deliver treatments that they believe in and should be able to convey that belief to their patients. Patients who believe in the credibility of the treatment they receive are more likely to get positive outcomes (Norcross & Lambert, 2018).

Regardless of the specific treatment chosen, good interventions for suicidal patients

- should empower patients. This involves more than just having a good informed consent process. It means listening carefully to the concerns of

---

[2]Evidence also suggests that cognitive therapies can be effective for the inpatient treatment of suicidal behavior (e.g., Ghahramanlou-Holloway, Neely, & Tucker, 2015).

patients, directly soliciting their input throughout management and treatment, and explaining procedures (Jobes, 2016; Joiner et al., 2009).

- should value the psychotherapeutic relationship. Not only is this a feature of all effective treatments, it is especially important in reducing the social isolation that suicidal patients often feel. Effective psychotherapists also ensure cultural competence (e.g., Hayes, McAleavey, Castonguay, & Locke, 2016).

- should motivate patients to engage in, support, and adhere to treatment (Bryan & Rozek, 2018).

- should develop and implement effective crisis intervention and suicide management plans. This includes skills to reduce distress and access supports when necessary (Bryan & Rozek, 2018).

- should teach patients to regulate their emotions (Bryan & Rozek, 2018).

- should address suicide-related behaviors in psychotherapy, such as suicide attempts that occur during treatment, responding to time or event contingent suicidal threats, and so on.

These themes overlap. For example, psychotherapists who respect patient autonomy and engage patients in treatment decisions will be more likely to motivate them to adhere to the treatment goals.

This chapter looks at the first four of the six factors identified previously: patient empowerment, treatment relationships, and suicide management, which includes motivating them. Chapter 4 looks at the last two of the six factors identified previously: how psychotherapists can teach patients to regulate their emotions and how to address suicide-related behaviors that occur in psychotherapy.

PATIENT EMPOWERMENT (INFORMED CONSENT)

As noted in the discussions on principle-based ethics in Chapter 1, respect for patient autonomy or patient decision making is one of the overarching ethical principles that is especially applicable to health care. This has sometimes been called the shared decision-making model (J. Park, Goode, Tompkins, & Swift, 2016) and involves patients in the treatment processes and goals as much as is clinically feasible. Cramer et al. (2013) identified the development of a collaborative treatment plan as one of the core competencies when treating suicidal patients.

Respecting patient autonomy most obviously occurs in the informed-consent process, although it can be manifested throughout all aspects of psychotherapy. Psychotherapists who believe that respecting patient autonomy only occurs through the informed consent process are missing many opportunities to improve patient care. Psychotherapists can also respect patient autonomy by trying to understand their patients' perspective on their issues and explaining the reasons behind treatment recommendations (Joiner et al., 2009).

Empowering patients has several advantages. Patients will be more likely to follow through with treatment programs that they helped create and felt invested in it. In addition, an attitude of respecting patient autonomy recognizes that patients are the experts on their own experiences, lives, and emotions. Patients "are the undisputed expert on themselves" (W. R. Miller & Rollnick, 2013, p. 15). They have the essential information that will make the difference between a good and a poor treatment plan. Anything that encourages patients to share their insights increases the likelihood that a good treatment plan will be developed. Patients tend to prefer the shared decision-making approach (J. Park et al., 2016). There is some evidence that supports the importance of shared decision making. Psychotherapy outcomes tend to be better when patients and psychotherapist have a consensus on the treatment goals (Norcross & Lambert, 2018).

Some psychotherapists may, perhaps out of anxiety or lack of experience, adopt a more directive stance with suicidal patients than they would with other patients. By doing so, they risk getting into a power struggle with patients or starting to argue with them. Arguments against suicide could be countered with arguments as to why suicide is a good idea. A dynamic may develop wherein psychotherapists argue implicitly that they have the answers to their patients' problems. A cooperative approach takes a different perspective. As expressed in the CAMS philosophy, "the answers to your struggles exist within you—we will find those answers together" (Jobes, 2016, p. 54). Another advantage of an empowering approach is that it aligns itself with the drive for autonomy, one of the essential human needs identified by self-determination theory (Ryan & Deci, 2008). Any treatment strategy that aligns itself with a human need is likely to motivate patients. In rare situations it may be necessary to temporarily become more directive. This may occur, for example, if patients are too demoralized to participate fully in treatment.

The attitude of respecting patient autonomy can strongly influence the nature of treatment. For example, when working with suicidal patients, psychotherapy is more effective when the psychotherapist "lets go of controlling the patient—[and] disengages from the potential power struggle of denying the patient his or her suicide option" (Jobes & Ballard, 2011, p. 59). When this happens "the typical patient usually feels relieved, less compelled to take his or her life and more interested in collaborating in potentially lifesaving treatment" (Jobes & Ballard, 2011, p. 59).

This emphasis on patient empowerment is a major contribution of the CAMs approach. In this approach, psychotherapists do not argue with the patients but listen carefully and try to understand their experiences. Psychotherapists might say, "Let us see if together we can find a viable alternative to suicide to better deal with your pain and suffering" (Jobes, 2016, p. 54). To further emphasize the collaborative nature of the treatment, psychotherapists often sit right next to the patient while they fill out the CAMS forms together.

Another advantage of empowering patients is that it reduces ambivalence among patients about treatment. When patients feel that their autonomy is respected, they will be more likely to adhere to and engage in treatment. Engagement means that patients participate freely in treatment decisions, disclose their thoughts, assert their preferences, and inform their psychotherapists of what appears to be effective or not. The importance of engaging patients is illustrated in the following vignette.

Patients and Treatment Goals

One psychotherapist told me that he used to be frustrated that his patients did not follow through with the treatment goals he had carefully crafted after a painstakingly thorough evaluation. But he reported that he was amazed at how well these patients responded to treatment when they got to choose their own treatment goals!

Empowering patients also means being candid with them about the reasons for the treatment recommendations and conceptualization about their presenting problem, including the specific diagnosis they are given. The purpose of giving the diagnosis is not simply to reveal a term to patients, but to explain what that diagnosis means and link it to the treatment plan. For example, the term *borderline personality disorder* has now entered the vocabulary of many laypersons and has the connotation of having disruptive and unpleasant behaviors. Therefore, simply telling patients that they have a borderline personality disorder runs the risk of offending without enlightening. It would be better to explain that, despite what laypeople might say about borderline personality disorder, it is a treatable disorder characterized by a great deal of emotional pain and quick shifts into unpleasant emotions. Psychotherapists can then explain how the specific strategies can reduce the patient's painful emotions.

At the minimum, respecting patient autonomy includes giving essential information about the nature of psychotherapy, which is called the *informed consent process*. Informed consent should take place at the start of psychotherapy or "as early as feasible" in the psychotherapeutic relationship (*Ethical Principles of Psychologists and Code of Conduct*, Standard 10.01 (a); American Psychological Association, 2017). When treating suicidal patients, it is sometimes necessary to defer some of the elements typically given in the informed consent process to ensure that time is spent focusing on the patient's immediate safety. Sometimes psychotherapists can give the information out in segments depending on the patient's need. For example, when treating suicidal patients in a crisis it may be indicated to cover exceptions to confidentiality in the first session because that may be relevant to the patient's willingness to share information. Other information commonly included in the informed consent process, such as policies concerning use of social media, credit cards, and so on, can be deferred to when the crisis has passed.

Informed consent in mental health care differs from informed consent in physical health. Mental health care often requires more active participation and patient investment than physical health care. Whereas some patients who receive physical treatments simply must take pills or agree to an operation, patients who receive mental health treatment must invest their time and energy into the treatment process over a period of months or more. Psychotherapy is not a spectator sport, but an activity that works best when patients are actively engaged in the process. Just as the patients retain the ultimate responsibility for whether they live or die from suicide, patients also retain the ultimate responsibility (and credit) for living a more productive life.

The informed consent process helps patients understand what to expect in psychotherapy. It also articulates what the psychotherapists expect from their patients. All patients should be informed about the general nature of treatment, limits of confidentiality, risks involved, and the opportunity to ask questions (Rudd et al., 2009). Often it is good to supplement the discussion of informed consent with a written document. This book recommends the informed consent document developed by the Trust.[3] It is in the public domain and may be modified to accommodate the unique features of one's own practice. Whatever informed consent document is used, it is important that it addresses some of the major points identified by Jobes (2016), Joiner et al. (2009), and Wenzel, Brown, and Beck (2009):

- the potential involvement of family members, if appropriate;

- the potential for a referral for medication;

- the potential need to share information with professionals providing mental and physical health care;

- expectations that the patients will comply with the conditions of psychotherapy—patients will be expected to attend psychotherapy (or arrange for a new appointment if they need to miss one for a good reason) and to participate fully and voice feelings and ideas honestly;

- although psychotherapists will strive to make psychotherapy as comfortable as possible, it may involve discussions of stressful events and may evoke unpleasant emotion;

- noncompliance could be grounds for terminating treatment; and

- an agreement that one of the goals would be to prevent future suicide attempts and to address the life circumstances that lead patients to consider suicide as an option.

Often it is necessary to go over these points in more detail, give examples, and respond to patients' questions. Efforts should be made to describe the conditions of treatment in positive terms. Informed consent is not a one-time event but continues through treatment as new interventions are added or as

---

[3]The Trust is a major professional liability insurer for psychologists. The informed consent form can be downloaded (https://parma.trustinsurance.com/Resource-Center/Document-Library).

the treatment plan change. It is appropriate to give patients a rationale for the treatment recommendations. If a psychotherapist decides, for example, to offer dialectical behavior therapy to a patient, then it is appropriate to explain the scientific evidence that supports the use of this type of psychotherapy for certain disorders. If a psychotherapist decides to require homework as a part of offering acceptance and commitment therapy (ACT) for depression, then it is appropriate to explain why homework improves outcomes with ACT.

Some patients may feel put off by the statement that their failure to comply with psychotherapy could be grounds for termination. However, psychotherapists can express that concept positively. Here is how a psychologist could express this concern:

> I value your time and well-being too much to offer you a treatment that lacks a reasonable chance of success. I know that these treatments have a very high likelihood of success. However, this only occurs if you keep appointments, do homework assignments, be open with me about what is on your mind, and so on. If you don't cooperate in therapy, then its likelihood of success is greatly diminished. You are too important to me to get second-rate therapy. You deserve only the best that I can give.

Issues dealing with treatment adherence are discussed in more detail in Chapter 4.

THE PSYCHOTHERAPEUTIC RELATIONSHIP

Effective psychotherapists develop alliances through listening attentively to their patients and expressing empathy with their situation (Wampold, Baldwin, Holtforth, & Imel, 2017). They also respect patient autonomy as described previously. Building and maintaining a good relationship is one of the core competencies that Cramer et al. (2013) identified when working with suicidal patients.

Years of research have demonstrated that various factors in the treatment relationship, such as collaboration, goal consensus, development of an alliance, and expressions of empathy and positive regard, are demonstrably effective in improving patient outcomes. In addition, congruence, cultivating positive expectations, promoting treatment credibility, managing countertransference, and repairing alliance ruptures are likely effective in improving outcomes (Norcross & Lambert, 2018).

Suicidal behavior is influenced by the quality of the psychotherapeutic relationship (Dunster-Page, Haddock, Wainwright, & Berry, 2017). Patients who feel valued by their psychotherapists are less likely to attempt suicide. One sample of patients reported that knowing that their psychotherapists cared about them was the most common reason why they did not kill themselves (Montross Thomas et al., 2014). At times psychotherapists may decide to protect the relationship even if it means getting less information than they would want to estimate the likelihood of suicide. At times it may be more helpful to allow the patients to tell their stories, even if it means that psychotherapists will not have the opportunity to ask questions that would gather information more directly related to the risk of suicide.

The psychotherapeutic relationship helps reduce the loneliness that suicidal patients may feel. Although patients may be talking to their psychotherapists only for 1 hour a week, the relationship helps fulfill affiliation needs because it tends to be more honest, emotionally meaningful, and reliable than most other relationships. Patients have reported that just having a psychotherapist who was willing to sit with them while they expressed their pain was often very helpful (Dunkley et al., 2018). Another advantage of focusing on the relationship is that it aligns itself with affiliation needs, one of the essential human needs identified by self-determination theory (Ryan & Deci, 2008).

Some suicidal patients may have difficulties in forming or maintaining close relationships. For example, depressed patients may distort the nature of their interactions with others that confirm their views of themselves as unworthy. Or they may annoy others with excessive attempts for reassurance or may actively avoid interpersonal conflicts (Joiner et al., 2009).

Building relationships also means refraining from harmful behaviors. Norcross and Wampold (2011) and Castonguay, Boswell, Constantino, Goldfried, and Hill (2010) identified several behaviors associated with poor outcomes, including having negative confrontations (hostile, pejorative, critical, or sarcastic statements), neglecting patient needs or their perceptions of their needs, giving too many or premature interpretations, and failing to modify treatments to accommodate patient needs.

These harmful behaviors have an authoritarian tinge and place too much control in the hands of the psychotherapists. Also, these behaviors convey to patients that they are not valued or are not important. Even minor behaviors that, in isolation, may appear harmless enough could diminish the quality of the treatment relationship. Consequently, psychotherapists should, for example, return phone calls promptly, keep appointments on time, and ensure that the time in treatment is being used productively. Psychotherapists who have good reasons for being late or for having to take an urgent phone call during a session should apologize for the inconvenience and reiterate the importance of the time that spent together.

Psychotherapists need to be especially careful with patients who belong to groups that have historically faced prejudice or stigmas because of race or ethnicity, sexual orientation, physical appearance, excess weight, or other factors. Prejudice is a source of chronic stress (Simons et al., 2018) and may lead to self-stigma, psychological and physical strain, and an increase in all-cause mortality. Some patients may have internalized the societal rejection or developed less-than-optimal interpersonal strategies to deal with the stigma.

Effective psychotherapists consider *intersectionality*, or how race, ethnicity, and culture mix with gender, educational level, sexual orientation, religion, or socioeconomic status. As stated by Rosenthal (2016), intersectionality highlights the importance of attending to multiple, interacting identities and ascribed social positions (e.g., race, gender, sexual identity, class) along with associated power dynamics, as people are at the same time members of many different social groups and have unique experiences with privileges and disadvantage because of those intersections. (p. 475)

For example, the experiences of a Black male one generation removed from the Caribbean who has a college education, a good income, and a professional career differ substantially from the experiences of a Black male of the same age who is a high school dropout, lives in poverty, and has spent time in prison.

Culturally competent psychotherapists have better outcomes than psychotherapists who are not culturally competent. Hayes, Owen, and Bieschke (2015) found that psychotherapists differed in their ability to be effective with racial or ethnic minorities. "Cultural competence can be distinguished from general therapist competence" (p. 312). Later, Hayes, McAleavey, Castonguay, and Locke (2016) opined that "it is possible to identify multiculturally expert therapists who evidence competence with both REM [racial and ethnic minorities] and White clients" (p. 261).

Conscientious psychotherapists will be attentive to the potential that they may hold implicit biases that reduce their effectiveness in building good relationships. Effective psychotherapists sometimes check with their patients to ensure that they are understanding them correctly and that the patients feel heard and understood. They might say, "Did I capture your feeling correctly?"

THE THREE MS OF MANAGING SUICIDE RISK

Management strategies keep patients alive until psychotherapy has a chance to work. Management strategies keep patients from going into a suicidal crisis or allow an easier disruption of the suicidal crisis until psychotherapy reduces the patients' high baseline of dysphoria, and teaches them how to prevent suicidal crises. Suicide management plans should be tailored to the needs of the patients and involve as much patient input as is clinically feasible. The most salient management strategies are the three Ms: *m*otivating the patient (commitment to life), *m*eans safety, and *m*onitoring. Other options will be presented (breaking confidentiality, psychiatric hospitalizations, involuntary psychiatric hospitalizations, and the use of emergency rooms) that are sometimes indicated but must be used with discretion.

Psychotherapists should have a rationale as to why they chose, or how they implemented, each suicide management strategy. Some psychotherapists, perhaps reflecting an alarmist attitude, will proudly proclaim that they will "do everything they can" to protect a suicidal patient without considering whether "everything" is needed or helpful. The "kitchen sink" strategy has problems. It involves recommending every possible intervention just so psychotherapists can say, "I threw all my resources at the problem: even the

TABLE 3.2. Strategies to Manage Suicide Risk

Management strategy	When indicated
Motivate	For all suicidal patients
Means safety	For all suicidal patients who have identified how they intend to kill themselves
Monitor	For all suicidal patients, at varying degrees depending on risk, ranging on a continuum from keeping regular appointments to psychiatric hospitalization
Breaking confidentiality	To be used selectively when it is not possible to secure the immediate safety of a patient without notifying a third party
Psychiatric hospitalization	For all suicidal patients who need close monitoring for safety or for medication management
Involuntary psychiatric hospitalization	For all suicidal patients who need close monitoring for safety or medication because of an imminent risk of suicide and the benefits of hospitalizing the patients outweigh any harm from hospitalizing the patient
Emergency room referral	To be used selectively when it is urgent that patients receive an immediate evaluation and there are no other options, or the patients need immediate medical attention

kitchen sink." More is not necessarily better. For example, psychotherapists may decide to inform a family member of the suicidal thoughts of their patients because they believe it is important to "do everything I can." Although involving family members is usually therapeutically indicated, the decision needs to be based on the patient's needs, not based on the psychotherapist's goal to prove that he or she "did everything I could."[4]

Psychotherapists should use the management strategies that are likely to help their patients. Table 3.2 presents a general guide that psychotherapists can use to decide which management strategies to use with which patients. It is appropriate to use motivational strategies with all suicidal patients, including those who have suicidal ideation alone, but no plans. Motivational strategies are especially important with patients who have ambivalence about being in treatment. Monitoring should be used for all suicidal patients, with the degree of monitoring adjusted to the risk of suicide. Means safety (means restrictions) should be used with patients who have suicide plans. The final management strategies—disclosing patient information without their consent, psychiatric hospitalizations, involuntary psychiatric hospitalizations, and emergency room referral—should be used selectively because they have the potential to harm patients. These management strategies are essential components in several well-regarded interventions (e.g., Jobes, 2016; Joiner et al., 2009; B. Stanley & Brown, 2012; B. Stanley, Brown, Brenner, et al., 2018).

---

[4]All material in this paragraph is from "Ten Questions to Promote Excellence When Working With Patients With Suicidal Thoughts," by S. Knapp and B. Schur, 2019, *The Pennsylvania Psychologist, 79*, pp. 1–3, 5–7. Copyright 2019 by the Pennsylvania Psychological Association. Adapted with permission.

Motivating Patients

Sometimes patients with strong suicidal ideation feel hopeless and do not believe that psychotherapy, or anything, will help them. A first step is to motivate the patient for treatment.

When I worked with suicidal patients, I spoke with confidence about their ability to feel better and to connect with their will to live a meaningful life. It was a confidence born out of my experience with many suicidal patients. Patients' expectations concerning the outcome of treatment are positively related to good patient outcomes (Norcross & Lambert, 2018).

Consistent with the recommendations of Jobes (2016), it is useful to talk with patients about reasons for living (this is covered in more detail in the section on commitment to life agreements) and the costs of suicide. It can often help to ask patients to adopt a long-term perspective. For example, it may be profitable to ask them the following:

- What if you are wrong and things did get better?
- What meaningful activities would you likely miss out on?
- What people would you miss?
- How will your relatives or loved ones remember you? (Ellis & Newman, 1996)

Even if patients adopt a pessimistic perspective and insist that nothing will ever change or that no one would ever care, it may be worthwhile to ask them to suspend that thought and consider the chance that they might be wrong. It may be worth pointing out that many persons who once felt the same way recaptured meaning in their lives.

I have known some patients with serious and pervasive disorders who did not respond well to treatment, even when it was delivered compassionately and competently. It is understandable that psychotherapists may feel discouraged at the prospect of taking on such patients and adjust their expectations downward. Nonetheless, I have also seen some such patients make substantial improvements, despite a history of poor responses to treatment. The conclusion I drew was to show more humility about my predictions. Although the word *humility* is often evoked to keep psychotherapists from being too confident in their optimistic predictions, it could also be evoked to keep psychotherapists from being too confident in their pessimistic predictions as well. This point was well represented by an event at the outpatient facility where I was working.

A Competent Intern

An intern was assigned a patient who had struggled for several years with numerous emergency room contacts and several psychiatric hospitalizations. The patient had been seen by two other experienced psychotherapists, with negligible improvement. Ordinarily an intern would not be assigned such a case. But when the regular staff person suddenly had to take a temporary medical leave, an intern was selected to provide interim treatment until the regular psychotherapist could return. However, 3 weeks into treatment with the intern, the patient began to improve substantially. The emergency room contacts stopped, and he never had another psychiatric hospitalization. No one on the treatment team had expected such positive results, especially in such a short period of time!

Sometimes psychotherapists will hear the statement "You cannot stop a patient who really wants to die from suicide." As noted in Chapter 1, this may be literally true, but it becomes problematic if it leads psychotherapists to become less energetic, hopeful, or confident in their ability to save lives. Every psychotherapist has some influence, even with the most suicidal patients, that may greatly increase the likelihood that they will live. Good suicide assessment, management, and treatment saves lives.

Even patients who "really want to die" feel some ambivalence about killing themselves, and this ambivalence makes them receptive to the feedback of their psychotherapists. One psychologist asks patients, "If you were not suffering so much, would you still want to die?" They almost always say "no," to which she replies, "I think I can help you with that" (Whiteside, 2016).

Psychotherapists can explain that with evidence-informed treatment, a high majority of patients feel better and are able to address problems successfully or at least see solutions other than suicide. Psychotherapists can explain that depression or anxiety can impair one's problem-solving abilities and that when their depression or anxiety begins to lift, it becomes easier for them to solve their problems. Psychotherapists can explain the process of breaking larger problems into smaller components to make them more manageable.

It is reasonable to ask patients to give treatment a try. One psychotherapist bluntly tells patients, "I don't do good psychotherapy with dead patients" (Taube, 2018). A psychotherapist might say, "If you are dead, you lose the chance of getting better." Jobes (2016) will sometimes even tell a patient that if treatment does not work, you can always kill yourself, so you have nothing to lose. Some psychotherapists respond very negatively to this comment, but I urge them to think of the advantages of such comments. First, it would not be necessary to make this comment to all patients, but with patients who feel deeply ambivalent about living or feel skeptical that psychotherapy will help them.

Second, the statement is not delivered sarcastically or meant to come across as dismissive. Instead, it is delivered with frank sincerity and is meant to be taken literally. It acknowledges that psychotherapists can never guarantee that treatment will work. However, psychotherapists can promise to deliver good quality service with data supporting its effectiveness.

Furthermore, the statement only reflects what the patient is already thinking. Deeply ambivalent patients might already be telling themselves, "If this does not work, I can always kill myself." Consequently, the same statements by psychotherapists are benign in that no patient ever died from suicide by having their psychotherapists talk about suicide candidly.

Finally, many patients feel relief that their psychotherapists are speaking candidly. Psychotherapists are not using euphemistic language, minimizing the seriousness of the situation, ignoring the realities, or denying the fact that the patient considers suicide an option. Readers may recall the importance of respecting patient autonomy, which includes their participation in important decisions. This statement only acknowledges that the patient ultimately decides whether to live or die.

No-Suicide Contracts

Some agencies and individual psychotherapists still routinely use no-suicide contracts. The nature of no-suicide contracts varies, but generally they require patients to sign a prewritten document stating that they will not kill themselves. Although a few patients have reported that such no-suicide contracts helped ensure their safety, evidence does not support their use (Edwards & Sachman, 2010). Indeed, if they are forced on patients as a not-so-hidden-way to protect practitioners from liability, they can impede treatment. One patient who refused to sign such a contract said, "Don't worry, I will drop out of treatment for a few weeks before I kill myself, so you won't be sued." One psychotherapist told me that she, acting on the directive of her agency director, spent an entire hour badgering her patient to sign the contract. "She did not want to sign, but eventually I broke her down." Instead of helping the patient in this time of crisis, the session was spent in an unproductive power struggle.

In addition to their clinical limitations, no-suicide contracts provide no legal protection for psychotherapists if a patient were to die from suicide. In the event of a lawsuit, a court would evaluate the behavior of the psychotherapists according to the prevailing standard of care. These standards are informed by experts who rely on learned texts or peer-reviewed publications (Chapter 5 discusses standards of care in more detail). The psychotherapists who rested their defense on the use of a no-suicide contract would be hard pressed to find any authority on suicide to support them.

Some psychotherapists recognize that no-suicide contracts have no intrinsic value but claim that the failure of a patient to sign a no-suicide contract indicates their degree of suicide intent. Those who fail to sign such agreements, it is argued, lack confidence in their ability to control their suicidal impulses. However, no evidence supports that assumption. Patients may decline to sign the contract for many reasons (McKeon, 2009). Some patients may just have a healthy resentment against being bullied.

Other psychotherapists will provide a middle ground in which they offer a no-suicide contract but use it only as a vehicle of discussion without being pushy or intrusive. This avoids some of the ethical and clinical problems associated with pushing no-suicide contracts on patients, but psychotherapists can do even better if they consider the commitment-to-life or commitment-to-treatment agreements alternative described next.

Commitment-to-Life Agreements

Commitment-to-life agreements (sometimes called commitment-to-treatment agreements) represent a healthy alternative to no-suicide contracts (Rudd, Mandrusiak, & Joiner, 2006). The focus of the productive commitment-to-life agreement is on what patients *will do* during times of emotional turmoil. In contrast, the focus of the unproductive no-suicide contract is on what patients *will not do* (Jobes, Rudd, Overholser, & Joiner, 2008).

Ideally, a commitment-to-life agreement will reflect an ongoing process that involves the patient in the development and implementation of the treatment plan. Part of respecting patient autonomy is to ensure that patients know that they have choices, including the choice of what should be in that agreement. Psychotherapists can also respect their patient's autonomy by explaining why they are making certain recommendations.

Commitment-to-life agreements are indicated for all patients except if the patients are at an imminent risk of suicide and efforts are being made to seek a higher level of care, if the patient is psychotic or appears incompetent, or if the patient is illiterate or has trouble reading. Often psychotherapists can estimate literacy by noting the educational level of their patients, although this is not a foolproof method. Also, some patients that do not have English as a primary language may be proficient in speaking English but have poor reading skills in English.

The commitment-to-life agreement may be either a written document or an app that patients can put on their smartphones. The commitment-to-life agreement can include a list of reasons for living, a list of warning signs (e.g., negative emotions associated with an increased risk of suicide), a list of activities or individuals to seek out because they inhibit suicidal behaviors, and a crisis intervention plan. Much of the document can be written in the patient's own words.

Patients can also create a hope or survival kit that includes photographs of loved ones, lists of reasons for living, music, or other objects that encourage hope. It could be a shoebox or a simply an envelope. Psychotherapists who use the survival kit may wish to review with patients the objects that they place there and their lifesaving value. Men tend to prefer the term survival kit as opposed to a hope kit (Bryan & Rudd, 2018).

One app, the Virtual Hope Box, can be used as a commitment-to-life agreement. This app could include photographs or music in addition to written statements. It is in the public domain and can be accessed at https://msrc.fsu.edu/funded-research/improved-virtual-hope-box. Bush et al. (2017) reported that suicidal service members who used the Virtual Hope Box reported a significantly greater ability to handle upsetting emotions and thoughts than controls who only received printed materials on coping with suicidality.

Reasons for Living

The first parts of the commitment-to-treatment agreement could list the reasons for living. Interesting research by Bryan, Rudd, Peterson, Young-McCaughan, and Wertenberger (2016) suggested that the will to live and the will to die might not be a single dimension, but two dimensions, and some evidence suggests that the will to live might be more responsive to treatment than decreasing the will to die (although methodological issues weakened the strength of this finding). Nonetheless, if this finding is accurate, then it reinforces the value of having patients identify reasons for living.

Patients can often identify important relationships or salient values. The more detail patients can give the better. It is better for patients to write that "my religion considers suicide to be a violation of the Ten Commandments" or "God's goal is that I promote life and seek ways to do His will on earth,"[5] rather than to write that "suicide is a sin." If patients are using an app, this list may be supplemented by inspirational songs, religious symbols, or pictures of loved ones. Pictures and songs can activate positive emotions that written words cannot always do.

Anything is appropriate as a reason for living. It could be as lofty and meaningful as "living to see my granddaughter grow up," or it could be as mundane as "find out if the Cleveland Indians are going to have a winning season this year." If patients have difficulty identifying a reason for living, then psychotherapists can ask them for the reasons they had for living before they got depressed, or what would they like to have as a reason for living. It could be phrased as, "What do you like to do?" "What did you used to like to do?" "What did you like to do before you got depressed?" or "If you could have a reason for living, what would it be?" Or they could say, "Name someone you admire. What do you think are their reasons for living?"

Warning Signs and Activities

When interviewing patients, psychotherapists should get information about the warning signs associated with their suicidal crisis state. A goal is to try to reduce harmful emotions and to prevent (or at least interrupt) a crisis that could lead to a suicide attempt. Here the data derived from the screening and assessment process can help identify some of the warning signs that are likely to lead to the acute crisis. Readers may recall that the questions about suicidal ideation, attempts, and plans tried to elicit information about the external and emotional circumstances that led to a suicide attempt because it is likely that the external and emotional circumstances that led to past attempts will lead to future attempts. At times it could be appropriate to explain the fluid vulnerability theory to patients and the role of warning signs.

Psychotherapists may need to educate some patients on the importance of monitoring their emotional state and responding to emotional distress before it gets too out of control. One of the major challenges is to identify the emotional states of patients immediately before they attempted suicide. Emotions can get out of control very quickly (Kleiman et al., 2017). O. R. Simon et al. (2001) found that 24% of those who attempted suicide made the decision to act less than 5 minutes before the act, and 70% made the decision in less than an hour before the act.

Consequently, it appears important to know what could happen in the daily lives and experiences of patients that could move them quickly into a

---

[5]Many conservative religions often use the masculine when referring to deity, despite recent efforts of many to use gender-neutral or gender-inclusive language. However, psychotherapists should allow patients to decide how to phrase the statement.

suicidal crisis. This information can help circumvent the development of the suicidal crisis and can be used to develop a crisis plan. In the experience-sampling methodology, suicidal patients or research participants are asked to identify their thoughts, feelings, or behaviors at various points in time during the day.

No one set of emotions or behaviors occur with every patient. In addition to the emotions and behaviors found in the ASAD, SCS, or CAMS (e.g., social withdrawal, hopelessness, entrapment, self-disgust, agitation, irritability, insomnia, nightmares), suicidal patients may feel other emotions or display other behaviors as well such as sadness, anxiety, fear, or impulsivity. These intense emotions, when coupled with the desire to die and an acquired capability for death, may precipitate a suicide attempt (Ribeiro, Silva, & Joiner, 2014).

Psychotherapists can identify the precipitants of the suicidal crisis by looking at the sequence of events that led up to the suicidal thoughts, including the outward events and inward reactions to the events. Readers may recall that psychotherapists were urged to learn details about their patients' suicidal ideation, past suicide attempts, and suicidal plans, including the feelings and behaviors associated with them. It may even help to chart these events or to ask patients to describe what happened as if they were relating the scenes in a television show (Brent, Poling, & Goldstein, 2011). Through a series of these chain analyses, psychotherapists and patients may be able to discern patterns of thinking and reactions. According to the script protocol, the sequence could start with having patients describe the events that led to the suicidal crisis, then identify their thoughts, and then behaviors. Detail can be important, such as asking patients to describe their eye movements, gestures, posture, and so on. Then psychotherapists and patients can review the chart and decide if the patients could have engaged in activities that could have circumvented the suicidal thoughts (Joiner et al., 2009).

Bagge, Littlefield, and Glenn (2017) found that acute interpersonal crises occurred within 6 hours for about one third of those who attempted suicide, a finding that is consistent with the findings of Nock, Hwang, et al. (2010) that interpersonal fights often precipitated suicide attempts among adolescents. Of course, the precipitants and likely reactions (or warning signs) would be unique to every patient. Nonetheless, these studies suggest that patients should be alert for the potential for interpersonal conflicts to lead to suicide.

Wichers, Wigman, and Myin-Germeys (2015) identified some patterns that may be relevant here. Often dysphoria is caused not so much by a major event, but by the reaction to many smaller events. A negative response to one event may persist into subsequent events. "Psychopathology arises over time as the result of a cascade of smaller short-lived changes in affect and behavior that reinforce each other over time" (Wichers et al., 2015, p. 364). A vicious cycle occurs when one negative state influences the patient's reactions to other negative states. A tipping point may occur after a small event starts a cascade of emotions that leads to an intense crisis. In addition, the likelihood of moving into these distraught states can be heightened if patients have a background of poor sleep, nightmares, fatigue, or physical pain that make them more vulnerable to unproductive emotions or thoughts.

As this applies to suicidal patients, it may help to monitor and circumvent the small negative emotions that could precipitate a suicidal crisis. Psychotherapists might use the metaphor of a dam preventing a flood. The dam could overflow because of one very large rainstorm or several smaller rain storms over a short time period.

Patients can also monitor their emotional distress by taking their emotional temperature periodically. On a scale of 1 to 10, they can identify the extent of their global sense of well-being. Or they can take their emotional temperatures at times that they expect to be stressful, such as during a stressful workday.

Patients may need guidance on handling suicidal thoughts. Some patients may avoid or try to suppress unpleasant thoughts. But suppressing thoughts risks that they will arise again in unwanted situations. Psychotherapists can explain that the attempts to suppress thoughts can lead to the *white bear phenomena*, whereby trying to avoid thinking about a topic, such as a white bear, paradoxically increases the mind's focus on it (e.g., Wyland & Forgas, 2007).

Ideally patients will come to the point where they reappraise suicidal thoughts as welcome warning signs that something in their lives is not going well. The idea of welcoming suicidal thoughts may seem counterintuitive for most patients. However, if the thoughts are viewed as a lighthouse or traffic sign that warns the patient of danger, patients can consider the suicidal thoughts as a signal that they need to stop; observe their thoughts, feelings, and behavior; and determine what is underlying their sense of discontent. One survivor wrote that she was eventually able to

> see the suicidal thoughts as an early warning system. I must not take the thoughts literally, believe them, or obey them. What the suicidal urge is showing me is that something about how I have been living needs to die. . . . The suicidal thought is now my cue to stop. To tend. To seek solace. (L. Harris, 2018, pp. 5–6)

In the short term, however, psychotherapists can encourage patients to distract themselves or postpone the thoughts by identifying a time of day when they can "plan" to have those thoughts. Or patients may be taught to accept the suicidal thoughts without judging them. When later in the day comes, the thoughts often lack the salience or strength that they had when they arose spontaneously. Suicidal thoughts can be viewed as passing events or phenomena that can be observed, but not something that needs to be taken literally or adhered to.

Some psychotherapists may want to assure their patients that they will become happy if they participate in psychotherapy. For many patients this is an appropriate comment. However, two caveats may be in order. First, there may be cultural factors to consider. For some cultures, being happy is not the default goal that it often is in the majority culture in the United States. Other cultures may give greater importance to contributing to the family or larger kin group, or to otherwise fulfilling obligations. This can have implications for treatment as, for example, psychotherapists may focus on the patient's goal of being a better parent, child, member of the community, and so on. Psychotherapists can explain that an excess of negative emotions can keep them from reaching their goals.

Second, emotional well-being does not mean only an increase in positive emotions, although such an increase is desirable. Instead, emotional well-being can mean an appropriate balance of emotions, so that negative emotions do not overwhelm the patient. Psychotherapists can explain that not all negative emotions are bad. They become harmful when they are in excess, cloud out positive emotions, or impede one's ability to address life problems. So, psychotherapists may rephrase the goal as one of getting the negative emotions into a proper proportion with positive emotions. As stated by Haines et al. (2016), "emotions are functional. . . . Yet in many situations they are adaptive only if appropriately regulated" (p. 1651).

Over time in psychotherapy, patients will become better at cognitive or behavioral relaxation skills that will help them lower the baseline of their arousal and therefore become less likely to get into a suicidal crisis. In the short run, however, the goal is to develop strategies to help reduce the likelihood that they will enter a suicidal crisis.

In addition to identifying personal warning signs, it would also help to identify or list activities that can short-circuit those suicidal thoughts. Going back to the metaphor of the dam, patients can prevent a dam burst (an overwhelming feeling of dysphoria leading to a suicide attempt) by reducing the amount of water on the lake (shortcutting negative emotions) or by increasing the strength of the dam (engaging in experiences that produce positive emotions or social connections). Patients do not have to be completely successful all the time. Any step that reduces the dysphoria in intensity or duration or that strengthens positive emotions will reduce the likelihood that the dam will burst.

These activities could distract the patient or reduce the patient's distress. The patient may be asked to view the dysphoria not as a state demanding escape at all costs but as a problem that needs to be solved. In creating this list of possible activities together, patients can review the activities, strategies, or social contacts that they used to stabilize their mood in the past, or activities, strategies, or social contacts to avoid because they may increase their emotional pain. For example, most depressed and suicidal patients found that talking with peers, exercising, or doing things with others helped them reduce suicidal thoughts (although for a minority of patients these activities do not help; G. E. Simon, Specht, & Doederlein, 2016). Suicidal thoughts are more likely to occur when patients are doing nothing and less likely to occur when they are at the home of a friend or family member or engaging in another social activity (Husky et al., 2014). Sometimes it can help to include contingency plans. If going for a walk is generally helpful, what should the patient do if it is raining heavily outside (Homaifar, Bahraini, Silverman, & Brenner, 2012)?

The following sample list of potentially helpful activities comes from Jobes (2016), Joiner et al. (2009), B. Stanley, Green, Ghahramanlou-Holloway, Brenner, and Brown (2017), and my experience. These include distracting activities such as those that involve movement or involvement of the senses:

- exercising by walking, jogging, or going to the gym, or through a group activity, such as tennis, basketball, or softball;
- going to a restaurant, going out for a snack, such as a specialty bagel, etc.;
- cleaning the house; or
- going shopping, buying new clothes or household accessories.

Often, effective activities that prevent or interrupt the suicidal crisis involve interactions with others, including pets. They could be

- taking the dog for a walk,
- visiting a friend,
- writing a letter or sending an email to a friend or relative, or
- doing a random act of kindness or volunteering to help someone.

Other activities including meaningful introspective activities, especially if they focus on values, could be helpful. But patients should avoid anything that leads to rumination. Some of these activities could include

- listening to music, watching TV, going to a movie, going to a concert;
- writing in a journal, drawing, or painting;
- reading a book or a magazine; or
- meditating, listening to meditation tapes, praying, or going to church.

Good activity plans include more details. For example, a more perfunctory activity statement might simply list "calling a friend" when upset. A better activity statement might list "call John at 555-1212" (Gamarra, Luciano, Gradus, & Wiltsey Stirman, 2015).

Activities involving movement or interactions with others generally disrupt suicidal thoughts better than sedentary activities. Talking to a friend or taking a walk is generally better than watching TV. Social activities, such as talking to a friend or relative, can help for several reasons. Chapter 2 noted that patients may attempt suicide for different reasons, such as to end suffering, communicate their distress to others, relieve feelings of loneliness, or stop feelings of shame (S. S. O'Connor, Comtois, Atkins, & Kerbrat, 2017), but that all the reasons involve intense emotional suffering. Patients who involve themselves with others may find the activities distracting, but they may also be an opportunity to reinforce reasons for living. For example, a patient may interact with a caring person who can recognize their degree of suffering or relieve feelings of loneliness, or a patient may encounter a friend who shows caring and respect that is incompatible with the patient's feelings of self-loathing.

If sedentary activities are used, then it may help to pick ones that engage many senses such as taste and smell (going to a good restaurant), touch (getting a massage), or sound and sight (going to a concert). Activities that focus on values (e.g., prayer, mediation) may strengthen protective factors against suicide by linking patients to a religious group or to religious doctrines that promote life. Some activities such as cleaning the house or engaging in artwork may help in so far as they can give the patient a sense of accomplishment when they are finished. "Buying new clothes" could be beneficial, if it is linked to an effort to improve one's self-presentation, although for some patients it might just represent impulsive buying and not be that worthwhile of an activity. A few patients reported taking street drugs as a distraction (G. E. Simon et al., 2016), although such activities should be discouraged.

The theory of *implementation intentions* may help explain how to make these strategies successful. The general idea of implementation intentions is that psychotherapists and patients will spell out "if–then plans" in advance. Patients can anticipate feeling unpleasant emotions, and when they do, they will know to implement a plan to reduce those unpleasant feelings. Implementation strategies have been used with a wide range of mental health problems, such as anxiety, schizophrenia, depression, and attention-deficit disorder (Toli, Webb, & Hardy, 2016), and have been incorporated as a component of different treatments such as ACT (Ivanova, Yaakoba-Zohar, Jensen, Cassoff, & Knäuper, 2016) and cognitive behavior therapy (Fritzsche, Schlier, Oettingen, & Lincoln, 2016).

As it applies to distracting activities, when patients begin to feel the dysphoria or distress that often precedes or accompanies suicidal thoughts, they will know to respond with the agreed-on action. Eventually patients will develop a strong mental link between the "if" (dysphoria) and the "then" (agreed-on activities designed to reduce the dysphoria). Ideally patients will develop confidence in their ability to reduce the frequency, duration, and intensity of their dysphoria.

Psychotherapists can improve the effectiveness of these plans by spending enough time with patients to make the options meaningful, rehearsing or reminding patients to use their strategies, reviewing these strategies during psychotherapy sessions, identifying obstacles to implementing them, and being willing to modify the strategies as new information comes to light.

All the activities designed to interrupt the suicidal thoughts and behaviors have an additional benefit. Patients tend to respond well to interventions that align with the essential needs identified by self-determination theory. Teaching patients skills help them develop mastery, which is the third need according to self-determination theory (Ryan & Deci, 2008).

Crisis Plan

A crisis occurs when "an individual is experiencing intense thoughts about suicide, combined with dysphoria and the subjective experience that he or she cannot cope effectively with these emotions, and will act on his or her suicidal thoughts" (Joiner et al., 2009, p. 84). In other words, they have entered a suicidal crisis and are not certain that they can get out of it. The commitment-to-life agreement can include a crisis response plan or a detailed step-by-step procedure for the patients to follow when they are in an acute suicidal crisis. Some suicidal crises can be anticipated, especially if the patients are experiencing some of the same stressors that precipitated past crises.

The goals of crisis intervention are to help the patients understand their feelings, deactivate their suicidal thoughts, and if necessary get emergency care (Joiner et al., 2009). The details of the crisis plan can be put into the commitment to treatment agreement, and patients can also put them on a brief card to carry with them for easy access. The crisis information (either or both as a stand-alone 3×5 card or as part of a commitment-to-life document) could first include activities likely to disrupt the suicidal crisis. One rule of thumb may be to instruct patients to use the activities in their suicidal plan once. If that fails, they should repeat the activities a second time or look for different activities to reduce their emotional turmoil. If that fails, then they should identify themselves as having a crisis and move to the next step.

The crisis plan could also include the after-hours number of their psychotherapists and crisis numbers to call. Psychotherapists who undertake the treatment of suicidal patients should make themselves available for after-hour calls. However, it is prudent to have a backup if their psychotherapists are unavailable for some unforeseen reason. Psychotherapists can add another number such as a local crisis intervention service or the National Suicide Prevention Lifeline number (1-800-273-8255 or 1-800-273-TALK). Psychotherapists can assist patients in entering the phone number in the patient's phone to increase ease of access. Psychotherapists can also give texting information (HOME to 741741) to access trained counselors from the Crisis Text Line. Sending patients to the emergency room should be the last option.

The three steps on the 3×5 note card are do activities, call crisis line, go to emergency room. For example, a card might read

1. Activities: call John (555-5555), go for walk, listen to Mozart, ice cream.

2. Dr. Smith: 555-5551; National Hotline (1-800-273-8255)[6] or crisistextline.org.

3. Anytown hospital ER: 1000 Maple Street, 555-5511.

Psychotherapists can ask patients about the extent to which they believe that they will follow the plan on the activity card. "Tell me on a scale of 1 to 5, how likely will you be to engage in one of these activities if you get upset?" If patients express a low intention of using the plan, it can start a conversation about how to make the activities more useful. It may also be indicated to review the steps in the plan with patients to ensure that they understand the plan.

Psychotherapists who receive crisis calls should listen carefully to their patients and try to elicit their feelings. The immediate goal is to help the patient feel understood and, in the process, to understand their own feelings.

---

[6]Its full name is the National Suicide Prevention Lifeline.

Psychotherapists can validate the feelings—acknowledge the patient's pain—without necessarily accepting the premise. The psychotherapeutic relationship involves working things out together and exploring things together. The attitude that the psychotherapists should convey is that "we can work this out together."

Psychotherapists can also review with patients if they have any suicidal plans. Even patients who did not previously reveal suicidal plans may have developed them recently. If the patients have plans, then it is time to revisit the issue of means safety to ensure that the patients do not have access to the means to kill themselves. If psychotherapists are unable to deactivate the suicidal thoughts of their patients, then consideration needs to be given to more intensive monitoring, including the possibility of a hospitalization.

Collaboratively made commitment-to-life agreements have value. Similar plans are part of the evidence-based CAMS protocol (Jobes, 2016). In addition, Bryan, Mintz, et al. (2017) found that patients who were offered a crisis response plan had fewer suicide attempts, fewer psychiatric hospitalizations, and less suicidal ideation than patients who were offered a no-suicide contract. Also, Zonana, Simberlund, and Christos (2018) retrospectively looked at outpatient mental health records and found that patients who had safety plans were likely to have more outpatient appointment, miss fewer appointments, have fewer emergency room visits, and have fewer suicide attempts. Finally, Gamarra et al. (2015) found that more specificity in such plans was associated with a reduced rate of psychiatric hospitalization.

Commitment to life or commitment to treatment are not static documents. They should be reviewed as needed and modified as necessary, especially if the life circumstances or the mental status of the patient has changed.

Means Safety Counseling

Means restriction counseling occurs when psychotherapists work collaboratively with patients or significant others to restrict patients' access to the deadly resources (Bryan, Stone, & Rudd, 2011). However, C. Chu et al. (2015) preferred the term *means safety* as opposed to *means restriction* because the goal is to promote the safety of the patients. The means safety term also avoids the word "restriction," which may have negative connotations for patients.

Means safety counseling is effective because it delays easy access to lethal means during the window when suicidal urges are high. Most patients have ambivalence about dying, and when the urge to die temporarily gains ascendance, they will use the means that is most readily available to them. The suicidal impulses will ordinarily pass by the time the patients figure out a second way to kill themselves (Yip et al., 2012).

Means safety plans can save lives whether it is by restricting the ease of obtaining poisonous carbon monoxide gas or deadly pesticides (M. Miller, 2012) or restricting access to firearms. If patients are considering taking an overdose of medications, then physicians can be contacted and informed to keep the prescriptions for medications at a sublethal level. Also, patients can be asked to turn over excess drugs to trusted family members or friends.

If patients are considering shooting themselves, then patients can be asked to restrict their access to their guns. Access to firearms is a special concern because those who attempt to die by shooting themselves are more likely to die (Anestis, 2016). Firearms account for only 5% of all suicide attempts, yet 50% of all suicides. This is because attempts with firearms almost always result in death. Access to firearms increases the risk of death by suicide regardless of the age or gender of the patient. Restricting access to firearms may be the single most important step that psychotherapists could take to protect the lives of their patients.

Asking patients if they own firearms might not be sufficient. It can also be necessary to ask whether the patients have access to firearms owned by others or have plans to purchase a firearm. Most gun owners have more than one gun, so it is necessary to restrict access to all guns. One psychotherapist told me that his patient had promised to get rid of all his guns. Months later he revealed that he had kept one gun back, "just in case."

Some critics may argue that taking or removing the weapons from the possession of the patients will only cause them to seek out other ways to kill themselves. However, data do not support this assumption. Removing access to firearms reduces suicides (Stroebe, 2013).

Often patients do not appreciate the close link between firearms accessibility and suicide. Those who did not believe in the link between firearm access and suicide were less likely to store weapons safely (Anestis, Butterworth, & Houtsma, 2018). Consequently, it may help to educate patients or loved ones about the way that suicide thoughts can come quickly and the goal of safe gun storage, which is to provide temporary safety until the likelihood of entering a suicidal crisis has decreased substantially.

If patients turn firearms over to a trusted family member or friend, R. I. Simon (2007) recommended that psychotherapists directly contact the individual who has temporary possession of the weapons to ensure that the transaction occurred. This is such an important intervention that efforts must be made to ensure that patients follow through as they promised.

Often suicidal patients will agree to give up their guns temporarily, consent to use gunlocks, agree to store ammunition and weapons separately, or disassemble their firearms (C. Chu et al., 2015). Psychotherapists should not accept guns directly from their patients. First, it would appear to complicate whatever transference issues that the patient may have. Making psychotherapists the custodian of the guns gives them too much apparent power and would put them in the position of having to decide when to give the guns back to their patients, possibly increasing liability if patients attempted suicide. One patient I know of brought his guns into the psychotherapist's office without notifying the psychotherapist ahead of time. The psychotherapist gave the guns to the county sheriff, who became the temporary custodian of the weapons.

Lockwood (2018) noted that some states restrict the transfer of weapons from one person to another. The laws vary considerably: Some states have no restriction on gun transfer, whereas others permit transfer between some relatives with no restriction but do not permit transfer of guns to other persons without having the other person go through a background check. There is no substitute for knowing the laws in one's state or province. If psychotherapists live in a state that restricts the transfer of guns, then psychotherapists can consider other options such as the removal of ammunition from the house or the use of gun locks.

Jobes (2016) considered the restriction to firearms so important that he reserved the option to terminate treatment (with a referral) with suicidal patients who refuse to restrict their access to firearms. He wrote, "I reserve the right to assert a basic ground rule in order for therapy to proceed. I do not want to clinically compete with the temptation of a gun" (p. 82). All this would occur in the context of a detailed informed consent process whereby the patient has agreed to fundamental rules of psychotherapy. The failure to abide by this rule, according to Jobes, constitutes going back on their agreement to participate in good faith in psychotherapy.

When discussing means safety with patients, it is usually indicated to allow them to generate ideas for means safety. Helping them get some distance may be indicated, such as by asking, "If you had a close friend at risk to die from suicide by firearms, what would you advise him to ensure his personal safety?" Some of the initial ideas that the patients come up with might not be very good, but that is only the start of the conversation where psychotherapists and patients can weigh the benefits and shortcomings of different options.

Some patients may resist giving up their guns. They may feel that they are being bullied or pressured into doing something that they do not want to do. Cultural factors may be involved here as well, as "firearm ownership can be seen as linked to membership in a particular culture" (Betz & Wintemute, 2015, p. 449), although individual gun owners may have different reasons for possessing weapons. Some gun owners may perceive that their psychotherapists hold negative beliefs about guns (or gun owners), which are being played out in psychotherapy. If patients refuse to secure their weapons, it is not profitable to argue with them. Limited self-disclosure could be indicated here. Psychotherapists who own guns or who have lived in families where guns are owned can acknowledge the value that gun ownership has in their own families.

Psychotherapists can also consider techniques from motivational interviewing (W. R. Miller & Rollnick, 2013). *Motivational interviewing* is a "person centered counseling style for addressing the common problems of ambivalence about change" (W. R. Miller & Rollnick, 2013, p. 410). It requires sophistication and skill to do well, so this section will only review some of its basic premises and refer readers to other sources for more detail on how to implement it properly.

Motivational interviewing is based on the premise that change is more likely to occur when patients are adequately motivated. The goal is to help patients decide whether or how to change. Arguing with or trying to persuade ambivalent patients often does not produce the desired outcome. When psychotherapists argue for one side, the ambivalent patient is likely to defend and counter with arguments from the other side. To circumvent that dynamic, motivational interviewing involves two processes. The first is developing a relationship and the second is promoting *change talk* ("any client speech that favors movement toward a particular change goal"; W. R. Miller & Rollnick, 2013, p. 406). Change talk is more likely to occur after asking open questions or giving reflections and less likely to occur after asking closed questions or giving information. Psychotherapists can allow patients to guide the discussion and offer their opinions only if the patients ask them or if the patients give their permission for them to offer their opinions. Nonetheless, psychotherapists will only give their opinions after the patients have had the chance to express their feelings and thoughts (Britton, Bryan, & Valenstein, 2016). Motivational interviewing can be combined with any number of psychotherapeutic orientations.

Monitoring

It is indicated to periodically monitor patients when the risk of suicide is high. Monitoring treatment progress is one of the characteristics of effective psychotherapists. However, here monitoring refers to keeping track of the patient's suicidal thoughts and plans.

The levels of service chart introduced at the beginning of the chapter gives psychotherapists a methodology to evaluate the necessary level of service according to the need for external control.

Psychotherapists and patients should work together to determine the optimal level or method of monitoring. Monitoring involves contact by others to ensure the short-term safety until patients can effectively monitor themselves. Psychiatric hospitalization is the most intensive monitoring that can be used if the risk of suicide is very high.

The monitoring of outpatients is far less intrusive. If the monitoring occurs in the context of outpatient treatment, then psychotherapists should ask patients about their suicidality at every session if there is a risk of suicide. Simply asking whether they currently have suicidal thoughts might not be sufficient, because some patients might have had strong suicidal thoughts earlier in the week but have none at the time of the appointment. Consequently, it is preferable to ask patients about the frequency, intensity, and duration of suicidal thoughts since the last meeting. If the risk is high, psychotherapists can see the patients more than once a week or ask patients to call the office between sessions to give an update on their status. Or patients may simply call the office and leave a phone message that does not necessarily require a callback, on the days between sessions.

The goal of asking about thoughts is to get a gauge of the risk of a suicide attempt. In addition, asking about suicidal thoughts can be an informal barometer of emotional well-being. Failure to ask about suicide may lead some patients to assume that their psychotherapist does not care about this issue, does not want to be bothered, or does not want to have an apparent increase in liability from learning that the patient is suicidal.

Most but not all patients answer accurately when they are asked about thoughts of suicide. Nonetheless, about 75% of patients who died from suicide denied suicide thoughts at their last health care visit (Berman, 2018). Consequently, psychotherapists should evaluate the response considering the totality of the patient's progress. A patient who denies suicide thought but still has a high level of dysphoria and stress may still need careful monitoring.

Although the self-report of suicidal thoughts is very important, such self-reports have their limitations. Patients may feel more relaxed or comfortable while in the presence of their psychotherapist whom they trust and respect. That feeling of comfort may lead patients to underreport the frequency, strength, and duration of their suicidal thoughts. It is unlikely that the patients are lying (although this could occur at times), but more likely that the therapeutic setting has positive or uplifting features that may influence patients to underreport their suicidal urges.

If patients show a high risk of suicide, it might be indicated to ask them permission to view their social media postings. The manifest content of the posting, including reactions to stress, appraisals, or events, and so on, may provide leads on suicide-related themes considered by the patient since their last appointment.

To compensate for the limitations of self-report, it may be prudent to use a brief suicide screening instrument to supplement the patient's self-report of suicidal ideation (see Chapter 5 for more detail on how it fits into a more comprehensive quality enhancement strategy). This may be the same instrument that the psychotherapists used during the initial evaluation of the patient. This screening instrument provides a check or second source of information on the patient. A side benefit of using the same screening instrument is that psychotherapists can keep a record to show the patients their progress based on quantifiable data in case they ever felt discouraged about their progress.

For patients with a serious risk, the monitoring may involve a spouse, a friend, or another family member as part of a team who will check in with the patient periodically and provide a second source of data on the patient's suicidal behavior. The monitoring arrangements can be part of the commitment-to-life agreement.

Enlisting Family Members Into the Team

Family members or friends may be used as supports or team members (the term *team member* appears preferable to *monitors*). Cramer et al. (2013)

identified notifying and involving other persons as a core competency when treating suicidal patients. Psychotherapists should rely heavily on the input of their patients on the option of engaging loved ones as team members. Psychotherapists should have a clear clinical rationale for countermanding a patient's wishes concerning eliciting team members (see next section on disclosing patients' information without their consent).

Nonetheless, engaging family members or friends can be a very important step in preventing a patient suicide. Draper, Krysinska, Snowdon, and De Leo (2018) reported that 90% of the next of kin of a suicide decedent were aware of the warning signs of suicide compared with only 45% of the patient's health care professionals. In addition, families were more likely to reach out to health care professionals than health care professionals were to reach out to them. Involvement of the family is an underutilized strategy that could substantially help the patient.

Most families have good intentions and will be strong allies on the recovery of their loved ones. However, psychotherapists should not automatically assume that is the case. A study by the Center for Collegiate Mental Health (2018) found that 10% of college counseling students strongly disagreed with the statement "I get the emotional help and support I need from my family" (p. 36). Although this response does not mean that the families will never turn out to be a helpful part of a treatment team, it does suggest that psychotherapists should not assume that patients would welcome the involvement of their families. Psychotherapists should ask for details about the nature of the family relationships before deciding whether or how to involve them in treatment.

It is not sufficient just to invite family or friends as team members; it is important to socialize them into their role. Psychotherapists should be certain that team members understand what is expected of them, what they can do that would be helpful, and what they could do that could be harmful.

Two sources of information suggest the importance of preparing family members for their roles as team members. First, George-Levi et al. (2016) found that the amount of adherence to medication for cardiac patients varied by the style of caregiving of the patient's partner. Applying these findings to suicidal patients, some well-meaning team members may engage in counterproductive overmonitoring to the point that patients feel that they are under constant surveillance. These concerns found some support in a qualitative study, wherein suicidal men reported tensions with loved ones who sometimes appeared too vigilant in their monitoring, overinterpreted what behavior constituted a risky behavior change, or wanted to impose restraints on their behavior (Fogarty et al., 2018).

Also, family members who express hostility or criticism can impede the success of psychotherapy (Chambless et al., 2017) and that should be addressed by the psychotherapist. Some team members may—unless they are properly socialized—adopt a dismissive or harsh approach. For example, they may want to argue with the loved one or adopt a "tough love" approach and tell them to just snap out of it or just get over it (Ellis & Newman, 1996). Other family members may mistakenly believe that suicidal people will always find a way to kill themselves despite their efforts to prevent a suicide. Still other family members may deny that the patient is mentally ill or even discourage them from taking their medications (R. Simon, 2011).

Also, the importance of means safety should be explained to the team members. About one third of the public believes that efforts to restrict means would not be effective because the patients would just find other ways to kill themselves (M. Miller, Azrael, & Hemenway, 2006). This misconception needs to be addressed quickly.

Education is the optimal way to address potential problems. Family members can be told that suicidal behavior almost always arises out of a mental illness that is treatable—it is not simply a matter of will power. Death by suicide is not inevitable. About 90% of those who survived a suicide attempt eventually died from other causes (M. Miller & Hemenway, 2008).

Some family members may be very disturbed themselves and incapable of helping the patient (R. Simon, 2011). For example, some family members may become very distraught at learning of the suicidal potential of their loved ones. Their fear may add another layer of burden to the patient. At times, it may be necessary to refer family members for psychotherapy themselves.

Being a member of the patient's team does not mean that the support person will supervise the patients or assume responsibility as to whether the patient lives or dies. Having family members keep constant surveillance on a family member is fraught with problems, including the fatigue on the part of the support person. A patient who needs around-the-clock supervision should probably be in a hospital (R. Simon, 2011).

However, team members can have some tasks or goals developed by patients and their psychotherapists. For example, the team member may be available to help patients circumvent an emotional cascade by helping to engage them in pleasant or distracting tasks, allowing them to vent, or helping them to problem solve. Or, psychotherapists can provide information concerning the crisis plan and help the patient follow through with it if necessary.

Families can help their loved ones by planning activities that involve connections with others including friends or members of the extended family. Psychotherapists can also explain the importance of means safety, the value in limiting alcohol or other recreational drugs, and how certain activities can help disrupt a suicidal crisis. Psychotherapists can explain how suicidal thinking can lead to distortions of situations and a reduced ability to think through problems. Furthermore, psychotherapists can stress the importance of adhering to treatment, including taking medications if any were prescribed and keeping psychotherapy appointments, and also what the family should do if there is a suicidal crisis. It may be productive to write down the crisis instructions for the family as it may be difficult for them to remember these instructions if a crisis occurs. Finally, family members can share information with the psychotherapists, with the consent of the patient, concerning their perceptions of the patient's progress and alert the psychotherapists if the patient appears to be deteriorating, is talking more about suicide, or is engaging in worrisome behavior such as giving away precious items or making a will.

The effectiveness of these strategies requires good communication between patients and their team members and the active involvement of the patient. Men, who are often too embarrassed to talk about their feelings, may need assistance in informing family members on when and how to support them and when to back off. One psychotherapist working with an older man considered to be the patriarch of the family explained the support-seeking activities in terms of the "instructions" he was giving family members.

OTHER OPTIONS FOR MANAGING SUICIDE RISK

The other methods of managing suicidal risk are disclosing information about patients without their consent (breaking confidentiality), seeking a psychiatric hospitalization, seeking an involuntary psychiatric hospitalization, and going to an emergency room. One of the core competencies for psychotherapists working with suicidal patients is to know the laws in their jurisdiction regarding such options (Cramer et al., 2013). According to these laws, psychotherapists may disclose information without the consent of their patients to protect the life or safety of an individual or society, although states and provinces vary on how they describe this exception. In addition, psychotherapists or family members may involuntarily hospitalize individuals who are imminently suicidal, which typically requires having a serious mental illness and a high risk for a suicide attempt. States and provinces vary on how they define "high risk"; some require an actual suicide attempt to justify an involuntary psychiatric hospitalization. There is no substitute for knowing the exact wording of the laws in one's state or province.

Some options, such as disclosing patient information without their consent (breaking confidentiality), and involuntary psychiatric hospitalization contradict the wishes of the patients. Psychotherapists should proceed with such actions with caution, although they can be used in limited circumstances as described in the following section.

Disclosing Information Without Patient Consent (Breaking Confidentiality)

Psychotherapists will sometimes encounter patients who do not want their friends or family members to know about their suicidal thoughts or do not want family members to participate as part of a treatment team. In these situations, psychotherapists must decide whether the benefits of notifying the family outweigh the harm.

Recent years have seen litigation on this issue on college campuses. Several psychotherapists in college counseling services have been sued for failing to notify parents that their children had suicidal thoughts. One could easily imagine a scenario in which psychotherapists who failed to notify family members were making a huge mistake. On the other hand, one could just as easily imagine a scenario where psychotherapists who did inform family members were making an equally huge mistake. After a patient has died from suicide, it is easy to look back and claim that the psychotherapists should have notified (or not notified) family members. Consequently, psychotherapists should clearly document the rationale for their decisions.

Disclosing patients' information without their consent (breaking confidentiality) runs counter to the principle of respecting patients' decisions. On the other hand, some psychotherapists may argue that it may be the only way that they can ensure the safety of their patients and adhere to the overarching ethical principle of beneficence (promoting the well-being of their patients). Consequently, it appears that two or more ethical principles are in conflict. A psychotherapist cannot adhere to one ethical principle without violating the other.

Principle-based ethics can guide psychotherapists on how to balance two or more overarching ethical principles that appear to collide. The founder of principle-based ethics, W. D. Ross (1930/1998), anticipated conflicts between moral principles and offered a methodology to address these conflicts:

> When I am in a situation . . . in which more than one of these prima facie duties is incumbent on me, what I have to do is to study the situation as fully as I can until I form the considered opinion (it is never more) that in the circumstances one of them is more incumbent than any other. (p. 268)

The decision on which ethical principle gets more weight depends on the "considered opinion" of the psychotherapists. In other words, psychotherapists should give priority to the ethical principle that appears most important. The *Canadian Code of Ethics for Psychologists* (Canadian Psychological Association, 2017) states that the ethical principles of patient well-being trumps other principles, but even then, it acknowledges that there may be exceptions to the generality.

Beauchamp and Childress (2009) expanded on the methodology proposed by Ross (1930/1998) and presented several steps to follow when a moral agent considers allowing one moral principle temporarily to trump another. The most salient steps are (a) to determine if the proposed intervention is likely to succeed; (b) to determine if the person has better reasons for acting on behalf of one overarching ethical principle than the other; and (c) to minimize the infringement to the offended moral principle. That is, "the form of the infringement selected is the least possible commensurate with achieving the primary goal of the action" and "the agent seeks to minimize any negative effects of the infringement" (Beauchamp & Childress, 2009, p. 34).

In the following paragraphs, a principle-based analysis is applied to situations in which psychotherapists must determine whether to notify a family member against the wishes of the patient. Here the principle of beneficence (promoting the well-being of the patient by notifying the family) appears to conflict with the overarching ethical principle of respect for patient autonomy (respecting the wishes of the patient and not notifying the family). When any action appears to violate an overarching moral principle, psychotherapists should slow down their thinking and reflect carefully on their choices.

First, psychotherapists must determine that notifying a family member or another person would help the patient. Sometimes notifying families can substantially harm the patient. Although most families are responsive and caring for their loved ones during this time, a few families have a high degree of pathology and may respond in a way that increases the risk of suicide. It is important that psychotherapists have accurate information when making these decisions. This requires honest and accurate communications between patients and their psychotherapists, which is more likely to occur if there is a good treatment relationship and the patients perceive that their psychotherapists are acting in their best interests.

Also, psychotherapists need to determine if the benefits of notifying the family outweigh the harm. One benefit might be that the family members could help patients to prevent or interrupt the suicidal crisis or respond better in an emergency. On the other hand, disclosing might harm the patient. If patients feel offended by the disclosure, they may drop out of treatment or, if they stay in treatment, become less forthcoming about their suicidal thoughts and plans. In the short run, disclosing might help protect the patient. But in the long run, disclosing might have increased the overall risk of suicide by ending psychotherapy or greatly reducing its effectiveness.

If psychotherapists determine that notifying a third party, such as a family member, is necessary to ensure the safety of the patient, then beneficence (patient well-being) would temporarily trump the ethical principle of respecting patient autonomy (honoring the patients' wishes to keep their confidentiality). However, principle-based ethics also require moral agents to try to minimize harm to the offended moral principle, which in this case is respect for patient autonomy. If it is necessary to inform a third party of the patients' suicidal intent, then it is preferable that psychotherapists explain to their patients why they are making this decision and to involve the patient in making decisions as much as possible. For example, psychotherapists might say, "I need to inform your spouse of the strength of your suicidal thoughts. I know that she is in the waiting room and I am going to ask her to come in and talk with us. Would you like me to tell her about your suicidal thoughts, or would you want to do it?" If the patient says that he would like the psychotherapist to do it, then the psychotherapist can say, "this is generally what I would say . . . does this make sense to you? Would you like me to change anything that I say?" The information shared should be the minimum necessary to fulfill the purpose of the disclosure.

Psychotherapists can refer to their informed consent discussion at the beginning of psychotherapy when they discussed exceptions to confidentiality. That review should include the statement that information within psychotherapy is confidential with some exceptions, including when patients present an imminent risk to harm themselves or others. Psychotherapists can explain that this is one of the situations involving a risk of harm to self and confidentiality is no longer absolute.

Often patients do not tell their loved ones about their suicidal thoughts because they do not wish to burden them or because they feel ashamed of the thoughts. I have no data on the outcome for such disclosures, but psychotherapists have told me that the family members who receive this information often appreciated hearing it and felt relief because they sensed that something was very wrong.

Psychotherapists will make better decisions if they reflect on their decision-making processes. For example, some psychotherapists may feel anxiety at making these decisions and adopt the first *just-good-enough* solution that they come across. Although it is not the optimal solution, it appears minimally adequate, and it reduces the anxiety of the psychotherapists to at least have a decision. However, unless the need for a response is imminent, it is best for psychotherapists to slow down their thinking, involve the patient and team members in the decision, and consider alternatives (Knapp, Gottlieb, & Handelsman, 2015). Psychotherapists might say, "Help me think through this issue." "How can we keep you safe, and still respect your wishes not to involve your family?" Perhaps patients might be willing to inform (or allow their psychotherapists to inform) one family member, but not another. Or perhaps patients may be willing to divulge (or allow their psychotherapists to divulge) some information to family members but withhold other information that is embarrassing and not essential for them to know.

Psychiatric Hospitalizations

It is indicated to send some patients to a psychiatric hospital. During a 3-year period, my colleagues and I facilitated about 130 psychiatric hospitalizations for suicidal behavior in the rural Northern Appalachian county where we worked (Knapp, Dirks, & Magee, 1982). In hindsight, I think most were justified, although we had no way to monitor patient outcomes over time.

The most common reason for a psychiatric hospitalization would be if the patient did not appear capable of surviving outside of the hospital. This process for determining this can be made using the level of care charts described in the beginning of this chapter where the patient has an acquired capability to die, access to means, a high baseline of distress, and a likelihood of entering a suicidal crisis. In addition, patients may be hospitalized if they are psychotic, if they need medication but have complicated pharmacological or serious comorbid medical issues that require close monitoring, or if they need electroconvulsive therapy (ECT). Although ECT has been overused in the past and retains a public stigma, recent evidence has suggested that it can have good outcomes for depression if used selectively (Fink, 2014).

However, some psychotherapists mistakenly believe that hospitalization is the standard of care for suicidal patients. It is not. It is indicated for some patients and contraindicated for others. When our team assumed responsibility for psychiatric emergencies, the total number of hospitalizations decreased by about one third from the previous years, because we emphasized outpatient treatment. During that time, the local state hospital continued to discharge many long-term patients into the community. If these newly discharged high-risk patients were removed from our data set, I suspect that the rate of hospitalizations would have decreased even more. We worked to keep many patients out of the hospital because we thought that they could get better treatment outside of the hospital than in the hospital.

Bastiampillai, Sharfstein, and Allison (2016) argued that the increase in suicide rates in the last 20 years may be attributable, in part, to the decline in the number of psychiatric beds that has occurred during this period. Perhaps the lack of psychiatric beds is one reason, out of many, for the increased rate of suicide. However, the authors failed to highlight several important facts.

First, as most psychotherapists who have ever tried to hospitalize a patient know, that process can be stressful for patients and psychotherapists. It may mean waiting hours (and sometimes days) for a bed in an appropriate facility to become open. It may mean waiting for hours in the emergency room or taking seemingly countless phone calls from hospitals reporting on the bed availability. Getting patients hospitalized can be especially difficult if they lack health insurance or are only insured through policies with poor benefits, as are often found in medical-assistance policies. The reimbursement rates for medical assistance tend to be low, and many psychiatric hospitals will not admit them as patients or will only accept a limited number of them. Psychotherapists appropriately include the stress of getting a hospital bed into the equation of whether to seek a hospitalization.

Second, the quality of service in psychiatric hospitals varies considerably. Some patients receive good services in hospitals. It sets them on the path to stability and positive psychological health. Other patients do not receive meaningful services in hospitals beyond a safe environment. Psychotherapy rarely occurs in some psychiatric hospitals. I had a patient in one hospital complain to me that he was receiving no substantive treatment: There was one generic group therapy session each day, and the physician saw each patient for about 10 minutes a day. "Doc, I am not getting any help here," he told me. This patient got more treatment as an outpatient.

Also, hospitalizations are often contraindicated for persons with chronic suicidal thoughts. Unless the danger of suicide is imminent, these patients are usually better off trying to handle their lives outside of the hospital. Otherwise their lives run the risk of becoming a continual revolving door between home and hospital with little progress.

In addition, the milieu of the hospital can be stressful. Depending on the unit, patients may observe or interact with frightening, aggressive, psychotic, or highly disorganized patients. One patient entered a psychiatric ward voluntarily and while on his way to his room, witnessed attendants attempting to subdue a violent patient, became frightened, and immediately signed himself out.

Also, psychiatric hospitals frequently restrict the freedom of patients. They may only allow patients to use plastic knives, take away their cell phones, or even take away belts or sharp object. Patients may be subject to 24-hour surveillance or 15-minute checks. Often these restrictions are needed to ensure the safety of patients, but they do offend many patients who want greater autonomy (Chung, Ryan, & Large, 2016). I do not criticize the use of these restrictive measures but only note that they do come at a psychological cost.

Furthermore, a hospitalization itself can cost the patients money both through the cost of the hospitalization and through the loss of income, and they can disrupt the patient's connections with work or family. A hospitalization often brings social stigma. Also, patients feel that they are in a protective bubble when they are in a hospital. When they are discharged they return to the same interpersonal stressors, loneliness, and daily hassles that had precipitated their suicidal thoughts in the first place (Owen-Smith et al., 2014). Large, Ryan, Walsh, Stein-Parbury, and Patfield (2014) claimed that these stressful experiences of getting into or being in a psychiatric hospital may contribute to the suicide of some patients who would still be alive if they had stayed at home.

Finally, referring psychotherapists should be sensitive to issues surrounding discharge and follow-up care. If psychotherapists do not intend to take the patient back after discharge, they should tell the hospital as soon as possible so that it can make other treatment arrangements on discharge.

Psychotherapists should carefully monitor patients who have recently been discharged from psychiatric hospitals because suicides tend to increase shortly after discharge from a hospital. Patients who made the most extensive planning and preparation for their attempts in a prehospitalization attempt are at the greatest risk for a suicide attempt after discharge (Jordan & McNiel, 2018).

Hospitals often do not adequately plan follow-up services with discharged patients. Most health care systems report Healthcare Effectiveness Data and Information Set (HEDIS) on many performance measures, including the number of patients with psychiatric hospitalizations for depression who receive outpatient appointments within 7 days or 30 days of discharge. The percentages are astonishingly low, even though postdischarge is a high-risk period for suicide. Across commercial insurers, about 50% of patients discharged with mental illnesses did not receive appointments within 7 days of discharge, and about 30% received no appointment within 30 days of discharge. The percentages were lower for Medicaid and Medicare patients (NCQA, 2017).

Although the ideal is to make the discharge decision cooperatively with the patient, insurance company oversight into the hospitalization process strongly influences the decisions of mental health professionals and patients. Hospitals sometimes feel economic pressure to discharge patients because managed care companies threaten not to pay for extended hospital stays.

Again, hospitalizations are indicated for some patients; the point here is that the decision needs to be based on the needs of the patient, the type and quality of services offered in the hospital, and a consideration of the downside of hospitalizations. Ideally, psychotherapists will know something about the hospital to which they refer patients and have realistic expectations about the services offered.

Involuntary Psychiatric Hospitalizations

Some patients urgently need hospitalization to save their lives but refuse to go. During my 3 years working full time in emergency services, my team facilitated 61 involuntary psychiatric hospitalizations for suicidal behavior. Even in retrospect, I think almost all these were justified. However, my team made these decisions very carefully.

Here again psychotherapists can rely on principle-based ethics to guide their decisions. The principle of beneficence (promoting the well-being of the patient by ensuring that they do not die from suicide) appears to conflict with respect for the patient's decision-making ability (to stay out of the hospital). Psychotherapists need to ask if less intrusive means to protect the patients have been exhausted and, if not, ask if the benefits of the hospitalization outweigh its harm and try to implement the hospitalizations as humanely as possible. Each of these topics will be discussed in more detail in the next section.

Have Less Intrusive Means Been Exhausted?

Involuntary hospitalizations should only occur if other, less intrusive means have been ruled out. Psychotherapists should consider whether the patient could be treated as an outpatient or whether the patient would go to the hospital voluntarily. Often psychotherapists can secure a voluntary hospitalization if they carefully explain the benefits of the hospitalization to the patients. It can help to walk the patients through the steps of a hospitalization from their arrival at the hospital until they get up to the unit. This step seems so obvious, yet some psychotherapists accept without contention the first response of a patient who says "no" to a psychiatric hospitalization. If the need for a psychiatric hospitalization is imminent, then the "no" just represents the first step in a conversation.

Readers may argue that the refusal of psychotherapists to accept the answer that the patient first gives violates the norm of respecting patient autonomy. But the issue is more complex. Are patients making autonomous decisions if they lack all the facts necessary to make an informed decision or if they are responding to inaccurate stereotypes? Are patients making autonomous decisions if they are responding during a state of emotional crisis without the opportunity to rationally think through their decision? Even if it is assumed, for argument's sake, that the patients are acting autonomously, according to principle-based ethics, one overarching ethical principle may trump another, if it is appropriate to do so and an effort is made to minimize harm to the offended moral principle.

I once had a patient who refused to go to the hospital. Later in the conversation I learned it was because she did not want the neighbors to see her leave in an ambulance; we arranged for her to go in her daughter's car, and she then went willingly. Another patient did not want to go to the hospital. As we spoke, I learned that she assumed that she would be sent to the hospital where her late husband died. The very thought of going to that hospital filled her with dread. I suspected that she might have posttraumatic stress disorder (PTSD), or some subclinical variation of PTSD related to her husband's death. She went willingly to another hospital.

On several occasions, I have spent 2 hours or more talking with patients about their need to be in a hospital. One such patient told me that she still did not think she needed to go to the hospital, but because it seemed so important to me, she was willing to go. Another patient said, "You are not going to stop talking until I agree to go, are you?" We laughed together at his comment, but he went to the hospital. Of course, these patients could have simply left at any time, but the fact that they allowed me to continue talking to them indicated some ambivalence on their part. Motivational interviewing can be indicated in some of these situations (basic information about motivational interviewing was covered earlier in this chapter in the section Means Safety Counseling).

Often third parties can help turn a likely involuntary hospitalization into a voluntary one. I have had several patients who refused to go until they first spoke to their family physician. The opinions of these family physicians carried great authority with the family. As soon as the family physician said they should go, they went voluntarily. Sometimes clergy have similar influence.

Of course, a few patients will be in an acute psychotic state with a diminished capacity to process information carefully. But even psychotic patients fall along a continuum. I have spoken to psychotic patients who were so bizarre and aggressive that my immediate goal was to get out of the interview without being assaulted. On the other hand, I have spoken to other psychotic patients who were disturbed by their hallucinations yet willing to talk about them and consider treatment options.

Often psychotherapists must decide about an involuntary psychiatric hospitalization quickly under less-than-ideal circumstances. Patient emergencies can come at inconvenient times. Over a weekend or after hours it may be easier to spend the necessary time with a patient without interruptions. However, if the emergency occurred during a work day, it may be necessary to balance the needs of the suicidal patients with those of other patients who have scheduled appointments.

I have intervened with patients in chaotic situations. When conducting a home evaluation of a woman with a strong risk of a suicide attempt, I continually had to deal with intrusive family members or neighbors who believed that it was essential for me to receive their opinions on the matter. They had nothing of value to say and kept me from developing a good conversation with the woman at risk. At the same time, I was receiving phone calls from the hospitals alerting me as to whether they had a bed available (most did not). The experience left me quite frazzled. Ideally, I would have had the time to talk with the woman at risk without interruption. However, that was not the case. Ideally, I would have thought through the issue with calm deliberation and received consultation. But the urgency of the situation prevented me from doing so. I had to act quickly. In this case the woman at risk had dealt with me once briefly during a previous crisis, trusted my good motives, and eventually agreed to a hospitalization voluntarily (although she had strongly refused to go when her husband had asked—or ordered—her to go).

This was one of the more stressful hospitalizations I have had to deal with, but other interviews often included obstacles that prevented a thorough evaluation and an optimal intervention. These types of emergencies require *hypervigilant decision making* wherein psychotherapists must "conduct a less-than-exhaustive information search, do an accelerated evaluation of the data, consider a limited number of alternatives, and come to rapid closure on a decision" (Kleespies, 2014, p. 39). My only advice to professionals in those situations is to do the best that they can, recognizing the limitations created by the situation. Because of the difficulties in making these decisions, some states only apply higher negligence standards (called *gross negligence*) in involuntary hospitalizations than are applied when delivering health care in other venues. Professional negligence is discussed in more detail in Chapter 5.

Do the Benefits of an Involuntary Hospitalization Outweigh the Harm?

Psychotherapists need to determine if the hospitalization will further the overarching ethical principle of beneficence (promoting patient well-being). This requires balancing risks and benefits. Unfortunately, no formula exists for precisely estimating the risk of suicides in the short term. Nonetheless, some patients have risk factors so high that it appears that their lives are in imminent risk, and a hospitalization would appear indicated. Typically, they would fall in the imminent risk category according to the levels of service chart described earlier in the chapter.

I have evaluated psychotic patients who were hearing voices ordering them to kill themselves. I did not think these patients would live very long outside of a hospital. My team initiated an involuntary psychiatric hospitalization against one nonpsychotic patient who was so intent on suicide that she had hid lethal doses of drugs in her vagina. Fortunately, the hospital staff was alert to her extreme suicidality and did a cavity search.

Although an involuntary psychiatric hospitalization can be necessary, it often occurs at a cost. In their review of psychiatric hospitalizations, Kallert, Glöckner, and Schützwohl (2008) found that patients who had been involuntarily hospitalized had a higher rate of suicide postdischarge than voluntary patients. They were more dissatisfied with treatment and more likely to believe that the hospitalization was not warranted. These findings are hard to interpret. They might suggest that the involuntary nature of the hospitalization may account for the poorer outcomes compared with voluntary hospitalizations, although it is possible that involuntary patients had more risk factors for suicide to begin with.

Nonetheless, it is important to consider some of the shortcomings of psychiatric hospitalizations as described in general previously, including their potential to disrupt social relationships, disrupt work schedules (or even losing a job), embarrass the patient, and so on. Furthermore, involuntary psychiatric hospitalizations incur additional risks. Sometimes the police must implement the order. I have seen police act with extreme tact and skill in these circumstances, and I have heard of situations where they used force unnecessarily. Even when police act with maximum courtesy, the experience of being taken away in handcuffs can humiliate some patients.

Also, an involuntary psychiatric hospitalization can sometimes cause patients to lose faith or trust in their treatment providers (Wortzel, Matarazzo, & Homaifar, 2013). Even when released, some suicidal patients may simply stop treatment or, if they continue treatment, be quiet about their suicidal thoughts. Furthermore, patients may lose the right to own firearms, which can very important for those who are hunters, recreational gun users, collectors, or who perceive the need of fire arms for personal protection.

Because involuntary hospitalizations have the potential to harm the treatment relationship, they may increase the long-term risk of suicide for some patients. Consequently, involuntary psychiatric hospitalizations should be initiated only in rare circumstances where the life of a patient is seriously threatened, and the professional has no other way to diffuse the danger.

Effective Implementation of Hospitalizations
Ordinarily it is recommended that family members agree to the involuntary psychiatric hospitalization. This increases the likelihood that the family will invest in the benefits of the hospitalization and continue to recognize the serious needs of their loved one. It also reduces the likelihood of future splitting, wherein the family aligns itself with the patient against the psychotherapist whom they claimed initiated the hospitalization. If the patient returned home and began to complain about the hospitalization, the family members might agree (or say they agree) with the patient's perspective to avoid conflict. Thus, the family members who once begged the psychotherapist to hospitalize the patient may later mispresent their role in the hospitalization and shift all the responsibility on the psychotherapist.

In the state where I worked, the involuntary hospitalization process included a petition that, if executed by the proper authorities, would mandate that the individual receive an evaluation by a physician who could decide whether to admit the patient involuntarily. The petition included a section where the reasons for the request for the examination could be written down. Whenever possible, I asked the family to write down the reasons on the petition in their own handwriting, to ensure that they stood by the decision. In only a few rare occasions did I write down the reasons for the hospitalization myself.

Whenever a referral is made for a hospitalization, whether it is for voluntary or involuntary hospitalization, the referring psychotherapists should attempt to communicate the reasons for the hospitalization recommendation to the physician who is evaluating the patient for admission. I know of situations where psychotherapists assumed that the evaluating physician would easily see the need for hospitalization, only to have the patients sent home. Once a psychotherapist spent a lot of time convincing patients of the need for hospitalization but failed to inform the evaluating physician that the statutory grounds for an involuntary psychiatric hospitalization existed. The patient changed his mind about being admitted, was sent home, and attempted suicide that night.

It changes the dynamic of an interview when a physician has received a message from a psychotherapist giving good reasons why the danger of suicide is imminent. Before receiving this information, physicians look for justifications to admit the patient. After receiving this information, physicians now feel that they must look for justifications to reject the admission.

Emergency Rooms

Certainly, it would be appropriate to send suicidal patients to a local emergency room if they had sustained physical harm and needed immediate medical attention. It could also be justified if psychotherapists believed that a psychiatric hospitalization had to be initiated immediately and had no other way to secure an admission. Some emergency rooms have good mental health staff and provide quick and effective treatment. Many others do not have such resources. Unless psychotherapists know that the emergency room delivers high-quality care, it could be indicated to send a suicidal patient to an emergency room only for medical purposes or when other crisis intervention options are not available. Readers may recall that the crisis intervention card discussed earlier in this chapter put going to the emergency room as the last option. Emergency rooms are often crowded and unpleasant. The wait times can be long and often the emergency rooms do not have a psychiatrist or psychologist on call. Even if a psychiatric admission is indicated, patients may often have to wait in the emergency room for many hours until a bed becomes available.

In addition, psychiatric patients in emergency rooms risk encountering unsympathetic staff. Jobes (2016) described a situation where he and the patient heard emergency room personnel complain that the patient was taking up space needed for real patients. I had a similar experience where a patient told me that she overheard the emergency room staff complaining about the bed she was taking in the emergency room. My interpretation is that some emergency room staff often lack the expertise for the psychiatric problems that they encounter. Some evidence supports this interpretation. Tanguturi, Bodic, Taub, Homel, and Jacob (2017) found that the residents in the emergency room varied considerably in their documentation of suicidal patients and often failed to document information that would be very important in determining the risk of a suicide. Betz et al. (2018) found that 85% of the charts of suicidal patients contained no documentation that the physician had assessed the patient's access to lethal means.

The best way for me to express my concerns about emergency rooms is to ask the readers to describe their last experiences in an emergency room. Did they get a lot of attention? Was the service prompt? Did they feel the examination was thorough? Often the answer to all those questions is no.

Frequently psychotherapists in solo or small group practices will have a voicemail on their answering machines instructing patients with "true emergencies" to go to the emergency room. Commercial insurance companies may require such messages, and they may be sufficient to alert individuals who are not yet patients and mistakenly assume that psychotherapists in an outpatient practice can respond immediately to an emergency from a nonpatient. However, ongoing patients should be given more detailed instructions concerning emergencies, which would include the option of emergency rooms only under limited circumstances.

4

Interventions Part Two

Suicide-Informed Psychotherapy

This chapter continues the discussion of the elements of effective interventions with suicidal patients. Chapter 3 covered the initial stages of interventions, including the informed consent process, the importance of the treatment relationship, and suicide management strategies. Effective psychotherapists will continue to use the suicide management strategies as needed throughout treatment. This chapter covers suicide-related issues that arise in psychotherapy, and ways to reduce the symptoms commonly found among suicidal patients. The recommendations suggested herein should apply regardless of the theoretical orientation of the psychotherapist.

SUICIDE-RELATED TOPICS THAT ARISE IN PSYCHOTHERAPY

Psychotherapists can help maintain an effective treatment relationship by being flexible in their scheduling and helping patients adhere to treatment. In addition, psychotherapists will refer to psychopharmacologists as needed, coordinate services with other health care providers, help patients navigate suicide-related websites, learn to address threats of time-contingent suicide, and respond to suicide attempts that occur during psychotherapy. Also, psychotherapists can offer strategies to reduce the emotional pain of their patients and can address religion or values in psychotherapy. Finally, they can end psychotherapy with discussions of relapse prevention and continued patient growth.

http://dx.doi.org/10.1037/0000145-005
Suicide Prevention: An Ethically and Scientifically Informed Approach, by S. J. Knapp

Flexibility in Scheduling

It is reasonable for psychotherapists to establish limits on the times that they are available to meet patients, but suicidal patients require more flexibility. It may be necessary for psychotherapists to see patients more than once a week, depending on the risk. Psychotherapists may have made extra appointment times available after or before their normal working hours to ensure that they can see their suicidal patients, at least temporarily. In extreme cases it may be necessary to shorten the time spent with other patients (or sometimes even cancel appointments) to respond to a patient in a suicidal crisis. Fortunately, these accommodations will be rare for most psychotherapists.

Psychotherapists who treat suicidal patients must ensure the availability of after-hour services. Psychotherapists should give local or national emergency numbers as a backup when they are not available, but it is preferable that psychotherapists make themselves directly available for emergency calls. Ironically, a policy of restricting access to after-hour services may backfire. One study found that psychotherapists who gave patients the option of calling them after hours had fewer after-hour patient calls than psychotherapists who did not present that option (Reitzel, Burns, Repper, Wingate, & Joiner, 2004). The reasons for the finding are not clear, although it is possible that the psychotherapists who offered after-hours services had done a better job in socializing patients on how to use the after-hours services responsibly.

It is true that a few patients may attempt to abuse this access. In such cases it may be indicated to review the definition of a crisis call and when it can be used. If they still abuse the access, then psychotherapists can restrict such calls to a brief evaluation of the immediacy of suicidal risk (Linehan, 1993).

Helping Patients Adhere to Treatment

Most patients are conscientious and keep appointments, pay bills, and cooperate in psychotherapy. Other patients are less conscientious, or they may feel too demoralized and discouraged to fulfill their commitments. A few may demand special privileges, request exceptions for themselves, or have mistaken ideas about what psychotherapy means. It is important to set the expectations for psychotherapy clearly. If, for whatever reason, a patient fails to cooperate, despite efforts to motivate the patient, the psychotherapist can refer to the original informed consent document that identifies the conditions of psychotherapy. The informed consent agreement becomes crucial in establishing and maintaining reasonable standards of therapeutic care.

The ultimate form of nonadherence is to drop out of treatment. Swift and Greenberg (2015) estimated that one fifth of patients drop out of treatment prematurely. However, for suicidal patients, the risk of dropping out can be life threatening. Hom and Joiner (2017) found that suicidal patients who dropped out of treatment had lower global assessment of function ratings, had more comorbid diagnoses, and were more likely to have substance abuse disorders than those who did not drop out of treatment. Those who need psychotherapy the most appear to have the greatest difficulty staying in treatment. Also, the factors that drive persons to suicide are sometimes the same factors that make it difficult for them to participate fully in treatment.

At times, patients do not adhere to treatment if they feel discouraged because they have not made sufficient progress in treatment. Psychotherapists can anticipate and address this discouragement. First, they can acknowledge that treatment may be difficult. This can be part of the role induction that occurs during the informed consent portion of treatment where psychotherapists describe the process of treatment.

With patients who present with serious disorders or complex comorbid problems, it is important to be honest and accurate about appropriate treatment. Ideally, psychotherapists will offer hope to patients in the role induction process. Psychotherapists can explain how most suicidal patients go on to live good and productive lives and how the treatments selected have evidence and professional experience behind them designed to maximize patient recovery.

Second, psychotherapists can ensure that they focus on what is important to their patients. Patients who enter treatment may have a general sense of dysphoria without having a clear sense of how to address these feelings. After a few sessions, however, patients may be better able to identify specific goals for treatment. Psychotherapists can normalize this shift and better clarify goals as progress, in so far as patients are better able to identify the antecedents of the dysphoria or parse out the specific emotions they feel.

To avoid a mismatch on patient goals, some psychotherapists will ask patients to write out their agendas for the session ahead of time, thus ensuring that their psychotherapists know what is on the patient's mind. This helps patients to identify and articulate what is important to them. Other psychotherapists will routinely ask patients at the end of each session about the extent to which the session met their goals (Maeschalck & Barfknecht, 2017). This gives psychotherapists an opportunity to learn about the effectiveness of treatment, and also to learn about and accommodate reasonable patient preferences.

Even patients who are making progress may sometimes feel discouraged. However, it can motivate patients if the psychotherapist can show them data from the start of treatment that indicates a steady progression toward improvement.

Also, effective psychotherapists monitor patient progress vigilantly. Patients who respond early in psychotherapy tend to have better outcomes. Patients who do not improve early in psychotherapy have an increased risk of treatment failure (Lambert & Shimokawa, 2011). Psychotherapists should address the lack of response to treatment early (this is discussed in more detail in Chapter 5).

Furthermore, Swift and Greenberg (2015) claimed that having a regularly scheduled appointment helps provide continuity for patients. If patients miss a session, it is often desirable to call them shortly thereafter and offer an opportunity to reschedule. This will assure patients that the psychotherapist is not angry about the missed appointment.

In addition, consideration needs to be given to the timing and modality of psychotherapy. Often suicidal patients have had traumas in their backgrounds. Dealing with traumas should be delayed until the suicidal crises have passed, the treatment relationship is strong, and the patient has expressed a desire to delve into these unpleasant past events. Group psychotherapy may be effective for many patients, but patients who are suicidal need more monitoring and individual attention than group psychotherapy alone could provide.

Psychotherapists should not terminate patients who have an imminent risk of suicide. The decision to terminate a patient should not be taken lightly. On the one hand, the factors that make it difficult for patients to participate in treatment may be some of the same factors that contribute to their risk of suicide. Psychologists do not want to appear to be punishing patients for their symptoms. On the other hand, continual noncompliance threatens the quality of services. I concur with Jobes (2016) that psychotherapists should retain the option of terminating patients who are noncompliant with treatment. It does not constitute abandonment if psychotherapists make an appropriate referral. A central issue is whether patients are benefitting from treatment, which is not the same as improving from treatment. Patients can benefit if the psychotherapy keeps them from getting worse. However, psychotherapists should keep open the option of terminating patients who are not benefitting from treatment, if efforts to get treatment on track have failed, and if referrals for other treatment options have been made.

The decision to terminate patients against their wishes could be made by relying on principle-based ethics. On the one hand, the overarching ethical principle of respect for patient autonomy would suggest that psychotherapists should continue to honor the patients' wishes and keep treating them. On the other hand, the overarching ethical principles of beneficence and nonmaleficence would suggest that patients are receiving no benefit by continuing in ineffective treatments and that treatment should be terminated. Continuing in the ineffective treatment is wasting the patient's money and keeping them from seeking out treatments that could be more useful. In addition, patients who are participating in ineffective treatments may conclude that all psychotherapy is ineffective and therefore become discouraged from getting any psychotherapy, even if the failure is due to their noncompliance.

When two or more overarching ethical principles collide, it is indicated that one principle be identified as the most important, but harm to the offended moral principle be minimized. If the decision is made to terminate the patients against their wishes, then psychotherapists need to take steps to minimize harm to respect for patient autonomy. They may, for example, be very clear about the reasons for the termination, offer suggestions on alternative services, or offer to take the patients back if they ever decide that they could comply with the conditions of treatment. If the decision is made to continue to treat the patient, then psychotherapists would need to take steps to minimize harm to beneficence or nonmaleficence. They may, for example, be very clear that the patients are receiving a watered-down form of treatment that has a reduced likelihood of success because the patient failed to engage fully in treatment.

Psychotherapists vary considerably on how they respond to these situations. Some psychotherapists have discharged patients reluctantly. Other highly competent psychotherapists have told me that they would never discharge patients against their wishes. I defer to the judgment of individual psychotherapists but suggest that they structure the informed consent process to leave open the possibility of termination for noncompliance.

Medications

Rudd et al. (2015) found that the suicidal patients they treated in their study used an average of 2.1 medications. About 60% were on antidepressants, and others took sleep hypnotics, benzodiazepines, or antipsychotics. Referrals for medication should be made to a psychiatrist or psychopharmacologist[1] if it is clinically indicated to do so, even though they might not reduce the short-term risk of suicide.

Medication referrals are almost always indicated if patients have bipolar or psychotic disorders. It has been reported that lithium reduces suicidal risk in patients with bipolar disorder, but strong evidence for this is lacking (Bryan & Rudd, 2018). Nonetheless, evidence suggests that clozapine can reduce suicidal risks in patients with schizophrenia (J. J. Griffiths, Zarate, & Rasimas, 2014).

Referral for medications may be indicated if patients have nightmares that they appear unable to control, although nonpharmacological interventions, such as imagery rehearsal therapy, can effectively reduce nightmares. Outcome studies have consistently found that prazosin has also been effective for nightmares arising from posttraumatic stress disorder (PTSD; Nadorff, Lambdin, & Germain, 2014). Medications may also be indicated for extreme agitation.

On the surface, it would appear reasonable to assume that the drugs that reduce depression should also reduce suicidality in the short term. However, the support for that assumption is anecdotal, not empirical.[2] Often antidepressant medications reduce the risk of suicide in the long run, but psychotherapists

---

[1]Ideally this would be a psychiatrist or a prescribing psychologist. However, most psychotropic prescriptions are written by physicians and sometimes advanced practice nurses or physicians assistants. Given the shortage of psychiatrists and prescribing psychologists, psychotherapists can only try to do the best they can in terms of getting someone willing to prescribe psychotropic medications.

[2]Research on the use of antidepressants for treating suicide contains many methodological issues. Most studies with antidepressants screen out individuals with a high risk to die from suicide. Furthermore, the base rates for suicide tend to be low to begin with, making any effort to look at patients who died from suicide difficult because of the low numbers. Some studies have found that antidepressants will reduce suicidal ideation, but suicidal ideation is not necessarily the optimal dependent variable because it is not the same as dying from suicide.

should not adopt a false sense of security. Some medications can take days (or weeks) to become effective; multiple medications may have to be tried before an effective one is found. The risk of dying from suicide while on anti-depressant is highest in the first 28 days of starting the medication and in the first 28 days after stopping the medication (Coupland et al., 2015).

It is possible that antidepressants may increase the risk of suicide in the short term because they give suicidal patients sufficient energy to implement their suicidal plans. There is some evidence that lethargy associated with high levels of depression may protect patients against a suicide attempt (Rogers, Ringer, & Joiner, 2018). On the other hand, some patients retained a level of suicidality that did not diminish or only diminished slightly during the early stages of drug treatment. In any event, starting a patient on antidepressant medication does not immediately decrease the risk of suicide. Taking a pill does not remove a gun from the house. Medications should be used in concert with other suicide management strategies.

Many suicidal patients are treated jointly by a psychiatrist or another prescriber and a psychotherapist in a process called *split treatment*. The psychiatrist will typically do an initial evaluation of one-half hour to an hour and then have periodic medication checks that last for 10 or 15 minutes. The frequency of the medication checks will vary depending on medical necessity. Psychotherapists, on the other hand, will typically spend much more time with patients and have made a more comprehensive evaluation of suicide risk. Sometimes the psychiatrist and psychotherapist will work for the same agency or institution, but often they do not. This split treatment works best when the two treaters view each other as part of the same treatment team (Meyer, 2012). The parties should ensure that they have regular contact with each other as needed.

Patients should sign releases to allow communication between their health care professionals. I have only had one patient refuse to sign a release of information form. She had personal issues with the physician that we were able to talk through and resolve. However, I have consulted with psycho-therapists who have had patients who refused to sign such authorizations to exchange information between treating professionals. This raises serious concerns. In the worst-case scenario, a patient could be telling the psycho-therapist that she is suicidal and ready to take her life, but then denying any such thoughts to the prescribing psychiatrists who is, out of ignorance, prescribing potentially lethal doses of medication. If patients refuse to sign a release with the treating psychopharmacologist, then psychotherapists need to have candid conversations with their patients about the reasons for the refusal and, if possible, try to accommodate reasonable concerns. If these steps do not resolve the issues, the failure of a patient to sign a release is a major issue in nonadherence with treatment and would be grounds for the ethical decision analysis concerning termination without patient consent.

The prescriber should know the degree of suicide risk and the factors used to determine the risk, the diagnosis, the symptoms used to justify the diagnosis, the treatment plan and how it is progressing, and any other information relevant to treatment. For example, most psychotherapists will ask patients about all medications that they are taking, including herbal or over-the-counter medications. This information should be conveyed to the prescriber. Although the prescriber may also ask the same questions, it should not be assumed that patients will give the same responses and may withhold information because they fear that the psychiatrists will criticize their use of nontraditional treatments.

Psychotherapist–prescriber communication ensures that patients with a risk of suicide are not being prescribed potentially lethal doses of medication. This could be an especially important issue if patients are receiving different prescriptions from other physicians for medical purposes, thus increasing the risk that patients might make a lethal mix of medications.

Sometimes psychotherapists and prescribers may differ on their perception of the degree of suicide risk or the optimal treatments. Such differences should be viewed as an opportunity to learn from each other and not a power struggle. With patients who have serious personality disorders, treaters need to be aware of the possibility of splitting, or a situation in which treaters are pitted against each other through the exchange of misinformation or distorted information.

Patients may differ on how they approach medication. Some patients want medication; others claim to be medication phobic. Perhaps they had a trial of medication that did not yield good results or that resulted in bothersome side effects and little benefit. This can be viewed as a problem to be addressed cooperatively with, of course, patients having the final decision about whether to take the medication.

Other patients do not want to depend on medication or view it as a crutch or a sign that they have a mental illness. This is an opportunity for psychotherapists to explain that medication alone seldom resolves these problems, that it is an ally, and that recovery requires the cooperation of the patient. For example, an antidepressant may help patients control emotions and think through social problems more clearly. However, it cannot repair a strained relationship.

If patients take medication, they should be committed to complying with the treatment. Nonadherence is a major cause of medication failure. Patients may not understand how the medication will help them or have inaccurate beliefs about medication (e.g., it can get them addicted). Some patients believe that they only need to take their prescribed medications when they feel especially poorly, in the same manner that they take an aspirin when they have a headache. Other patients will discontinue medications when they first experience side effects. They may have looked up the drug online and become overly sensitive to the possibility of side effects. Still others do not cognitively understand the instructions given to them.

Psychotherapists should address issues of compliance with their patients. They can start by asking patients what they think about being prescribed the medication, how much they think it will help them, and to review the medication instructions given to them. Compliance can be improved by explaining the purpose of the medication, the importance of taking the medication as prescribed, and how it will help them reach their treatment goals, and by offering practical suggestions on how to improve compliance (e.g., putting the medication for the next day in a pill box next to the bed or putting a reminder on their smartphone).

Psychotherapists can ask patients about their experience with taking medications in the past. It may be useful to think of taking medication as a stable habit that persists over time and across treatment providers (Glombiewski & Rief, 2013). Ideally, the assessment of their habits of taking medications will be done before or soon after they have been prescribed the medication.

Some patients cannot afford the medications. I have had several patients who took half the dose of medication prescribed because they could not afford to fill the next prescription. One can sympathize with patients who need to balance compliance with economic realities. But it is best that they talk this over with the prescribing psychopharmacologist and reach some accommodation. Prescribers may be able to switch to a generic or give out sample drugs. Some drug companies will enroll patients in low-cost drug programs ("Patient Assistance Programs for Prescription Drugs," n.d.).

Working With Other Health Care Professionals

It can be important to work cooperatively with other treating professionals. Many suicidal patients are being treated by physicians for physical disorders that may involve chronic pain or limitations on their activities of daily living and that may increase their perceptions of pain and perceptions of themselves as burdens on others.

Psychotherapists can sometimes assist patients to get better quality health care or to use their health care professionals more effectively. For example, patients may not have expressed the extent to which they feel pain to their physicians or their caregivers. Or they may have depressive symptoms that limit their motivation for rehabilitation services. Or, older adults or their caregivers may have adopted ageist beliefs and assume that patients have limitations greater than what would be warranted by the objective evidence.

In addition, it may be profitable to review the extent to which patients are adhering to the medical regimens as prescribed. Discouraged patients often do not keep appointments, do not exercise as instructed, do not take medications as prescribed or even get prescriptions filled. Reasons for nonadherence should be discussed and addressed. It can help to have patients reflect on their values and how self-care can be a component of value-driven behavior.

No data support the consistent effectiveness of cognitive pain management strategies in reducing suicidal behaviors. Nonetheless, Racine (2018) opined that there are promising indications that strategies that target mental defeat, pain catastrophizing, and hopelessness related to pain may indirectly address suicide-related thoughts. A reasonable conclusion would be to refer patients for cognitive pain management when indicated for pain relief. Any generalization to suicidal behaviors would not be assumed but could be a welcome side benefit.

Special Issues With Serious Personality Disorders

Effective treatments for patient with borderline personality disorder (BPD) are available. Psychotherapists who have mastered these skills will eschew false, dysfunctional, and potentially lethal assumptions about patients with serious personality disorders. They recognize the important role that trauma has had in the etiology of many of these patients. Dialectical behavior therapy (DBT; Linehan et al., 2015) is one of several therapies shown to be effective in treating BPD (see the review by Cristea et al., 2017), although it and the Collaborative Assessment and Management of Suicide (CAMS; Jobes, 2016) are the only ones with strong evidence that they can reduce suicidal risk among patients with BPD (Andreasson et al., 2016).

It is beyond the scope of this book to describe DBT or the other psychotherapies used to treat BPD. They require extensive training to perform with fidelity, and handling suicidal thoughts or threats is an integral part of those psychotherapies. Nonetheless these treatments help psychotherapists to establish and maintain a good relationship with such patients. Although it might be harder to establish a good working relationship with such patients, the benefits of doing so are important as patients with BDP had fewer suicide attempts if they perceived a good working relationship with their psychotherapists (Bedics, Atkins, Harned, & Linehan, 2015).

As noted in Chapter 2, suicidal ideation for some patients with BPD may represent a means of communicating distress. It is appropriate for psychotherapists to discuss the suicidal thoughts of their patients, what events preceded them, symptoms of their distress, and so on. Skilled psychotherapists balance monitoring of suicide risk with teaching new skills and addressing the patient's life problems. Low levels of chronic thoughts of suicide need to be monitored because they can suddenly morph into a high risk for a suicide attempt. In the parlance of the fluid vulnerability theory, these patients have a high baseline for suicide risk.

Hospitalizations can be appropriate for acutely suicidal patients if their safety cannot be ensured. However, the outcomes for multiple hospitalizations with patients with BPD have not been that good. Psychiatric hospitalizations could become clinically contraindicated, and treatment could devolve into a continual cycle of outpatient discussions of suicide, threats or attempts, hospitalizations, outpatient discussions of suicide, threats or attempts, hospitalizations, and so on.

Websites as Adjuncts or Adversaries

Many patients will go to websites to find information about health issues, including suicide. Unfortunately, they may also find prosuicide websites. These websites vary in their content, but they sometimes give patients information on how to kill themselves, including what combinations of medications will be effective and how to do so painlessly. The websites may go into detail and offer a step-by-step approach. Other websites may romanticize suicide or make it seem fashionable. Still other websites contain chat rooms where others will encourage a person to attempt to kill themselves. These chatrooms are problematic because discussions with other suicidal persons may lead a patient to perceive that suicidal thoughts are normative or even desirable.

The Darknet is a form of the Internet that is harder to access, is anonymous, and contains a high amount of criminal activity. Although there are no systematic studies of the amount of suicide-related content on the Darknet, there are reports that it can be used to access lethal poisons used for suicide (Mörch et al., 2018).

Psychotherapists can talk openly with patients about the content of these prosuicide websites. Although they may use phrases such as "promoting choice," the surface marketing may be misleading (Biddle et al., 2016). Some appear to be using the suffering of others as a source of personal entertainment. Informal reports have suggested that there is a lot of insensitivity, voyeurism, and sadism underlying the content. Patients can make real choices when they are free from extraordinarily intense emotions that can cloud their judgment. Psychotherapists can speak to their patients about Internet bullying and exploitation.

Psychotherapists can also refer their patients to positive resources on the web. The National Alliance for Suicide Prevention has an online publication, *Your Life Matters*, that includes inspiring stories. Other well-respected organizations such as the American Association on Suicide Prevention or the American Foundation for Suicide Prevention also have information that may supplement the positive and hopeful messages that psychotherapists are trying to promote.

Suicide Attempts During Psychotherapy

Some patients will attempt suicide while they are in psychotherapy. Because suicide attempts are more common than suicides, it is more likely that a psychotherapist will see a patient after a suicide attempt than to have a patient die from suicide. In their outcome study treating suicidal behavior, Rudd et al. (2015) found that 40% of patients in the treatment-as-usual condition and 15% in the cognitive therapy condition had attempted suicide during treatment. Leitzel and Knapp (2017) found that 23% of the members of the Pennsylvania Psychological Association reported that at least one patient had attempted suicide while in treatment in the past year.

These attempts can generate a lot of fear on the part of the psychotherapists and cause them to second guess their decisions and case formulation. For some patients, it may precipitate feelings of shame in that they allowed feelings of despair to overwhelm them.

A few psychotherapists believe that they should terminate patients who attempted suicide because such an attempt violated the psychotherapist patient no-suicide agreement, or because the patients "lied" when they said they were not suicidal at the last treatment session. Such terminations are misguided. First, as discussed in Chapter 3, no-suicide contracts are often useless and sometimes even clinically contraindicated. Those who treat the no-suicide contract like a business arrangement, akin to paying bills or purchasing a car, misunderstand the nature of psychotherapy.

Instead of blaming patients for "lying," psychotherapists should consider that some patients who rated the likelihood of a suicide attempt as low might not have adequately understood or appreciated the ease to which they could enter a suicidal crisis state. Suicidal impulses wax and wane over time. Some patients who were not suicidal at the last session may deteriorate quickly over a short period. Also, patients may fail to reveal suicidal thoughts for many reasons, including a lack of trust in their psychotherapists who might not have created a safe enough relationship with their patients so they could feel free to share their deepest thoughts.

Because the likelihood of a suicide attempt is especially high immediately after a failed attempt, the highest priority is to secure the immediate safety of the patient. It may be indicated to ask if the patient experienced any psychological trauma from the event itself, especially if they suffered physical trauma and had to receive medical intervention.

Also, a decision needs to be made concerning the adequacy of the current treatment and safety plans. New clinical information may have come to light after an attempt that would necessitate a review of the treatment plan. In some cases, this may require a referral to a different psychotherapist or a higher level of care, such as a partial hospitalization program (Ramsay & Newman, 2005). But in most cases psychotherapists should be able to continue with patients even after a suicide attempt.

Psychotherapists and patients need to review the events that led to the suicide attempt and how to change the management and treatment to reduce the likelihood of a future attempt. Psychotherapists should consider that the patient who attempted suicide the week before may be different from the patient who is before them now. Also, psychotherapists may need to do more to educate the patient on how to interpret or implement the crisis plan. It may be appropriate for psychotherapists to disclose their reasoning in making certain decisions in the treatment plan and to accept input from patients as to the reasonableness of these decisions or assumptions. It may be indicated to go through the events leading up to suicide attempt. What were your thoughts? What appeared to precipitate them? Were activities to interrupt the suicidal crisis state tried? If not, why? If activities were tried, then why did they fail? If the crisis number was not called, why?

For some patients, it may be appropriate to review the ground rules for psychotherapy and clarify expectations or responsibilities. If friends or family members are not currently part of the patient's treatment team, then it may be indicated to consider their participation in the process (Ramsay & Newman, 2005). If friends or family members are part of the patient's treatment team, then it may be indicated to review their roles.

These discussions require close attention to the feelings of the patients. Sometimes patients feel ashamed, and psychotherapists should try to minimize their embarrassment. Other patients feel disappointed or angry that their psychotherapists were not able to do more to prevent the attempt.

Sometimes psychotherapists need to respond to a suicide attempt in progress. For example, psychotherapists may receive phone calls from patients, informing them that they are in the process of attempting suicide (e.g., they reported that they just took a large quantity of pills, or are intending to do so immediately). I know a psychologist who received a call from a patient who said that she "just wanted to say good-bye," adding that she had just taken a large quantity of pills. Another patient swallowed a handful of pills right in front of his psychologist during a psychotherapy session. A mental health counselor told me that a patient pulled out a gun during a psychotherapy session, placed it to his head, and threatened to kill himself. The weapon discharged, although the head wound was not fatal. It is appropriate for psychotherapists to respond with emergency interventions (such as sending ambulances or the police) in these circumstances, even if the patients say they do not want the intervention. Involuntary psychiatric hospitalizations may be indicated.

Sometimes patients will send oblique messages with suicidal themes but without any other reference to suicide. Psychotherapists need to interpret these messages considering the totality of the information they have about a patient. For a few patients the messages may have been innocent enough. For other patients, the same comment may have the equivalence of a suicide threat.

Here the overarching ethical principle of beneficence (working to protect the well-being and life of the patient) appears to conflict with respect for the right of patients to make major decisions about their lives. Some might argue that respect for patient autonomy should trump beneficence and that patients should have the right to decide whether they should die.

But readers may recall that the issue of the right to intervene was raised in Chapter 1. The anti-intervention argument mistakenly assumes that a patient is acting rationally. It also assumes that this suicidal patient is conveying a rational and well-thought out plan of action while in the throes of great emotional turmoil. But, in this context, almost none of these patients are acting rationally. If patients wanted to die, then they would not have called their psychotherapists or crisis programs to announce their decision and create the option of a rescue. That very act demonstrates ambivalence on the part of the patient. So, any perceived conflict between beneficence and respect for patient autonomy is false. Although there may be moral justifications for rational suicide under limited circumstances, its determination should not be made through an emergency phone call, but rather thought through in a careful process that includes the opportunity for reflection, involvement of all concerned persons, and the input of impartial experts.

The American Association of Suicidology, which accredits crisis intervention programs, requires its centers to provide "rescue services" (e.g., police, ambulances) when callers present an imminent risk or actual act of suicide and refuse to accept interventions voluntarily. These unwanted interventions are very rare (Mishara & Weisstub, 2010).

Time- or Event-Contingent Suicide Threats

Some patients may report that they intend to kill themselves at a specific time or if a specific event occurs. A woman may claim that she will kill herself if her husband leaves. A college student may say he will kill himself unless he gets admitted into an elite graduate school. Oncology units have reported situations where family members say that they will kill themselves if their loved one dies, and sometimes family members carry through with these threats (Peteet, Maytal, & Rokni, 2010). It is understandable that psychotherapists may become unnerved by such statements and may view them as a form of blackmail that keeps them always on edge.

Psychotherapists can step back and review these events from the standpoint of *conditional goal setting*. Conditional goals arise when "thoughts of achieving an important future goal is seen as necessary and sufficient to attaining normal levels of future well-being" (Coughlan, Tata, & MacLeod, 2017, p. 434). Those who have engaged in deliberate self-harm are more likely than controls to view their happiness as contingent on certain events (Coughlan et al., 2017). Suicidal behaviors are more likely to occur if individuals see these goals as unattainable, thus leading them to see themselves as trapped in inevitable hopelessness and unhappiness. This makes sense from the standpoint of ideation-to-action theories of suicide wherein the feelings of hopelessness, defeat, entrapment, or humiliation could prompt a person with suicidal desire to attempt suicide.

Time- or event-contingent threats of suicide represent a variation of conditional goal setting. Suicidal persons with time- or event-contingent threats of suicide are like "ordinary" suicidal patients in that they often feel hopeless. They differ in that they have not entirely given up hope that their goals may come true, and they may be more rigid in focusing on the event.

Psychotherapists should keep some options in mind in these situations. First, they should treat these patients largely the same as they would their other suicidal patients. They should not alter the basic approach to suicide assessment, management, and treatment. A focus on a specific time or event most likely represents a cognitive distortion or an overgeneralization of the meaning of the event and should be a target for psychotherapy. Nonetheless, psychotherapists should not assume that the contingent event or future date is the only factor that could precipitate a suicide attempt.

Second, as with some other suicidal patients, it may be prudent to explicitly acknowledge that patients always have the option of killing themselves (Gutheil & Schetky, 1998). Also, it is prudent for psychotherapists to delineate their roles. It is permissible for psychotherapists to tell patients that they will use involuntary hospitalization laws to restrain them if the necessary conditions are met. Here psychotherapists need to ensure that they understand the laws of their state or province clearly. Some states or provinces only permit involuntary hospitalizations if a patient has attempted suicide. Furthermore, psychotherapists will typically have no way of knowing about suicidal acts unless patients tell them. Nor should psychotherapists present their positions as a threat. They are merely informing patients of their commitment to the healthier side of the patient. Indeed, the goal is to get patients to talk more about their suicidal thoughts, not to bully them into silence. Psychotherapists should not argue or plead. Arguing with patients about the wisdom of their decision is futile and counterproductive. Motivational interviewing may be indicated.

Psychotherapists should attend to the totality of the treatment relationship when time- or event-contingent threats are made. It is worth considering if patients want to influence the treatment relationship when they make such threats. Perhaps they can discern the impact of their threats on their psychotherapists. Do patients want to see their psychotherapists beg them to live? Do the patients want their psychotherapists to rescue them from their feelings? It is unlikely that psychotherapists would immediately be able to discern the motives of the patient, and sometimes patients may not be aware of the motives themselves. But psychotherapists need to consider this possibility.

ADDRESSING SUICIDE-RELATED THEMES

The following section suggests interventions that psychotherapists can use to reduce the distress of their patients, recognizing that any intervention needs to be tailored to the unique needs and preferences of every patient and integrated into the theoretical orientation of the psychotherapist. These interventions should promote emotional regulation and cognitive flexibility (Bryan & Rozek, 2018).

Psychotherapists should strive to find unity in the assessment, management, and treatment of suicidal risk. They should look for themes related to suicide risk identified in the assessment, consider them in managing suicidal risk, and address them during treatment. Patients may have many problems, and it may be difficult to determine which should have the highest priority. One rule of thumb would be to give the highest priority to strengthening social relationships (addressing thwarted belongingness or perceived burdensomeness). Of course, patients should ultimately decide which problems should be the priority.

TABLE 4.1. Reducing Drivers of Suicide

Symptom	Potential intervention
Social isolation[a]	Social activity scheduling, couple or family therapy, targeting prosocial values, educating patients on impact of a suicide on others; restructuring thoughts on perceived burdensomeness
Anxiety sensitivity	Psychoeducation to reduce rumination, rigidity
Self-hatred/shame	Values, cognitive restructuring, self-acceptance, self-compassion training
Hopelessness	Activity scheduling, values, cognitive restructuring Medication, relaxation, cognitive restructuring
Insomnia/nightmares	Sleep hygiene, imagery rehearsal, prazosin
Irritability	Cognitive restructuring, problem-solving
Impulsivity	Reduction of negative urgency by reducing stress and learning emotional self-regulation
Rumination and other harmful cognitive processes	Distraction, thought stopping, cognitive restructuring and selective attention

Note. [a]As manifested by social withdrawal, or indications of perceived burdensomeness, or thwarted belongingness.

The likelihood of entering into a suicidal crisis increases if a patient has a background of anxiety, depression, self-hatred, agitation, or other unpleasant emotions. A variety of techniques can be used to address these symptoms and lower the patient's baseline of distress (see Table 4.1). These suggestive techniques are not intended to be comprehensive. The following section will expand on several of these themes in more detail. Because the emotions and behaviors related to the suicidal crisis are so deeply intertwined, it is possible that targeting one set of problems may make other problems easier to deal with. For example, if patients with insomnia can sleep better, the interventions geared toward anxiety sensitivity or irritability may be more effective because the patients are better refreshed and less fatigued.

Social Disconnectedness

Suicidal patients often feel lonely or disconnected from others. They may lack the benefits that occur through day-by-day encounters with others. At times, the patient's social network weakened because of the death of loved ones or because of geographical moves that separated them from their family or close friends. At other times, there were arguments with loved ones. Because patients may feel unloved or unwanted, it can be difficult to motivate them to elicit social support from others.

Everyone feels lonely sometime. However, the loneliness for suicidal patients is accompanied by a sense of hopelessness and entrapment and a belief that they will always be lonely. These may result in feelings of perceived burdensomeness (i.e., they will always be a burden to others) or thwarted belongingness (i.e., they do not belong to a valued social group).

Loneliness can occur for many reasons, and interventions may need to be modified accordingly. It may be indicated to use interventions that encourage patients to engage in social activities, target maladaptive social beliefs, improve social skills, reduce social anxiety, or offer family or marital counseling.

Psychotherapists can encourage their patients to engage in more social activities and build a positive social support network. One suicide survivor, writing about her recovery, found that working with children with chronic and life-threatening illnesses led her to feel deep connections with others (Drouin, 2017). Psychotherapists can help patients to plan specific social events during their day or week.

Some patients may be difficult to motivate to engage in social activities. At times, disruptions involving conflicts or disagreements with loved ones have weakened the patient's social network. Often, with the benefit of helpful psychotherapists, patients can consider whether they misinterpreted the behavior of others, contributed to the problems through their own behavior, and might find it worthwhile to attempt a reconciliation.

Suicidal patients often have deficits in social problem-solving. They may respond passively when social disruptions occur or have little faith in their ability to rectify tense relationships. Problem-solving therapies may be indicated for such patients (C. Chu, Walker, et al., 2018). They may have difficulty identifying when offers of social support are being made, or they may fail to notice the positive aspects of social situations.

Sometimes patients may develop perceived burdensomeness out of a response to a serious physical illness. Believing that their families would be better off without them, they may fail to appreciate the enormous emotional pain that their suicide would have on their families. The pain of a suicide would greatly overshadow whatever burden that their illness caused. One way to address perceived burdensomeness is through self-distancing. Very few people advocate for the killing of helpless infants with disabilities or allowing disabled older adults to die because such an act or failure to act would offend fundamental beliefs about the sanctity of human life. Yet patients who perceive themselves as a burden are not applying the same logic to themselves.

Psychotherapists might ask patients to recall times that they have extended themselves to help others or to imagine how they would react if a friend or loved one asked for their help (Joiner et al., 2009). Along the same lines, it may help to appeal to their values and ask them to consider whether it is morally desirable for individuals to respond to the distress of others. The answer is almost always yes. Then the next step would be for the patients to apply that moral standard to themselves.

Perceived burdensomeness can be addressed in family or couple psychotherapy where family members can give feedback on their perceptions of the patient's value to them. Patients may have an overvalued belief in their perceived burdensomeness. They may perceive that their willingness to die is a "gift" to their loved one. Jobes (2016) stated that "I have seen this perception seem almost like a fixed delusion" (p. 70). Patients may initially argue with their loved ones, but the confrontation is a first step in breaking down this assumption on the part of the patient.

Psychotherapists may need to redirect patients toward their obligations to others. This perspective is easier to activate in those who have values or religious beliefs that identify obligations to others beyond themselves. Even those who have functional limitations and depend on others have obligations to their caregivers to express appreciation and to try to minimize the burden on their caregivers by doing as much as they can for themselves.

Joiner et al. (2009) recommended that psychotherapists should not argue with patients about whether they are a burden to others. But psychotherapists can ask patients to prove their beliefs. Because the consequence of the belief (suicide) is so high, it is important for patients to have complete confidence in that belief.

Finally, "anyone who is contemplating suicide needs to sit down and *carefully examine the profound impact that his or her death would have on others*" (Ellis & Newman, 1996, p. 53; italics in original). During the throes of their suicidal despair they may believe that the world would be better off without them. But Joiner et al. (2009) wrote that it may be worth reminding them that the average person who dies from suicide has six to 10 persons who experience extreme grief afterward. Studies of survivors suggest that Joiner's estimate is valid (Andriessen, Rahman, Draper, Dudley, & Mitchell, 2017).

When teenagers die from suicide, one out of three of their friends developed a clinical depression after the suicide, and those who were told about the plans or who had talked to the decedent within 24 hours of the death were especially affected. Most experienced high levels of grief up to 6 years later (Brent, Poling, & Goldstein, 2011). The death of a loved one from suicide may lead to posttraumatic symptoms and is associated with a lower quality of mental health among the survivors (Mitchell & Terhorst, 2017).

Military spouses who had a loved one die from suicide experienced poorer postmortem functioning than military spouses who had a loved one die in an accident or in combat (Aronson, Kyler, Love, Morgan, & Perkins, 2017). In civilian populations, those bereaved by suicide had higher rates of lifetime depression, self-blaming, and impaired social functioning compared with those bereaved by death from natural causes or an accident (Tal et al., 2017). Family members bereaved by a suicide experienced more physical pain and had poorer health than family members bereaved by other means of death (Spillane et al., 2017).

The "ordinary" process of grieving is complicated by guilt, and the social stigma associated with suicide may lead survivors to receive less social support. Pitman, Stevenson, Osborn, and King (2018) found that survivors would perceive a range of negative reactions from others, including blaming them (or their relatives), avoiding the topic, avoiding mentioning the late loved one, or sometimes showing a morbid fascination with the death. The survivors often concealed the cause of the death or revealed it only to a select few people or felt tension because of their fear that they would break down in public. Close friends often avoid them, do not express sympathy, offer aid, or make overtures for future contact following the suicide.

One survivor reported that her turning point in recovery came when she heard the story of a woman who lost her 20-year-old son to suicide. "For the first time in my life I understood the full scope of devastation and loss a survivor experiences" (Medeiros, 2017, p. 6). It may be indicated to suggest that patients read a book written by survivors of suicide. Two such books are *My Son . . . My Son: A Guide to Healing After Death, Loss, or Suicide* (Bolton & Mitchell, 1984) and *No Time to Say Goodbye: Surviving the Suicide of a Loved One* (Fine, 2000).

Anxiety Sensitivity

Anxiety sensitivity may be associated with an increased risk of suicide. *Anxiety sensitivity* is "fearing anxiety-related sensations due to misinterpretations that these sensations have negative cognitive, physical or social outcomes" (I. H. Stanley, Hom, et al., 2017, p. 95). The cognitive consequences may include fears of going crazy; the physiological consequences may include beliefs that they are having a serious physical illness such as a heart attack; the social consequences may include fears that others may notice signs of anxiety such as sweating (Schmidt, Norr, Allan, Raines, & Capron, 2017). Furthermore, anxiety sensitivity may greatly increase any stress reaction, thus possibly accounting for the part of the geometric increase in distress found in the acute suicidal affective disturbance. Capron, Schmidt, and others (e.g., Capron & Schmidt, 2016; Schmidt et al., 2017) have found that relative brief psychosocial interventions can help reduce anxiety sensitivity. The interventions can focus on specific symptoms, as well as harmful cognitive processes, such as rumination, mental rigidity, or selective attention.

Hopelessness and Self-Hatred

Many suicidal patients experience hopelessness, powerlessness, or a belief that their psychological pain will never change. They may believe that their future will be as gloomy as their present, and they interpret their past life as a series of failures. Individuals can exempt themselves from the risk of failure and the risk of disappointing others and themselves by thinking of themselves as condemned, worthless, or incompetent. If they put themselves out and try hard, they might fail—thus justifying their predetermined worldview.

Self-hatred or self-disgust also is implicit in thwarted belongingness and perceived burdensomeness. Patients may feel great shame over things they have done in the past (issues of moral condemnation are discussed in more detail in the section on Values and Religion later in this chapter). In addition, patients may feel shame at the presence of suicidal thoughts themselves.

Thoughts of hopelessness and self-disgust can become strengthened through *brooding*, a form of rumination that "involves a tendency to dwell on the negative consequences of one's distress" (Rogers & Joiner, 2017, p. 132).

Patients may overidentify with whatever misconduct they committed and fail to understand that mistakes are human and should be forgiven. Self-compassion may be indicated here. The components of self-compassion are mindfulness of suffering without being consumed by it, recognition of one's common humanity with others, and self-kindness. Self-compassion interventions include cognitive interventions as well as forms of loving meditation. Self-compassion is negatively associated with psychopathology (Muris & Petrocchi, 2017), and self-compassion interventions can help reduce distress (Germer & Neff, 2013), symptoms of depression (Ehret, Joormann, & Berking, 2018), and PTSD (Barlow, Goldsmith Turow, & Gerhart, 2017), and even help reduce rumination and hopelessness among suicidal persons (Chesin et al., 2016).

Nightmares and Insomnia

Nightmares can be an especially important marker of distress. Ribeiro, Bodell, Hames, Hagan, and Joiner (2013) found that two thirds of suicide attempters had frequent nightmares before their attempt and that the likelihood of an attempt increased in persons with frequent nightmares. The two interventions most commonly researched with nightmares are the medication prazosin (Breen, Blankley, & Fine, 2017) and imaginal rehearsal, which is a form of cognitive behavioral psychotherapy (Seda, Sanchez-Ortuno, Welsh, Halbower, & Edinger, 2015).

Because insomnia is often associated with suicidal thoughts, it may profit patients to learn about sleep hygiene. Such activities may include informing patients of the importance of establishing a regular sleep schedule, avoiding caffeine or vigorous exercise close to sleeping time, engaging in relaxing or soothing activities close to sleeping time, and so on. If the insomnia is chronic, the American College of Physicians recommends cognitive therapy, and if that fails, medications can be added (Medalie & Cifu, 2017). Medications may be indicated for acute insomnia (Buysse, Rush, & Reynolds, 2017).

The research on the relationship between insomnia and suicide is in its infancy, but evidence has suggested that psychological factors, such as social isolation, hopelessness, and a feeling of entrapment, may account for the relationship between insomnia and suicide (Littlewood, Kyle, Pratt, Peters, & Gooding, 2017). Working on cognitive appraisals, learning emotion-regulating strategies, and reducing social isolation should help to reduce insomnia. Decreasing negative emotions appears to reduce insomnia better than increasing positive emotions (Ward-Ciesielski, Winer, Drapeau, & Nadorff, 2018).

Patients who sleep better will be better able to address their life stressors and solve problems. From the standpoint of the fluid vulnerability model, their decreased emotional turmoil should reduce their baseline of distress.

Life Stressors

Sometimes patients feel overwhelmed by their challenges and obligations. They may believe that they can do nothing to address these concerns. Suicidal patients often have a restricted ability to address or solve their problems. In part this limited repertoire of solutions may be caused by the intensity of negative emotions. However, often patients increase their ability to think through problems when they are in psychotherapy. As they feel relief from sharing their problems with a caring and concerned person, their negative affect may begin to decline, and they find themselves open to solutions to problems that only minutes before seemed intractable.

Psychotherapists can help address this sense of being overwhelmed by asking patients to slow down and break down the tasks one by one and to identify specific behavioral steps that they can take to handle each obligation (Ramsay & Newman, 2005). Psychotherapists can also monitor their patients for "catastrophizing" or looking at the worst possible scenario for every event. Some events, such as a divorce or job loss, are beyond the ability of patients to control. However, "stuff happens." Psychotherapists can acknowledge the pain but refuse to acknowledge that the results will devastate their patients.

RELIGION AND VALUES

It can help patients to strengthen their protective factors by considering values, which are often, but not always, informed by religion. Frequently, suicidal patients will ask, "What is the meaning of life?" or "What is it all about?" Studies on the meaning of life have used many different measures and have been influenced by different religious and philosophical traditions, but typically they measure purpose or value.

However, those who are socially isolated or who have poor moods tend to report less meaning in life. Heintzelman and King (2014) suggested that there may be some psychological logic behind this finding because humans need social interaction to survive or thrive, and pairing pleasure with evolutionally helpful behavior may be nature's way of reinforcing life-sustaining activities.

This suggests that meaning in life will improve as patients become more socially connected and their mood improves. But the direction may go both ways: Focusing on values can also lead to an increase in social relationships and improved emotional health (R. Harris, 2008). This could mean asking patients to talk about what is important to them or what gives their life direction.

A *goal* is a completed task (e.g., getting an A on a test after studying), whereas a *value* is a direction (e.g., studying because it is enjoyable or a step toward a valued goal). Suicidal patients may be frustrated in reaching their goals, but attention can be given to their values. Ideally values would be self-chosen and not merely a recitation of socially acceptable phrases or expectations.

Unfortunately, during periods of internal turmoil, considerations of values often get put on hold. Consider this example:

Connecting With Values

When asked about her values, a patient quickly recited lengthy segments from the catechism that she had learned as a child. However, she had not connected these writings to her personal life, and she could not identify how they motivated, directed, or inspired her.

Focusing on values can motivate patients. Although pleasurable activities can be motivating, R. Harris (2008) warned against giving such activities too much attention. He stated that "pleasant feelings will come and go, just like every other feeling. So, enjoy them and appreciate them when they visit, but don't cling to them!" (p. 201). Values-driven activities are more motivating. People can endure a lot of pain and suffering for the sake of their values.

The treatment goal is to help patients identify and connect with their values in their daily lives (R. Harris, 2008). At times, it may be indicated to ask patients what prevents them from living their values. Sometimes the discussion can be direct, such as having patients write down their values, reflect on them, discuss them, and then rewrite them.

However, various exercises or instruments can be used as well. One way is to ask patients to consider various life domains (e.g., family, work, community) and ask what values they have in any of these areas (R. Harris, 2008). Often clients settle on an interpersonal value such as nurturing intimate relationships, parenting, or improving social connections. Patients may say that they have no values or that they care about nothing. Psychotherapists can ask, "What did you used to value?" or "If you could care about something, what would it be?" or "What would you value if you were not so depressed?"

Other exercises include asking patients, "What would be written on your tombstone?" "If you could be at your own funeral, what would you like people to say about you?" Patients can also be asked how persons would respond if asked about their impact on them: What did your wife (or husband, child, friend, e.g.) like about you? (R. Harris, 2008).

Patients can connect values to reasons for living. They may find that this involves contact with other people and that values are worth pursuing even when there is little hope of success. They may also find that they cannot be so worthless if they are acting in a way that promotes worthwhile values.

Integrating Religion Into Psychotherapy

Psychotherapists may wish to integrate specific religious rituals or religious perspective into psychotherapy. Before doing this, they should consider several factors, including whether they have examined the potential for their own biases or blind spots (Plante, 2014), whether they are competent to do so, and whether patients want to incorporate religion into psychotherapy.

Vieten et al. (2013) identified 16 required attitudes, knowledge statements, and skills for psychotherapists who want to integrate religion and psychotherapy. For example, one of the attitudes was that "psychologists view spirituality and religion as important aspects of human diversity, along with factors such as race, ethnicity, sexual orientation, socioeconomic status, disability, gender, and age" (p. 135); one of the knowledge statements was that "psychologists know that many diverse forms of spiritualty and/or religion exist, and explore spiritual and/or religious beliefs, communities, and practices that are important to their clients" (p. 135); and one of the skills was "psychologists help clients explore and access their spiritual and/or religious strengths and resources" (p. 135).

Competent psychotherapists understand their role. They should not use a religious-based intervention to prioritize a specific religious worldview at the expense of the patient's treatment goals or the treatment relationship. Nor should they confuse the role of being a psychotherapist with that of a religious counselor. The goal of the psychotherapist is to treat mental distress; it is not to strengthen faith, improve adherence to religious practices, or clarify religious questions.

Psychotherapists who integrate religion into psychotherapy should do so only with the consent of the patient. Skilled psychotherapists learn to determine when or how to integrate religion into therapy, and when not to do so. Some of the ways that religion can be integrated into psychotherapy include using prayer and meditation for relaxation or reflecting on religious/spiritual concepts to interpret events in one's life, and using a religious community for support (Pargament, 2007).

Religion can also encourage positive and healthy beliefs. Chapter 2 distinguished between life-protecting beliefs (it is a sin to kill oneself) and life-promoting beliefs (designed to improve the quality of life for oneself and others). Life-protecting beliefs tell patients what they cannot do (they should not die from suicide), whereas life-protecting beliefs tell patients what they can or should do (enhance the quality of their lives and the lives of others).

Psychotherapists should be happy to accept the life-protecting beliefs in the short run if they help keep patients alive. However, more sustained improvement occurs through life-promoting beliefs. Those who adhere to life-protecting beliefs alone often fail to appreciate that their life-protecting beliefs are not just arbitrary rules established by capricious authorities, but rest on the foundational belief that life has intrinsic value.

Life-promoting beliefs rest on values. People are willing to endure all kinds of hardships and failures if they are acting in a manner consistent with their values. Adapting the comments of Strosahl, Hayes, Wilson, and Gifford (2004), one could say that the goal of suicide prevention is, in a nutshell, to help patients identify their values and live consistently with them. Some of the life-promoting beliefs are self-compassion and positive religious coping. The protected role of values is also found in the three-step theory of suicide wherein connectedness could mean connectedness to a value system as well as a social group, and suicidal behavior only occurs when the pain and hopelessness overwhelm connectedness (Klonsky, Saffer, & Bryan, 2018).

Moral Injury and Self-Forgiveness or Self-Compassion

Some patients, such as veterans of military combat, feel intense guilt or shame. During combat, soldiers may perform or fail to perform acts that are inconsistent with the core beliefs they learned about protecting the well-being of others, resulting in moral injury. Many of the soldiers are young men and women (some as young as 18) who are put into life-endangering situations that would tax the psychological resources of the most morally mature individual.

Some acts may have been within the standards established by the military, but the ambiguity of the situation led to harm to civilians, nonetheless. Enemy combatants may use strategies designed to inflict moral injury, such as using a pregnant woman as a human shield. Although the rules of engagement permit killing the woman (because the failure to do so would lead to more loss of life), the events nonetheless greatly upset the soldiers involved. Or, even if the deaths or harm occurred only to enemy combatants, the reality of inflicting such harm may impact some soldiers in a way that they had not anticipated. Also, some soldiers performed acts outside of the norms established by the military that resulted in the deaths of civilians, such as when they engaged in revenge killings. They may believe that their offenses are so severe that they can never be forgiven (Frankfurt & Frazier, 2016).

One veteran adjusted adequately enough to civilian life until he had children. It reminded him of the children who were killed in a combat operation he participated in. He had a recurring thought that his children would be taken from him as punishment for his failure to protect the children who died during his combat operation.

Treatments that address moral injury may improve the outcomes for treating PTSD. Moral issues are not unique to veterans by any means. Civilians may feel shame because they acted poorly; perhaps they had an affair once, had pilfered money from their employer, or had done other immoral acts. Sometimes they overestimate the magnitude of their shortcomings. Consider this example of a woman who felt moral distress over what she believed were her past misdeeds.

A Guilty Mother

One patient castigated herself for being a failure as a mother. When I later met her adult children, they were bewildered by their mother's interpretation as they saw her as kind, supportive, and loving. The mother asked their forgiveness for specific things she had done to them in their childhood. The children did not even remember some events or had much more benign memories of the other events.

Positive and Negative Religious Coping

Religious beliefs influence how patients cope with difficult life events. For some, religion helps mitigate the harmful effects of stressful events. For others, religion exacerbates them. Religious coping strategies may be considered positive or negative.

Positive religious coping typically involves collaboration with God or the religious community or taking a benevolent reappraisal of the event (e.g., "God is reaching out to help me"). Some of the positive outcomes could include maintaining a loving supportive relationship to God, overcoming anger with God's help, working with God to solve problems, seeking to forgive others, or using religious beliefs to think through problems. Patients who use positive religious coping are more likely to believe that they have intrinsic value and draw on their religious community for resources or from their religious tradition for examples of fortitude during trying times. Because God is an ally, they feel more motivated to take actions to improve their lives.

In contrast, *negative* or *detached religious coping* involves alienation from God or the religious community or taking a malevolent reappraisal of the event (e.g., "I am being punished"). Some of the negative outcomes could include a failure to act on one's own to address the problem, failing to seek assistance from others, seeking revenge, failing to forgive, or perceiving the powerful forces of Satan in their lives. They believe that they have no intrinsic value, are isolated from their religious community, and have no religious tradition to strengthen them. Because God is responsible for their suffering, they may lose motivation to take actions to improve their lives. On the surface, one can see the link between negative religious coping and a sense of hopelessness or entrapment. Condemnation by God would appear to be the ultimate form of entrapment.

Distressed patients may slip into negative religious coping. They may latch on to Biblical phrases or elements of religious doctrine and interpret them in the most punitive ways. For example, a phrase often used is to "hate the sin but love the sinner." But distressed or suicidal patients often fail to make that distinction.

Michael Kierkegaard, the father of the melancholic existentialist writer Soren Kierkegaard, believed that he was condemned for eternity because once, during his youth, he cursed God. Matthew 12:31 states that all sins will be forgiven except the sin of blaspheming the Holy Spirit.[3] Some, like Michael Kierkegaard interpret this passage to mean that any act during a person's entire lifetime that could be interpreted as disrespectful to God, Jesus, or the Holy Spirit will result in eternal damnation, without exception. However, almost all theologians now interpret this to mean that a current state of resistance to spiritual sources will result in temporary separation from God or one's religious community.

Currier, Smith, and Kulhman (2017) found that negative religious coping was associated with an increased risk for suicide among Iraqi and Afghanistan American war veterans, a finding consistent with other studies. Most studies have found that positive religious coping leads to better psychological health when dealing with stressors or physical illness (Gall & Guirguis-Younger, 2013).

---

[3]"I tell you, every sin and blasphemy will be forgiven, but the blasphemy against the Spirit will not be forgiven" (Matthew 12:31, Revised Standard Version).

Although individuals may experience physical pain, grief, or sorrow, many can also find strength and gain valuable insights into themselves, develop closer relationships with others, or otherwise positively alter their perception of themselves or their environment after undergoing these stressful events.

Religion and Social Engagement

Psychotherapists can encourage patients to engage in the social aspects of their religious traditions, such as attending church, synagogue or temple, or religious education programs.

Religion not only offers solace and forgiveness, it also expects individuals to fulfill obligations to others. This means treating others with respect, forgiving them for their wrongdoings, and helping those who are less fortunate. During periods of depression or stress, patients often forget their obligations to others, and a desire to help others can be a life-altering event. Drouin (2017) reported that working with seriously ill children was an essential activity that reinforced her will to survive during a particularly stressful time. Stohlmann-Rainey (2017) reported that helping others often sustained her recovery. She volunteered at a suicide hotline: "Once I got on that hotline everything changed. I was whole again, and I could help people. That was the moment I knew I would live" (p. 4).

RELAPSE PREVENTION

As patients improve, psychotherapy can focus on termination. Although many patients may respond well to psychotherapy, relapses should be anticipated (Castonguay, 2013). When patients begin to show sustained improvement, it could be indicated to conduct relapse prevention interventions with them. Psychotherapists can discuss the confluence of events or life circumstances that led to past suicidal attempts or suicidal crises. They can discuss what events could lead to a loss of the psychotherapeutic gains and also to a return of suicidal thoughts. The events can be rehearsed in imagination. Those events that evoke the strongest emotions or are the most realistic may be the most helpful (Bryan & Rudd, 2018).

Suicides are the result of a confluence of many factors. The loss of a close relationship, a random accident, or an unanticipated decline in financial status may precipitate a suicidal crisis. But patients can create safety nets by cultivating close relationships, learning how to nurture them, and learning how to reduce their emotional arousal, and keep from overreacting to setbacks. Finally, they can identify resources for assistance if they perceive that they may be at risk of seeing a return of the suicidal crisis.

Psychotherapists can ask, "How will you know when the risk of suicide will return?" "How will you likely respond if thoughts of suicide reoccur?" and "Rate the likelihood that you would seek treatment again if suicidal thoughts returned." If respondents indicate a low probability that they would return to psychotherapy if suicidal thoughts returned, then this can be the basis for discussion.

Also, psychotherapists and patients can discuss ways that patients can improve the quality of their lives after they leave psychotherapy. After all, the goal is not just to prevent suicides, but to live a fulfilling life. This can be an opportunity for patients to think about how to live a life consistent with their values. The goal is to establish a positive outlook wherein patients live in accordance with their goals. The factors related to resilience are like the factors that improve an individual's quality of life: good social connections, healthy self-reflection combined with self-compassion, and a value-imbued life.

5

Professional Liability, Quality Enhancement, and Emotional Competence

This chapter first reviews the standards for determining professional liability. Of course, psychotherapists want to avoid being the subject of a malpractice suit or a disciplinary action, but this is best achieved by delivering high-quality professional services. This chapter also identifies several quality enhancement strategies that are based on overarching ethical principles. Finally, it addresses how psychotherapists can maintain and improve the quality of their services by protecting their own emotional well-being.

PROFESSIONAL LIABILITY

Many psychotherapists dread treating suicidal patients because they fear that their patients may die or they fear a lawsuit if their patients die from suicide or suffer harm from a failed suicide attempt while under their care. However, lawsuits for outpatient suicides are infrequent in part because courts understand that psychotherapists have limited control over the lives of outpatients. No outpatient psychotherapist can control the random events that could occur in the lives of their patients, such as an unexpected job loss or an unanticipated disruption in a social relationship. In contrast to outpatient treatment, lawsuits for inpatient suicides are more frequent because the hospital has more immediate control over the lives of their patients.

Psychotherapists can be subject to different disciplinary actions, such as malpractice suits, or complaints before licensing boards or ethics committees.

http://dx.doi.org/10.1037/0000145-006
Suicide Prevention: An Ethically and Scientifically Informed Approach, by S. J. Knapp

According to Dr. Jana Martin, CEO of the Trust,[1] about 20% of psychologists will have a disciplinary complaint filed against them, including about 5% who will have a malpractice suit filed against them sometime in their careers (K. Lee, 2017). Data on the frequency of malpractice cases for suicides are hard to determine because the data are proprietary and malpractice carriers do not share them. Nonetheless, the Trust listed suicide as the seventh most frequent type of malpractice suit against psychologists (Knapp, Younggren, VandeCreek, Harris, & Martin, 2013). It is a more common source of complaints against psychiatrists, however, because they prescribe medications and have control over inpatient admissions, discharges, and treatment.

The rules governing malpractice can be complex. This chapter does not review the rules concerning professional liability dealing with statutes of limitation, contributory negligence, the roles of fact and expert witnesses, and so on. Instead, this chapter reviews the features of malpractice that are most likely to inform psychotherapeutic practice.

Malpractice does not occur only because a patient suffered harm. Malpractice could occur if four conditions are met: the psychotherapist had a professional relationship with the patient and therefore owed a duty to the patient; the behavior of the psychotherapist deviated from an acceptable standard of care (usually defined as minimal standards of competence); the patient suffered damage or harm; and the actions of the psychotherapist directly caused or contributed to the harm to the patient. R. Simon (1992) called these the 4 Ds of malpractice (*duty, deviation, damage,* and *direct*).

The standard of care is "what most reasonable psychologists under similar circumstances do" (Sobelman & Younggren, 2016, p. 257). Practitioners who fail to meet the standard of care are called negligent. Courts determine the standard of care by relying on the testimony of expert witnesses during the trial. This standard, however, does not allow for unlimited variations or depend entirely on the idiosyncrasies of any one or two experts. Instead, these experts have their opinions informed by the enforceable standards of the profession's ethics code, the regulations of the state licensing board, applicable case law, and standards found in learned texts or peer-reviewed journals. The standards in courts might vary slightly from one to another, but they generally involve a consistent core of practices.

As noted briefly in Chapter 3, some states establish the standard of gross negligence (as opposed to ordinary negligence) for involuntary psychiatric hospitalizations. Gross negligence is a standard of conduct that is noticeably lower than ordinary negligence. This standard accurately reflects the difficulties involved in involuntary psychiatric hospitalizations where the involved professionals may not have the opportunity to get all the information to make this life-or-death decision because the patients do not or cannot cooperate with the interview. Also, the psychotherapists might not have access to other reliable sources of information; there is a need to decide quickly; and the

---

[1]The Trust is a major malpractice carrier for psychologists.

setting for the evaluation may be in a hospital emergency room, police station, or another location where there are frequent interruptions.

Psychotherapists can ensure that they are practicing at an acceptable standard of care by acquiring the competencies identified by Cramer, Johnson, McLaughlin, Rausch, and Conroy (2013) as delineated in Chapter 1 and explicated throughout the book, relying on the prompt list described later in this chapter.

The elements in the standard of care for suicidal patients include foreseeability, adequacy, and implementation. In determining standards of care, courts will ask if the psychotherapists should have foreseen the patient's suicide (or harm arising out of a failed suicide attempt), had developed an adequate treatment plan, and had implemented the treatment plan conscientiously. These three elements of the standard of care correspond roughly to three of the goals of assessment discussed in Chapter 2, which are to develop a diagnosis or describe the presenting problem, formulate a treatment plan, and use the data gathered in the assessment as a benchmark to measure progress. Psychotherapists who follow acceptable standards of care will use the data-gathering techniques known to identify suicidal behavior, develop a reasonable treatment plan based on an adequate assessment, and continue with or modify the treatment depending on the patient's response to treatment.

Some courts may find liability because the psychotherapist failed to foresee a suicide attempt because they did not use acceptable techniques to determine the risk of suicide. This could occur, for example, if the psychotherapist failed to even ask a patient about suicidal behavior or failed to follow up adequately when the patient expressed suicidal thoughts.

Other courts may find liability because the psychotherapist failed to develop an adequate suicide management strategy. This could occur, for example, if the psychotherapist had not attempted to restrict the patient's access to lethal means, failed to notified family members of the patient's suicidality when it was clinically indicated to do so, or relied too heavily on "no-suicide contracts" (Melonas, 2011).

Still other courts may find liability because psychotherapists failed to implement the treatment plan or failed to modify a treatment plan that they knew or should have known was not benefiting the patient or was unlikely to benefit the patient. This could occur, for example, if the psychotherapist failed to follow through with facilitating a psychiatric hospitalization as promised or failed to consider a referral for medication when it was clinically indicated to do so.

Licensing board complaints differ from malpractice suits in that a disciplinary action before a licensing board only requires that a psychotherapist violated a statute or board regulation. The regulations of licensing boards usually include the ethics code of the profession they regulate. Unlike a malpractice suit, in a licensing board complaint the patients (or the patients' representatives) need not prove that they were harmed; they only need to prove that a statute or regulation was violated.

If a licensing board determines that the psychotherapist violated a statute or licensing board regulation, it could issue disciplinary actions or require remedial steps such as requiring the licensee to take more continuing education. In extreme cases, it could suspend or revoke a license. Unlike a malpractice court, a licensing board cannot award damages to an injured party. In the case of suicidal behavior, it is more likely that the patients (if they survived an attempt) or their executors would file a malpractice suit as opposed to a licensing complaint.

It is also possible for psychotherapists to be brought before the ethics committee of a professional association. However, most of these associations, at least in psychology, now defer adjudications to their licensing boards, so they are becoming a less-common venue for disciplinary actions. In addition, disgruntled patients or relatives could complain to an institutional employer or an insurance carrier about the behavior of a psychotherapist. Such complaints could result in disciplinary actions or, in extreme cases, loss of employment or removal from an insurance panel.

Drivers of Complaints

The likelihood of a malpractice or licensing board complaint has only a moderate relationship to an objective determination of harm to the patient. Instead, complaints are often driven by patient or family anger at the treatment provider. Patients or their families who feel that their psychotherapists did their best and really cared about them are unlikely to file a disciplinary complaint. On the other hand, patients or their families who feel that their psychotherapists did not care about them, dismissed their opinions, or treated them with disrespect are more likely to file a disciplinary complaint.

When I was a staff member of the Pennsylvania Psychological Association, I collected data on the complaints made with our Ethics Committee. I was struck by how frequently complainants identified rudeness as one of their primary complaints. Several behaviors of psychotherapists such as hostile or critical confrontations, neglecting patient perceptions of their needs, and so on are linked to negative results (Castonguay, Boswell, Constantino, Goldfried, & Hill, 2010). These relationship-harming behaviors also increase the likelihood that patients or their families will file a malpractice or licensing board complaint. Conversely, many patients will forgive their psychotherapist's infractions if they believe that their psychotherapists cared about them and had their best interests at heart.

Special Areas of Risk

Two areas of professional practice, supervised practice and telehealth, need additional commentary as it applies to legal risk. Clinical supervision occurs when one professional controls the work product of a legal subordinate, such as a licensed psychologist who supervises a psychology intern or practicum student. Supervisors retain the ultimate responsibility for the quality of services provided. Supervisees have no legal authority to act without the consent of their supervisors. If the service falls below minimally acceptable standards of practice, the supervisor is legally responsible. This general rule has some exceptions, such as when a supervisee deliberately hides important information from the supervisor.

Supervision differs from consultation in that the consultee has the ultimate responsibility for the work product. The consultants may give their opinions, but the consultee retains the authority to make the final decisions. Often professionals confuse these terms, but from a legal perspective the concepts are clearly different. Supervisory practices are governed by several sets of rules including the professional ethics codes and regulations of state licensing boards. Effective supervisors know these rules and follow them closely.

It is beyond the scope of this book to review supervision in general, and readers who want more information are referred to other sources (e.g., Goodyear & Rodolfa, 2012). A body of literature has developed on how to supervise effectively and, although legally the supervisor–supervisee relationship is hierarchical, effective supervision involves a more cooperative and collaborative spirit.

As it relates to suicide, effective supervisors will ensure that their supervisees have basic competence in dealing with suicidal patients. Many mental health professionals have not had adequate training (Mackelprang, Karle, Reihl, & Cash, 2014; Schmitz et al., 2012). For example, the supervisees may have learned that hospitalization is the first line of intervention for patients with suicidal inclinations or may believe that a no-suicide contract should be used. Effective supervisors will review strategies for intervening with suicidal patients, perhaps using Cramer's competency standards covered in Chapter 1 as a guide.

In addition, even if students are well trained in suicide prevention, if they were trained out of state they would not know the relevant laws such as involuntary psychiatric hospitalization in the state where the training occurred. Finally, supervisors should review any unique institutional policies regarding suicidal patients.

Delivering telehealth services to suicidal patients may raise special risks, especially if the psychotherapy is being conducted across state lines. Practitioners who offer telehealth services may encounter patients who express suicidal ideation. This requires psychotherapists to be alert to some unique treatment problems even if the psychotherapists are practicing within legal standards.

Psychotherapists should offer telehealth services within the ethical and legal requirements of the profession. That is, psychotherapists should know and comply with state laws for the delivery of the service in the state where the patient is physically located, such as the laws concerning involuntary psychiatric hospitalization or permitted exceptions to confidentiality. Or, if the psychotherapists do not know the laws of the state, they should work in conjunction with a health care professional in that state who does know these laws. Psychotherapists who lack familiarity with the laws where the patients are physically located, or who fail to have a professional contact in that state willing to guide them in the event of an emergency, have put themselves in a precarious legal position and have jeopardized patient safety.

Psychotherapists using telehealth need to screen the patients appropriately. It is less of a worry when a psychotherapist treats a patient at a distant location whom they previously treated in face-to-face psychotherapy and had a good feel for the strengths and weaknesses of the patient. They can make better decisions about whether they can continue to treat the patient through telehealth safely. Even then, psychotherapists should ensure that they have a backup phone line if they lose contact with the patient and that they have local backup for emergencies, such as a family physician or a professional at a local mental health center (Luxton, O'Brien, Pruitt, Johnson, & Kramer, 2014). Consider how one psychotherapist appropriately handles these situations.

Obtaining Backup

A psychologist has become a minor celebrity because of some books he has written on marital therapy. He sometimes gets phone calls or emails from patients who want him to treat them even though they may live a thousand or more miles away. He regularly refuses to see them unless they can identify a mental health professional in their location who is willing to assume primary responsibility in the case of an emergency.

This psychologist wisely knows that he might interview a patient who seems well put together in the initial intake but in subsequent sessions will display problematic or even suicidal behavior. Then he would be stuck with a highly suicidal patient in a state where he does not know the hospitalization laws, has no contact with psychiatrists willing to see the patient, and does not know the local crisis services or even what local hospitals have psychiatric inpatient units.

EFFECTIVE AND FALSE RISK-MANAGEMENT STRATEGIES

Ethics consultants, malpractice carriers, and others have developed risk-management strategies to reduce the likelihood of a malpractice suit or licensing board complaint. These risk-management recommendations urge psychotherapists to think about how someone else might view their behavior in retrospect. One could say that these strategies are "a prospective assessment of [a] retrospective evaluation" (Sobelman & Younggren, 2016, p. 259).

Even though a bad outcome is not sufficient to establish liability in a malpractice case, it is only human that the decision makers will be influenced by *hindsight bias*. Knowing how something turned out can lead disinterested observers to conclude that they could have predicted the result. The hindsight bias is a universal phenomenon that occurs in a wide range of social situations. However, it can have an especially pernicious impact on a psychotherapist who has lost a patient to suicide. If a patient died from suicide or suffered from a suicide attempt, there will be a natural tendency to assume that the psychotherapist did something wrong. Therefore, psychotherapists should put themselves into a future mind-set and ask themselves, "What could go wrong?" "How would this behavior look in retrospect?" or "What would the best of my colleagues do in a similar situation?"

Asking these questions will help psychotherapists to deliver the best treatment that they can. After all, the best way for psychotherapists to reduce risk is to deliver and document good care. This emphasis on quality care is consistent with M. M. Silverman's (2014) concept of therapeutic risk management that is "patient-centered, supportive of the treatment process, and maintains the therapeutic alliance" (p. 375).

Effective risk-management strategies promote good patient care and are based on overarching ethical principles. So, the best risk-management strategies avoid harming the patient (nonmaleficence), promote patient well-being (beneficence), involve patients in their treatment (respecting patient autonomy), keep promises to patients (fidelity), and treat patients fairly (justice). If a purported risk-management strategy fails to meet that litmus test, then it qualifies as a *false risk-management strategy* and should be questioned.

False risk-management strategies purport to protect psychotherapists from malpractice, but do not. Often these false risk-management principles are based on dichotomous or simplistic thinking about complex clinical and ethical issues. Often they are peppered with absolutist terms such as *always* or *never.*

One such false risk-management strategy is that psychotherapists should never write down anything in detail because any crafty attorney can use it against them. The rationale is that if it is not documented, then the psychotherapist can always deny that the patient brought it up! However, lying about what happened in psychotherapy cannot be ethically justified.

Furthermore, the assumption that any crafty attorney can twist any words around is inaccurate. Courts assume that the clinical record is accurate. If a psychotherapist wrote that he asked the patient if she was thinking of suicide and that the patient said no, then the court will assume that the psychotherapist asked the patient if she was thinking of suicide and that the patient said no. No crafty attorney can undo that statement. Of course, problems can occur if the psychotherapist wrote incoherent or garbled sentences that make no sense. However, in high-risk situations, psychotherapists are urged to invest time to write thoughtful, precise, and detailed notes that address salient treatment issues such as suicide potential. Documentation is discussed in more detail later in this chapter.

Another false risk-management strategy is for psychotherapists to insist that their patients sign a prewritten no-suicide contract. As described in Chapter 4, no evidence supports the efficacy of such contracts (in contrast to commitment to life or commitment to treatment agreements, which are written collaboratively with the patient and are designed to promote their well-being). Even though noted suicidologists have strongly criticized no-suicide contracts, some agencies still use them.

Finally, I have heard psychotherapists say that they will do "everything they can" to protect a patient from suicide. On the surface, "doing everything they can" sounds like something a dedicated psychotherapist would do, and "doing everything" should be enshrined as a risk-management principle. However, as discussed in Chapter 3, some psychotherapists take an alarmist approach to suicidal patients and implement a wide range of interventions without thinking through the impact of those interventions on their patients. Instead, psychotherapists should do everything reasonable or helpful for their patients. Sometimes psychotherapists are urged to "CYA" ("cover your ass") when working with suicidal patients. Dr. Donald McAleer (personal communication, April 20, 2017) suggested that CYA should stand for "Can you articulate?" meaning, "Can you describe the clinical rationale for your decision?"

The best risk-management strategy is to deliver and document good patient care, guided by overarching ethical principles (Knapp et al., 2013). The best quality-enhancement strategies are grounded on overarching ethical principles, arise out of an attitude of humility, promote patient well-being, and reduce legal risks. The four strategies are (a) empowered collaboration (based on the principle of respecting patient decision making), which tries to maximize patient participation in the treatment process; (b) consultation (based on the principles of beneficence and nonmaleficence), which improves the quality of treatment by securing additional information or new perspectives; (c) monitoring progress or seeking redundant protections (based on the principles of beneficence and nonmaleficence), which measures progress or double-checks the information needed to guide service decisions; and (d) documentation (based on principles of beneficence and nonmaleficence), which provides legal protection and can also increase clinicians' acuity and self-awareness.[2] Some of the elements of these quality-enhancement strategies have been discussed in other sections in this book, but they are expanded here because of their importance. The quality-enhancement strategies arise out of an appropriate attitude of *humility* or a willingness to try to see oneself accurately (Davis, Hook, McAnnally-Linz, Choe, & Placeres, 2017).

Empowered Collaboration (Informed Consent)

Empowered collaboration is a concept that builds on and expands on informed consent. Whereas informed consent refers to respecting patient autonomy by seeking patient permission to start treatment, *empowered collaboration* refers to respecting patient autonomy throughout as much of the treatment process as is clinically indicated. Many of these ideas were already covered in Chapter 3 and are summarized briefly next.

Sometimes psychotherapist fear empowering patients because they fear that their patients may make the "wrong" choices, or that their desire to die will

---

[2]Dr. Eric Harris originally introduced these as risk-management strategies
(Bennett et al., 2006).

undercut any meaningful participation in treatment. Of course, if the patient is seriously depressed or demoralized, a psychotherapist may temporarily take a more active role in directing treatment. But, as much as clinically possible, psychotherapists should solicit meaningful patient input into decisions about safety plans, safety agreements, treatment goals, and so on.

As noted in Chapter 3, autonomy is one of the core motives identified in self-determination theory (Ryan & Deci, 2008). Patients are more likely to cooperate with a treatment that aligns itself with a fundamental human motive, such as autonomy.

In addition, respect for patient autonomy reflects healthy humility on the part of effective psychotherapists who know that their knowledge of the patient is inevitably less extensive than the patients' knowledge of themselves. Although psychotherapists may be experts on human behavior, their patients are experts on their own life experiences, histories, and emotions. Also, the more that patients invest in the development of their safety and treatment plans, the more likely that they will follow those plans. Patients are more likely to follow goals that they choose for themselves rather than goals chosen by others.

Psychotherapists can engage patients by listening carefully to their concerns and incorporating their perspectives into treatment. Furthermore, psychotherapists can empower patients by being transparent about their treatment methods, goals, and rationale. Empowered collaboration is most easily implemented when patients have a sense that their psychotherapists care about them.

Empowered collaboration is also useful when psychotherapists encounter a treatment dilemma. Sometimes psychotherapists will agonize about treatment decisions such as whether to involve the patient's family in psychotherapy or get a second opinion on medication. Often the best way to approach these decisions is invite patients as copartners in the decision.

Consultation (Expanding Resources and Perspectives)

According to science historian Steven Johnson (2010), good ideas come out of a network. That is, good ideas are more likely to occur when individuals exchange ideas with each other. Few scientific or cultural innovations were developed when individuals worked in isolation. Instead, scientists and artists were more likely to develop innovations if they interacted closely with others. History is replete with examples where huge advancements in culture and science occurred in specific locations and times, such as impressionist artists in Paris in the late 1800s, transcendentalist authors around Concord, Massachusetts in the 1840s, scientists at the Bell Laboratories in the 1950s, or innovators in the Silicon Valley today.

A similar process occurs in effective psychotherapy. Patients come into psychotherapy with sticky problems. If the problems were easy, then patients would have solved them long ago. Psychotherapy is more effective when patients and psychotherapists exchange information freely. One of the key ingredients of effective psychotherapy is to create conditions whereby patients can overcome embarrassment, shame, pride, or other emotions that keep them from sharing thoughts and feelings freely. Even then, psychotherapy can become stuck and the input of others may be needed to get it unstuck.

When treating suicidal patients, psychotherapists may need additional resources. This may require getting information, perspectives, or ideas from outside of the immediate patient and psychotherapist dyad, such as from members of the patient's family or friends, or from other treatment professionals including a primary care physician or a psychopharmacologist. It can also come from discussions with consultants.

Effective psychotherapists have a network of individuals or institutions to draw on for consultation. W. B. Johnson, Barnett, Elman, Forrest, and Kaslow (2012) described the importance of having a *competent community* or a network of colleagues, friends, or resources that help practitioners to offer good quality care. Ongoing consultations may occur between peers, sometimes as part of a group and sometimes as individuals. Often these are called "peer supervision" groups, although this is not technically accurate because supervision means a hierarchical relationship that cannot occur among peers. Professional associations or sometimes professional liability carriers (e.g., the Trust) can be part of that competent community in so far as they give important advice on legal or ethical issues.

Sometimes consultants do not provide new information, but instead they help psychotherapists think through their decisions. Often I have been consulted by psychotherapists and finished without offering any new information. Instead, I listened and asked questions, and often the psychotherapists reached a reasonable course of action on their own, without my having made a single substantive comment. Of course, if they had suggested something less than optimal or harmful, I would have spoken up and told them so. But the process of having to formulate and articulate one's concerns and talking it out appears to be all that some psychotherapists need to reach a good decision in many cases.

A collaborative approach is best where the consultant helps the consultee think through their goals and values (Knapp, Gottlieb, & Handelsman, 2017) and the reasoning behind their decisions. Rogerson, Gottlieb, Handelsman, Knapp, and Younggren (2011) noted that sometimes psychotherapists may use heuristics that would cause them to adopt less-than-optimal strategies. This may require consultants to tell the psychotherapists to slow down their thinking and attend to nonrational processes. Psychotherapists may adopt the first good-enough solution that comes to mind. Or psychotherapists may be victims of the *confirmation bias*, or the tendency to see new information that supports the decision makers previous judgment. This is a common psychological phenomenon that affects many decision makers, including health care professionals. It could occur, for example, if a psychotherapist decided that a patient had a major depression and then began to cherry pick or interpret subsequent information to confirm the diagnosis, when a more objective evaluation should have caused the psychotherapist to revisit the diagnosis (Knapp, Gottlieb, & Handelsman, 2015).

Effective consultation requires open communication between the consultant and consultee. Consultees benefit the most when they adopt a self-reflective attitude and show a willingness to accept feedback, even if it might be critical of their behavior. This is another example of the benefit of humility, or the willingness to see one's limitations.

Monitoring One's Work (Redundant Protections)

A redundant protection is any source of useful data about a patient in addition to the patient's self-report. Effective psychotherapists monitor their patient's progress carefully. Psychotherapists generally have a good sense of which patients are improving and which are not. However, psychotherapists tend to overestimate the number of patients who are benefitting from psychotherapy and underestimate the number who are deteriorating. Walfish, McAlister, O'Donnell, and Lambert (2012) found that psychotherapists estimated, on the average, that 3.6% of their patients got worse during treatment or less than an average of one out of every 25 patients. Yet a review by Castonguay, Boswell, Constantino, Goldfried, and Hill (2010) found that an average of 8% of patients got worse during treatment or an average of two out of every 25 patients. So, it appears that psychotherapists will fail to detect deterioration in an average of one out of every 25 patients. Psychotherapists who are vigilant about outcomes will take special steps to ensure that they can identify the one in 25 patients who have a trajectory toward deterioration that they might otherwise fail to identify.

To compensate for this risk of overestimating one's effectiveness, vigilant psychotherapists actively question the quality of their services. Appropriate humility—or striving to see one's self objectively—can lead to a higher level of services. They can take steps to ensure more accurate or complete information about their patients by monitoring patient progress and their own treatment processes.

Patient Monitoring

While patients are actively suicidal, psychotherapists should ask them about their suicidal thoughts during each treatment session. Or psychotherapists can consider giving them a brief screening instruments on suicidal ideation before each treatment session (see Chapter 3). These could be the same instruments that the psychotherapists used in the assessment process (see Chapter 2). These scales may pick up risks that would not be evident on the basis of the self-report of the patient.

In addition, effective psychotherapists make a special effort to monitor their patient's progress in psychotherapy. Typically, psychotherapists rely on the self-report of patients. However, given the seriousness of the condition, psychotherapists may wish to supplement those reports with other sources such as outcome instruments, or information from members of the patient's social network or other treatment providers. Ideally these additional sources will give clinical information that will help advance treatment goals.

Psychotherapists can use some outcome measures as a global indicator of patient change over the course of treatment. But simply instituting outcome monitoring in an agency will not necessarily improve outcomes (Wampold, 2015). Some psychotherapists dismiss data from outcome measures if they do not conform to their impressions of patient progress. Those psychotherapists who benefit from routine outcome monitoring are those who value it and use the information to inform their decisions.

In addition, psychotherapists can ask about specific dimensions of well-being. For example, Chapter 2 noted that psychotherapists can ask patients about the intensity, duration, and frequency of suicidal ideation. Psycho-therapists can continue to ask about those dimensions of suicidality throughout treatment and use it as a bell weather to measure progress. Similar questions can be asked about the patient's self-reported likelihood that they will die from suicide, their ability to sleep or avoid nightmares, and so on.

Even regularly asking patients about their overall well-being and response to treatment could be instructive. This could mean asking patients at the end of each session if the session was helpful for them, if they had a chance to talk about what was important, if the sessions included some parts that were not helpful, and so on (Maeschalck & Barfknecht, 2017). "Did you have a chance to talk about things that were important to you?" "What did we do today that was most helpful to you?" "What did we do today that was not helpful?" Specific questions tend to be more helpful than global or generalized questions.

Solicitation of feedback can occur very early in the process, even during the initial interview. One psychologist specializing in assessing children with autism routinely asks parents during the intake interview if he is understanding their child accurately or if there is important information that he is missing or misinterpreting. He will routinely ask the parents near the middle of the interview and toward the end as well.

The additional sources of information could come from the social network of the patient, such as family members and friends. Although the possible biases of the reporters need to be taken into account when interpreting the information, these family members and friends have access to information that the psychotherapists lack because they see the patient every day and under circumstances to which the psychotherapist is not privileged.

Involving the friends or family in the treatment can also reduce a patient's distress. Although conscientious psychotherapists put the welfare of their patients first, they are not oblivious to the needs of friends or family members. It is usually possible to promote their well-being by reducing their worry about their loved one.

Involving family in treatment has another advantage. If a tragedy were to occur and a patient were to die from suicide, those family members who had contact with the psychotherapist would know firsthand of the care and compassion that the psychotherapist showed. They would be less likely to sue, because they would not see the psychotherapists as anonymous individuals who failed in their duties, but as caring professionals who did their best.

If patients are not improving by the fourth session, then Knapp and Gavazzi (2012) recommended that psychotherapists use a prompt list (see Table 5.1). The prompt list includes a series of questions that psychotherapists can ask themselves (or their patients) to ensure that the quality of the services is adequate. It is not a checklist that requires an either/or response (either

TABLE 5.1. Prompt List

Patient collaboration (What does the patient say?)

YES ___ NO ___   1. Does the patient think you have a good working relationship?

YES ___ NO ___   2. Do you and your patient share the same treatment goals?[a]

YES ___ NO ___   3. Does the patient report any progress in therapy?[b]

YES ___ NO ___   4. Does the patient want to continue in treatment?[c] If so, does the patient see a need to modify treatment?

YES ___ NO ___   5. Does the patient believe that the risk of suicide is waning?

Additional reflections (What do you think about the patient?)

YES ___ NO ___   6. Do you believe you have a positive working relationship with your patient? (Does he or she trust you enough to share sensitive information and collaborate?)[d]

YES ___ NO ___   7. Is your assessment of the patient sufficiently comprehensive?[e]

YES ___ NO ___   8. Do you need to obtain additional information? Are you getting information from other family members or sources? Are you routinely asking about suicide? Are you using a suicide screening inventory to supplement other sources?

YES ___ NO ___   9. Do unresolved clinical issues of significant concern impede the course of treatment (such as Axis II issues, possible or minimization of substance abuse, or ethical concerns)?

YES ___ NO ___   10. Does the patient need a medical examination?

Documentation

YES ___ NO ___   11. Have you documented appropriately?

Other questions?

Note. From "Can Checklists Help Reduce Treatment Failures?" by S. Knapp and J. Gavazzi, April 2012, *The Pennsylvania Psychologist*, *72*, pp. 8–9. Copyright 2012 by the Pennsylvania Psychological Association. Adapted with permission.
[a]Do you understand your patient's goals and how he or she expects to achieve them? How do they correspond to your goals and preferred methods of treatment? If they differ, can you reach a compromise? Does the patient buy into treatment? Did you document the goals in your treatment notes? What did the patient say was particularly helpful or hindering about therapy? Have you incorporated your patient's perceptions into your treatment plan? [b]Do you agree on how to measure progress (self-report, reports of others, psychometric testing, nonreactive objective measures, etc.)? Does the patient need a medical examination? [c]If yes, why? [d]Can you identify what is happening in the relationship to prevent a therapeutic alliance? Does the patient identify an impasse? Do your feelings toward your patient compromise your ability to be helpful? If so, how can you change those feelings? Have you sought consultation on your relationship or feelings about the patient? If so, what did you learn? [e]Have you reassessed the diagnosis or treatment methods using the BASIC I.D., MOST CARE, or another system designed to review the presenting problem? Are you sensitive to cultural factors, gender-related status, sexual orientation, socioeconomic status, or other factors? What input did you get from the patient, significant others of the patient, or consultants?

I performed this activity or I did not). Rather it is a list of questions that prompt the psychotherapists to reflect on treatment and to talk to their patients (or consultants) about the progress of treatment and ways to improve.

Of course, the fourth session does not represent a hard-and-fast standard for using a prompt list. Psychotherapists can use the prompt list any time they suspect that a patient is not improving. Knapp and Gavazzi (2012) arbitrarily picked the fourth session because Lambert and colleagues had reported algorithms that could predict patient outcome with a high degree of reliability by the fourth session (Lambert & Shimokawa, 2011).

Monitoring patient progress and using the prompt list, if necessary, will help protect psychotherapists from falling prey to the *sunk-cost* effect whereby people are reluctant to discontinue an activity that they have invested heavily in, even if that activity does not appear to be helpful. Kahneman (2011) gave an example of the sunk-cost effect as driving to a concert through a dangerous blizzard because one has already paid for the tickets. Examples could also be found where people stayed with financial investments that were failing or marriages that were disastrous because they could not let go of an investment or a relationship that they had committed themselves to.

As it applies to psychotherapy, psychotherapists risk continuing with treatments that are ineffective because they have made a commitment to them. However, if psychotherapists routinely monitor patient progress or rely on a prompt list, they are more likely to identify a failing treatment program early and thus have less vulnerability to the sunk-cost fallacy.

Monitoring Treatment Processes

In addition to directly monitoring patient progress, it can also be useful for psychotherapists to monitor their own behavior. It is easy to lose track of all the factors that need to be considered when assessing and treating suicidal patients. While focusing on the immediate task of ensuring patient safety, it is almost inevitable that even highly competent psychotherapists will neglect to follow up on some important statement or ask all the recommended questions about certain aspects of suicide risk. Psychotherapists who use checklists will be less likely to forget to do some important tasks.

Some psychotherapists may strongly object to the use of checklists and argue that their job is so highly specialized and detailed that checklists oversimplify their tasks. The response is that this is exactly why checklists are needed. The tasks required are so complex and numerous that it is easy to forget to ask certain questions or perform certain tasks. In addition, working with suicidal patients can be emotionally stressful for psychotherapists, and that stress may, at times, impair their ability to attend to important details so that the quality of treatment may deteriorate, even if only slightly. Checklists have been used by many professionals such as airplane pilots and surgeons (Gawande, 2009).

This book recommends the use of aids to assist psychotherapists, such as the patient information form that contains the initial suicide question (see Appendix A) and a detailed checklist of questions (see Table 5.2) that

TABLE 5.2. Checklist

Initial Screening

> Did you ask patients about suicidal thoughts at least once, unless you can identify clinical reasons not to did so?
>
> Did you have a written question on suicide as well as asking patients directly?
>
> Did you follow up with patients who gave contradictory information in response to the written and oral questions?
>
> If the patients denied suicidal ideation but had high risk factors, did you follow up? Does the patient have passive thoughts of suicide (e.g., think that they would be better off dead, think that others around them would be better off if they were dead, etc.)?

Ideation, Past Attempts, and Plans

> Did you ask about the frequency, intensity, and duration of suicidal thoughts?
>
> If a patient indicated suicidal thoughts, did you elicit more detailed information on previous suicide attempts, their thoughts about surviving such attempts, plans for future attempts, if they know someone who died from suicide, or a history of suicide attempts in their family?
>
> Did you ask patients about the trigger, feelings, or behaviors (warning signs) that accompanied any past suicide attempt or that accompany thinking about suicide or making plans for suicide?
>
> If patients have suicidal thoughts, did you ask them the likelihood that they will die from suicide?
>
> Unless a patient indicated no or very low suicidal ideation or intent and/or did not have other high-risk factors, did you conduct a thorough suicidal evaluation?
>
> If patients have many risk factors and yet deny suicidal ideation, did you consider the possibility that they may be false deniers?
>
> Is the interview conducted in a caring and nonjudgmental manner?
>
> Did patients have an opportunity to tell their stories?
>
> Did patients feel that you care about them?

Detailed Suicidal Assessment

> When conducting a more detailed suicide assessment, did you gather data on the risk and protective factor for the patient?
>
> Does your interview cover the major topics: documenting demographic factors, social connectedness, life stressors and daily hassles, medical history, religion or spirituality, and emotional pain and mental illness?
>
> Does your interview elicit themes on thwarted belongingness, perceived burdensomeness, defeat, humiliation, entrapment, hopelessness, self-disgust, irritability, insomnia, nightmares, anxiety or agitation, and protective factors of values (religion), psychological resilience, and social connectedness?
>
> Did you understand the acquired capacity of the patients to kill themselves?
>
> Did you get an understanding of the patient's past emotional cascades or suicidal modes that accompany suicidal thoughts?
>
> Did you understand the triggers that could precipitate a suicidal crisis in the patient?
>
> Have you established a baseline for the patient's emotional functioning?
>
> Did you understand the capabilities of the patients in preventing a suicidal crisis or in short-circuiting such a crisis?
>
> Did the patients feel as if they had a chance to tell their stories?
>
> Did your patients sense that you care about them?

Screening Instruments

> If clinically indicated, did you use a screening instrument to further assess suicide risk?

(continues)

TABLE 5.2. Checklist (*Continued*)

Integrating Data

Can you describe the features of the patient's suicidal crisis state?

Can you describe the trigger that will likely move the patient into a suicidal mode?

What is the patient's baseline of emotional functioning?

What is the patient's degree of acquired capability of suicide?

Does the patient have access to the means of suicide?

Managing Suicidal Risk

Can you document a justification for the level of service (inpatient or outpatient) for the patient?

Did you motivate patients including a discussion of the reasons for living and harm that could occur to others if they were to die from suicide?

Did you create commitment to life agreement?

Did you create a crisis card that identified warning signs, distracting activities, and crisis number? Did you rehearse the crisis plan with your patient? Did you ask your patient about the likelihood that they would use the plan?

Did you restrict access to lethal means?

Did you refer patients for medication if clinically indicated to do so?

Did you follow up to ensure that your patients understood how to take the medication and that they are adhering to the treatment recommendations?

Did you establish a monitoring system appropriate to the needs of the patient?

Did you involve friends or family members if clinically indicated to do so, and if so, did you socialize them into their role? If you did not involve them, can you justify that decision?

Did you go through an ethical decision-making process if it were necessary to consider disclosing patients' information without their consent or instituting an involuntary psychiatric hospitalization?

Treatment

Did your informed-consent process address your expectations of the patient including adherence to treatment? Did you address noncompliance early? Did you try to understand the reasons why it occurred and how to motivate the patient to comply?

Did you create treatment goals cooperatively with the patients and try to involve them in important clinical decisions?

Did your treatment plan address the specific systems that are likely to put the patient into a suicidal crisis state?

Did your treatment plan address the factors that lead patients to have a high baseline of distress such as insomnia, isolation, self-hate, etc.?

Are you clear about how the patient is to respond if there is a crisis? Is the patient clear about how to respond?

Did your treatment plan address the patient's values?

Did you continue to monitor the patient's suicidal thoughts and keep means safety in place if there was a risk of suicidal behavior?

Did you document your interventions carefully, including being transparent about any decisions you made, and express your work clearly without using vague words?

Did you inquire into reasons for living and the patient's values?

Are you prepared to respond if the patient attempts suicide while in treatment, has made time- or event-contingent suicidal threats, or appears to be using suicidal behavior as blackmail?

Did you receive consultation if indicated to do so?

Note. From *The Assessment, Management and Treatment of Suicidal Patients: An Abbreviated Course,* by S. Knapp, 2016. Harrisburg, PA: Pennsylvania Psychological Association. Copyright 2016 by the Pennsylvania Psychological Association. Adapted with permission.

psychotherapists can ask themselves to ensure that they have covered the important issues in assessment, management, and treatment.

Documentation

Knowing how to document risks, plans, and clinical reasoning was one of the core competencies in treating suicidal patients identified by Cramer et al. (2013). Documentation serves several purposes. It fulfills legal requirements or requirements of insurers. It reminds treating professionals about what happened during psychotherapy. Documentation also helps patients if they see another professional in the future who needs to know what happened in psychotherapy. In addition, the creation of the documentation itself can be to an opportunity to reflect on the treatment. Finally, it can be a very effective form of risk management.

The general rule that courts use for evaluating information is that "if it is not written down, it did not happen."[3] Conversely, if it is written down, then the court will assume that it did happen. This final purpose of records is especially salient for psychotherapists who deal with high-risk patients. Unfortunately, some studies have found that many professionals who deal with suicidal patients failed to document the common predictors of suicide in their records (Alavi, Reshetukha, Prost, Antoniak, & Groll, 2017; Tanguturi, Bodic, Taub, Homel, & Jacob, 2017).

Treatment is routine for most psychotherapy patients. Most patients come in for short-term therapy, get better, pay their bills, say thank you, and are never heard from again. The documentation in such cases may also be routine and completed in the brief time between appointments. Treatment is not routine for suicidal patients. The documentation in such cases needs to be more extensive and detailed, and completed with more deliberation.

If a patient dies from suicide or suffers seriously from a failed suicide attempt, the family or surviving patient may question the level of care provided by the psychotherapist and initiate a malpractice suit. The suicide of a patient is a profound tragedy. However, there is no value in complicating that tragedy by having a lawsuit against a psychotherapist who acted conscientiously and competently. I know psychotherapists who delivered good care but nonetheless had to defend themselves in a malpractice suit because they failed to document services adequately. Conversely, I know psychotherapists who did not have to go to court because of the quality of their documentation. Consider the situation described in the following vignette.

Good Records Protect Psychotherapists

A mother initiated a malpractice suit against an outpatient practice following the suicide of her teenage son. After the mother's attorney received the psychotherapy

---

[3]Taken literally, this phrase is an overstatement. Courts will accept the testimony of health care professionals on content not covered in the medical record. However, the value of that testimony can be challenged as self-serving and has far less weight than the content of medical records.

notes as part of the discovery process, the case was dropped. The practice had documented numerous attempts on the part of the psychotherapist to get the mother to bring her son into treatment. Phone conversations were documented in the record, and copies of the two letters sent to the mother were included in the chart. The letters clearly identified the risk and almost seemed to be pleading with the mother to take the risk to her child seriously.

The general rule is that any subsequent health care professional should be able to look at the psychotherapy notes and have a general idea of what happened in psychotherapy. To reach that goal, psychotherapists should describe the information they gathered in determining suicide risk. In addition, psychotherapists should describe management strategies (e.g., commitment to life documents, efforts at means safety) and interventions. Also, psychotherapists should document all important decisions including the potential risks and benefits of those decisions.

Psychotherapists should write notes precisely. They should avoid using vague or confusing terms that do not have agreed-on meanings. For example, the words *suicidal gesture* is open to multiple interpretations and psychotherapists should not use them unless they define the term (Heilbron, Compton, Daniel, & Goldston, 2010).

Consider the differences between these two potential ways to write a psychotherapy note. One could write that the patient had a "suicidal gesture." Or one could write that "the patient had gathered more than 100 pills, placed them by his bedside, and had gone to the kitchen to get a glass of milk to swallow them when his parents came home and interrupted his attempt." It is obvious which note is more helpful.

The word *impulsive* may also be open to multiple meanings. Some psychotherapists may use it to refer generically to any attempt when the patient had not previously reported a plan to their psychotherapist. Nonetheless, others may use it to refer to a wide range of behaviors where the patient did not think about the consequences of their actions thoroughly.

Similarly, the word *manipulate* confuses readers. Does it mean that the patient deliberately took a nonlethal dose of medication, engaged in nonsuicidal self-injury, or expected to be interrupted in the suicide attempt? Also, James and Stewart (2018) found that psychotherapists sometimes blurred the distinction between the terms *self-harm* and *suicide*, suggesting a lack of a common understanding of the differences between the two terms. I have heard of psychotherapists who used the terms *nonfatal suicide* or *parasuicide*, which I guess meant an incomplete attempt. The problem is that the reader should not have to guess what was meant.

Effective care for suicidal patients requires an accurate understanding of past suicidal behavior. For example, if a patient put a gun to his head, fired the gun, and subsequently survived (perhaps the gun misfired), it would be important for future treating professionals to know this because it reveals the means and seriousness of the attempt. A simple phrase such as *nonfatal suicide* does not capture the important details and may mislead future treating professionals as to the seriousness of the attempt.

It is also useful to identify the sources of the information. Good psychotherapy notes are often peppered with phrases such as "the patient said," "the patient reported," "according to the patient," and so on. It can be helpful to use direct quotes from the patient. Professional opinions and interpretations should be labeled as such.

Efforts should be made to get past treatment records. Not only can these records inform the psychotherapists about what worked or did not work in psychotherapy, but they can also reveal crucial information. One psychotherapist received past treatment records on a patient who had denied ever having suicidal ideation. Because the patient showed no high-risk signs for suicide, the psychotherapist proceeded with treatment without inquiring further about suicidal behavior. Nonetheless, the past records revealed that the patient had at least one past serious suicide attempt. This information led the psychotherapists to learn more about the past event and to focus on current risks for suicide.

When I consult with psychotherapists about high-risk patients, I typically emphasize the importance of keeping good notes. Often psychotherapists tell me that they have not included important information their documentation. Psychotherapists should not alter treatment notes, although they may write addendums to notes and date them. If appropriate, the addendum may state that, on rereading the notes, the psychotherapist determined that the notes needed more information or more clarity. Consultations should be documented. Psychotherapists should also document that they checked the patient's level of suicidality at every session. If they decided that such suicide checks were no longer needed, they should document why they made that decision.

Psychotherapists should ensure that their treatment plan and treatment notes address all the problem areas identified in the assessment. If the psychotherapists documented in the intake that the patient has a problem with impulsivity, for example, then they should address impulsivity somewhere in their treatment plan and progress notes, or document why they no longer consider impulsivity to be a problem area. Perhaps the psychotherapists received information in subsequent meetings that led them to conclude that they had misinterpreted the degree or significance of any impulsivity problem. If so, the psychotherapists should document that in the record.

Some psychotherapists will use a symptom checklist as part of their intake process. This checklist might include a list of common symptoms where they simply check if the patient reported the symptom or if they saw manifestations of those symptoms in the session. Symptom checklists can be useful if they help psychotherapists to remember all the elements they need to look for. Nonetheless, if a symptom is checked, then it should be addressed in psychotherapy in some manner, or the reason that it was not addressed should be documented. If the psychotherapist checked a symptom, such as anxiety, but then never addressed anxiety in subsequent notes, it appears that the psychotherapist knew that anxiety was a problem but negligently ignored it.

Psychotherapists should keep copies of all emails that have clinical implications or at least summarize their content. There is no reason to keep mundane emails about routine scheduling or other administrative issues.

Salient events in psychotherapy should be documented, including patient noncompliance and efforts to increase patient compliance. Patient noncompliance is one of the major causes of treatment failure and needs to be taken very seriously.

If a suicidal patient suffered harm and a court ever reviewed the treatment decisions, psychotherapists would not be liable just because their decisions, in hindsight, were wrong. They would not be held liable for making a wrong decision that appeared to be the best decision given the information that the psychotherapists had at the time.

Psychotherapists would be held liable if they deviated from good standards of care and this deviation directly harmed or contributed to the harm to the patient. Ideally, the treating psychotherapist will have gathered sufficient information to make a good decision, and this information would include a detailed social history of the patient, a review of past treatment records, and conversations with family members or other treatment providers. However, ideal conditions seldom exist. Suicidal crises sometimes occur quickly, and psychotherapists often do not have the opportunity or time to gather all this information. Frequently past records are not available for review. Sometimes it is necessary to deal with the patient's immediate needs and to delay getting all the information that one "should" get. Here and with other decisions, patient welfare must come first. Psychotherapists would not be liable simply because circumstances prevented them from obtaining all the information that they ordinarily would want to get. In other words, sometimes allowing oneself to get incomplete information in an interview is the best clinical decision.

I have sometimes talked to suicidal patients for 2 hours or more and kept them on the phone or in the session until I felt that they were safe. But I always tried to monitor the patient's fatigue level and at times even asked their permission to continue the discussion. Often I ended a conversation based on my perception of their fatigue, even though I had not yet gained every bit of information that would be necessary in an ideal evaluation. I believed that the value of whatever additional information I might have gathered would be offset by the loss in the quality of the treatment relationship if I were to pressure the patient to continue past their comfort zone.

Documentation should be as transparent when making difficult decisions. Psychotherapists who treat suicidal patients often must balance the advantages and disadvantages of possible interventions. They can document what they did, why they did it, what other actions they considered, and why those actions were rejected (Taube, 2018). The levels of service formulae described in Chapter 3 may help inform those decisions. For example, psychotherapists may have to decide whether to recommend a hospitalization, or whether to notify a family member of the suicidal intentions of their patient, even if the patient does not give consent. Often these are not easy decisions, and the treating psychotherapist must determine if the benefits of an action outweigh the risks, perhaps by using the principle-based, decision-making model described in previous chapters.

However, a reader should be able to look at the notes and get a general impression of what information the psychotherapist was using and the reasons why a decision was made. Often, psychotherapists know that their decisions have risks to them. For example, a psychotherapist might have reason to believe that hospitalizing a patient would decrease the risk of a suicide in the short term but increase the risk of a suicide in the long run. If so, the psychotherapist should document the reasons for the hospitalization, the reasons against hospitalization, and the reason why the final decision was made.

ENSURING EMOTIONAL COMPETENCE

One of the core competencies in working with suicidal patients identified by Cramer et al. (2013) was ensuring emotional competence. Maintaining competence means more than just keeping up-to-date with the changing knowledge base and standards of care. Competence also includes maintaining *psychological fitness* or the "emotional or mental stability of a professional" relevant to their "capacity to practice safely and effectively" (W. B. Johnson et al., 2008, p. 590). Psychological fitness requires "self-care" or protecting and promoting one's physical or mental well-being.

Research from several authors has suggested that the rates of mental illness among psychologists approximate those of the population in general. For example, Follette, Polusny, and Milbeck (1994) found that mental health professionals had rates of personal distress similar to those of law enforcement officials. Norcross, Prochaska, and DiClemente (1986) found that the prevalence of psychological distress was no greater in psychotherapists than in laypersons. Blume-Marcovici, Stolberg, and Khademi (2013) found that on the Neuroticism scale of the Big Five, psychologists did not significantly differ from nonclinical samples (psychologists 5.1, compared with 4.8 for the population in general).

Although the rates of mental illness among psychotherapists may approximate the rates found in the population in general, psychotherapists face unique stressors, such as vicarious trauma, burnout, and compassion fatigue, and sometimes even harassment, stalking, cyberstalking, or even physical assaults (see review by Tamura, 2012). Psychotherapists have to deal with the risk of a patient suicide, and many will have patients die from suicide. J. Sternlieb referred to psychotherapy as "an emotional contact sport" (personal communication, June 15, 2018). It inevitably leads psychotherapists to experience a lot of emotions.

Burnout is a general term used to describe dysphoric feelings that occur when work experiences exceed an individual's ability or resources to handle them with emotional stability. It involves three dimensions: emotional exhaustion, depersonalization of patients, and a diminished sense of personal achievement (Maslach & Jackson, 1981). Burnout is correlated with several factors including working in a job with considerable administrative or paperwork obligations, working with difficult patients including those who have suicidal thoughts, and working in jobs with a reduced sense of control over one's work environment (Rupert, Miller, & Dorociak, 2017). Burnout tends to be more common among younger psychologists (Dorociak, Rupert, & Zahniser, 2017).

Compassion fatigue describes the elements of burnout related to emotional exhaustion and patient depersonalization. One can easily see how dealing with stressful suicidal patients could lead to burnout or compassion fatigue among psychotherapists who lack adequate training. It can be stressful enough for psychotherapists who are well trained. Often psychotherapists will expend a huge amount of energy trying to prevent a patient suicide (K. B. Webb, 2011), which can involve substantial worry, fear, and self-doubt.

Some negative feelings are an inevitable part of the life of a psychotherapist, including negative feelings toward patients. In working with patients, psychotherapists may also experience some forbidden emotions, such as sexual attraction, anger, disgust, or hatred. Because psychotherapists have a strong motivation to accept and heal others, it can be difficult for them to accept that they may feel negatively toward their patients. It is as if they had an internal voice that said "good psychotherapists do not feel angry at their patients."

However, ill feelings are inevitable when working with people. Psychologist Robert M. Gordon (1997) facetiously created a L (lie) scale that psychologists could use similar to the one found on the Minnesota Multiphasic Personality Inventory. Some of the questions could be, "Do you ever feel like cursing at a patient?" or "Did you ever have sexual feelings toward a patient?" (p. 19). Sometimes these feelings might be fleeting thoughts of little significance. At other times they may rise to the level where they may threaten to degrade the quality of treatment. If so, the best way to handle these emotions is to talk about them with a colleague, consultant, or one's personal psychotherapist. Suppressed emotions risk popping up at unwelcomed times. Sternlieb (2013) used the phrase *emotional leaks* to refer to the ways that unprocessed emotions can get expressed in countertherapeutic comments or behaviors on the part of the psychotherapist.

When negative emotions arise, it is necessary to ask if they were due to actions on the part of the patient that would aggravate any reasonable person or if they reflect some psychological vulnerabilities on the part of the psychotherapist. When sexual feelings arise it may be necessary to ask if the sexual attraction is reflecting an unmet need on the part of the psychotherapist.

Psychotherapists can sometimes use their emotional reactions to patients to alert them to problematic patient behaviors. When psychotherapists find themselves feeling annoyed at a patient it may represent a pattern of patient behaviors that are off-putting to others in the patient's natural environment. However, when psychotherapists are dealing with many unpleasant emotions unrelated to the patient's behavior, it can become more difficult for them to use their own emotions to analyze the significance of the patient's behavior.

Experiencing Traumas

Psychotherapists may elect to work with traumatized patients out of dedication to human welfare. But every psychotherapist risks encountering some patients with terrible stories of trauma or abuse. Some may have been survivors of political torture; survived rapes or assaults; participated in military combat; been involved in serious accidents; or otherwise been harmed, threatened with serious harm, or observed serious harm to others.

Some researchers believe that psychotherapists exposed to patient traumas develop a risk of developing traumatic symptoms themselves. Brady, Guy, Polestra, and Brokaw (1999), for example, found that psychotherapists with the most exposure to sexual abuse patients had the highest scores on a posttraumatic stress disorder (PTSD) inventory. Nonetheless, the evidence for secondary traumas has been inconsistent. It appears that the link between exposure to patient traumas and secondary PTSD is weak, although some psychotherapists do experience secondary trauma symptoms (Kleespies, Efe, & Ametrano, 2017). I may have been one of those psychotherapists.

Personal Experience With Trauma

I once had mini-PTSD symptoms from my work with a traumatized patient. What he had to endure was so horrible that it gave me nightmares, and I had intrusive and unwanted thoughts of the event. I never shared the content of the events with anyone else, including my wife, who is also a psychologist, because I felt I would just be spreading the horror to others that I love. Eventually, with the help of others I was able to compartmentalize the experience so that it no longer disrupted my life.

Patients Die From Suicide[4]

Psychotherapists find the death of patients from suicide to be very stressful (Chemtob, Bauer, Hamada, Pelowski, & Muraoka, 1989, p. 297). This event often triggers sadness, grief, and guilt, and the impact may be especially difficult for trainees (Gill, 2012). There may also be fears of a lawsuit or other disciplinary action against the psychotherapist. Such fears may cause psychotherapists to withdraw from contacts with others or inhibit them from talking about the events openly with their patients. Also, Ward-Ciesielski, Wielgus, and Jones (2015) found that the family survivors of the decedent often had ill-feelings toward the psychotherapist who was treating their loved one. Having a patient die from suicide is upsetting enough, but knowing that the family members blame you makes it that much harder.

---

[4] The entire section Patients Die From Suicide is from "Psychologists and Suicide: What if It Happened to Your Patient?" by S. Knapp, 2018, *The Pennsylvania Psychologist, 78,* pp. 4–5. Copyright 2018 by the Pennsylvania Psychological Association. Adapted with permission.

Psychotherapists who have survived a patient suicide have told me that the phone call they received about their patient's death struck them like a bolt of lightning. Frequently, they can repeat the exact words spoken to them, such as "Your patient is dead," or "You do not know me, but my brother always spoke highly of you." They can tell the time of day, where they were, and other circumstances of the event in detail. Baba Neal (2017) wrote,

> It was a Sunday night, and I was having dinner at a friend's house. I did not recognize the number that showed up on my phone. As soon as the caller introduced himself as a police inspector . . . I knew what his next words would be. (p. 174)

When I speak to such psychotherapists I always say, "I am sorry for your loss," recognizing that they are secondary victims of the suicide. Often they have called me for practical advice, such as how to respond to the family, what to tell the coroner, and so on. But I always ask them about their emotional well-being.

Talking with a colleague is perhaps the best response to these shocks. This allows psychotherapists the opportunity to vent, to express their concerns and regrets, and to receive emotional support. On the surface it appears that speaking to another psychotherapist who had also had a patient die from suicide would be especially helpful.

I have spoken to some excellent psychotherapists who have had patients die from suicide.

Sometimes the dreaded suicide was not unexpected. At other times it was quite unexpected.

One psychologist told me that the patient had denied any suicidal thoughts when he was asked about it during the first interview and showed no risk factors that would suggest a risk of suicide. I reminded the psychologist that as many people who die from suicide come from low-risk groups as come from high-risk groups.

Some psychotherapists work in institutions that review sentinel events such as suicide. These reviews are intended to look at what could have been done institution-wide to prevent such events, and ideally the review does not presume misconduct on the part of the psychotherapist. I have known psychotherapists who worked in independent practices who voluntarily submitted their records to a third party to get feedback on the quality of their services.

Handling Other Professional Stressors

What can psychotherapists do to ensure their emotional well-being and minimize the likelihood that they will be burdened by burnout, compassion fatigue, vicarious trauma, excessive grief over the suicide of a patient, or other disturbances that occur when working with suicidal patients? These profession-specific life events need to be put in perspective. Despite these painful events, most psychotherapists have rewarding careers (Dorociak et al., 2017).

Effective psychotherapists anticipate work stressors and develop strategies for handling them. They have taken seriously the recommendation of W. B. Johnson, Bertschinger, Snell, and Wilson (2014), who said that psychologists should "vigorously pursue self-care" (p. 71) and self-compassion. Many of the following strategies for ensuring self-care would be ones that could have been predicted from self-determination theory (Ryan & Deci, 2008). That is, the work will be more rewarding if psychotherapists feel a sense of accomplishment in their work (competence), have some control over the workplace (feel autonomy), and can develop good social relationships (affiliation).

The good news is that psychotherapists appear to have less burnout and better work-related emotional health as they age (Dorociak et al., 2017), although part of this may be due to an improvement in work conditions. Early career psychologists tended to report lower levels of emotional well-being. In part this may be because they engaged in fewer self-care activities. However, it may have also occurred because early career psychologists have more administrative demands and exposure to negative patient behaviors (Dorociak et al., 2017), are more likely to have institutional jobs where they have less control over their employment situation, and have more demanding caseloads. Some institutions follow evidence-based employee practices that ensure the well-being of their employees and service beneficiaries. However, I have also seen very shortsighted agencies that impose excessive work schedules and give little support to their employees.

Sternlieb (2014) claimed that self-care is a 50/50 proposition. One half of self-care is the ability to step back and find refreshment in day-to-day activities outside of work. The other half of self-care is the ability to process the emotional wounds that occur as part of the work of psychotherapists. This includes cultivating habits of self-care and taking one's emotional temperature to ensure that one knows when to seek additional help. Habits of practice that ensure a good overall lifestyle include getting enough sleep, eating healthy foods, exercising, attending to medical needs, and ensuring a productive social life. Meditation also appears to enhance one's overall well-being.

In addition, psychotherapists need to anticipate or address the unique emotional demands that will experience as psychotherapists. The first step might be to acknowledge that one has intense emotions generated by clinical work. Perhaps the ideal psychotherapists are those who can control their emotions and maintain psychotherapeutic distance. However, it is unrealistic to think that psychotherapists will always be able to reach that ideal. As Sternlieb (2013) stated, "You must see it to be it" (p. 21), meaning that one must first acknowledge that these emotions exist and then, "You must name it to tame it" (p. 21), meaning that one must think about the emotion sufficiently to consider its dimensions and label it.

It is frequently indicated to apply psychotherapist skills, such as problem-solving or mindfulness, to ourselves (Jergensen, 2018). Having cognitive strategies that help psychotherapists keep their work in perspective appears to help (Rupert et al., 2017).

A supportive work environment is associated with lower levels of burnout (Rupert et al., 2017). If upsetting patient behaviors occur, it will be important for psychotherapists to receive emotional support. When in difficult situations, it is important to "share the burden" or involve others in the critical decision making. Sternlieb (2013) said, "You must share it to bear it" (p. 21), meaning that sharing the burden helps reduce the emotional toll on the psychotherapist. Just the opportunity to express one's dismay can have healing effects and reduce stress. Indeed, Coster and Schwebel (1997) found that social support was rated as one of the key components of success among psychologists who were nominated by their peers as being well-functioning, and Dlugos and Friedlander (2001) found that peer-nominated, passionately committed psychologists continually sought feedback and consultation.

Health care professionals who are embedded in helpful social networks tend to deliver a higher level of professional care. They have created a competency constellation for themselves. For example, psychologists belonging to the Pennsylvania Psychological Association were significantly less likely to be disciplined by the State Board of Psychology than nonmembers (Knapp & VandeCreek, 2012). A follow-up study by Schultz (2018) reached the same conclusion. In addition, working in medical practices with strong social support systems was associated with fewer patient complaints (Klimo, Daum, Brinker, McGuire, & Elliott, 2000).

The reasons for the protective nature of these social groups are not entirely clear. Perhaps more competent professionals self-selected themselves into supportive professional environments. Or perhaps having professional contact with others increased the likelihood that the professional would receive more current information on trends in professional practice. Or perhaps the affiliations gave emotional support to the professionals or put them in an environment where others would watch out for them and protect their welfare.

In addition, psychotherapists can engage in other activities that could help improve their well-being. Bearse, McMinn, Seegobin, and Free (2013) found that 86% of psychotherapists have sought therapy at least once, and that 84% of them rated psychotherapy a 4 or higher on a 5-point scale of helpfulness (5 being the most helpful). In addition to helping relieve emotional pain, many psychotherapists reported that it helped them to appreciate better the role of being a psychotherapy patient.

Also, other professionals have found that participating in Balint groups helped them to better understand and process their emotions and their reactions to their patients. Michael Balint (1964) developed these groups in the 1950s to help primary care physicians better handle their emotional reactions to patients. Subsequent professionals have applied the Balint model to other professions including psychotherapists (E. Lee & Kealy, 2014).

Furthermore, psychotherapists can use expressive writing to help them better understand and process their emotions, including both the negative and positive feelings. One of the goals of expressive writing is to "promote the uninhibited articulation of thoughts and feelings" (Baddeley & Pennebaker, 2011, p. 87). Writing about these events is important, but it is even more helpful if writers have a chance to share their writings and reflections with others.

The most effective psychotherapists are those who take care of themselves and accommodate the emotional demands of the profession. The effort to prevent suicide requires a lifelong commitment to improving one's skill level, and this commitment cannot be sustained unless psychotherapists recognize and consider the emotional demands of their work.

Afterword

The rates of suicide have been increasing substantially in the past 20 years, and there is no reason to think that this trend will change any time in the near future. The need for a workforce that is well trained in suicide assessment and prevention is more critical now than ever.

The purpose of this book has been to help psychotherapists become better at helping patients at risk of dying from suicide. In doing so, I have tried to rely on basic and applied research on suicide, and to interpret it in an ethically informed manner. Of course, research is best applied and understood from the standpoint of how it impacts the day-to-day lives of patients and those who are trying to help them.

Over the years, I have treated suicidal patients, consulted with psychologists who are treating suicidal patients, and given professional presentations on suicide to psychologists and other mental health professionals. In my presentations and consultations, I balance being authoritative with being humble. I can be authoritative because I have studied and mastered the important concepts dealing with suicide prevention. But I must be humble because there is much that I do not know and much that no one knows about suicide.

In each of these presentations I try to learn something from the participants. I have had workshop participants tell me about suicides in opioid treatment centers, effective ways to engage suicidal adolescents, controversies concerning the role of medications in treating suicidal patients, and much

http://dx.doi.org/10.1037/0000145-007
Suicide Prevention: An Ethically and Scientifically Informed Approach, by S. J. Knapp

more. Each of these encounters has had a role in forming the final version of this book. But finishing this book is only the beginning of a continuing dialogue to advance the quality of service provided and our knowledge of suicide prevention. I look forward to continued discussions with scholars and practitioners on how to improve services to patients at risk of dying from suicide.

APPENDIX A

Patient Self-Report Sheet

Name _____ Date of birth _____

Address _____

_____

Home phone (___) _____ May we leave a message?   YES   NO

   May we text scheduling information to this number?   YES   NO

Cell/other phone (___) _____ May we leave a message?   YES   NO

   May we text scheduling information to this number?   YES   NO

Emergency contact _____ Phone _____

Please circle: Never married   Married

             Separated   Divorced   Widowed

Who referred you? _____

Briefly describe your goals for psychotherapy:

_____

_____

_____

From Patient Information Sheet by Samuel Knapp, 2011. Copyright 2011 by the
Pennsylvania Psychological Association. Adapted with permission.

Mental Health Background

Please list any psychotic medications (medications for your nerves) that you are taking (include prescription, over-the-counter, herbal, or illegal drugs).

Medication	Dose/frequency	When started?	For what symptom(s)?

List any previous mental health or substance abuse treatment (including any residential or hospital treatment) that you have received.

Date of treatment (approximately)	Name of treatment provider or agency	What was your problem at that time?	Were your treatment goals met?

Was there anything in your previous treatment that was particularly helpful or harmful?

_____

_____

_____

Over the last 2 weeks, how often have you been bothered by any of the following problems?	Not At All	Several Days	More Than Half the Days	Nearly Every Day
1. Little interest or pleasure in doing things	0	1	2	3
2. Feeling down, depressed or hopeless	0	1	2	3
3. Thoughts that you would be better off dead or hurting yourself in some way	0	1	2	3

Do you prefer to use your religious or spiritual beliefs to help you during treatment?

YES _____   NO _____

Medical Information

Name of Primary Care Physician or Provider _____

I may ask you to sign an "authorization" or "release of information form" that will allow me to send basic health care information (presenting problem, summary of treatment, etc.) to your primary care provider.

How would you describe your physical health? (please circle)

Excellent　　　　Good　　　　Average　　　　Poor　　　　Very Poor

On the average night would you say that your sleep is

Excellent　　　　Good　　　　Average　　　　Poor　　　　Very Poor

Please list any medical conditions that you have.

Medical condition or symptoms	Medications or other treatments. If drugs, include over-the-counter remedies and the dose and frequency

Please list any allergies or sensitivities to drugs, foods, or other substances.

_____

_____

_____

Do you smoke or use other tobacco products? YES _____ NO _____

During an average week, do you drink (please circle)?

Nothing　　1–2 drinks　　3–6 drinks　　6–10 drinks　　more than 10 drinks

Do you currently use recreational drugs such as marijuana, heroin, or other drugs?

YES ____　　NO ____

If yes, please indicate what you use and how much you use in an average week.

_____

_____

_____

Is there any other information that would be useful to know about you?

_____

_____

_____

Social History

Highest educational level (please circle one)

Did Not Finish High School   High School   Some College

College   Graduate or Professional School

Occupation _____

Current employer (or school) _____

How long have you worked there? _____

Please describe your social life (please circle one).

I often feel lonely   I sometimes feel lonely

I seldom feel lonely   I never feel lonely

Does your family have a history of mental illness or substance abuse? If so, please explain the nature of the problem, treatments they received, and the outcome of that treatment.

_____

_____

_____

Legal Information

Legal event		If Yes, give a brief description
Have you ever been arrested (include driving under the influence [DUIs])?	YES NO	_____ _____ _____
Have you ever been in prison?	YES NO	_____ _____ _____
Are you currently involved in any litigation?	YES NO	_____ _____ _____

Content Areas to Be Covered for Initial Interview and Additional Topics Relevant to Assessing Suicidal Patients

Presenting problems or reason for referral

1. Emotions likely to appear in the suicide crisis states including, but not limited to, entrapment, defeat, humiliation, perceived burdensomeness, thwarted belongingness, agitation, irritability, insomnia, self-disgust, and impulsivity

2. Acquired capability, including past suicide attempts and exposure to violence or suffering

Past psychiatric treatment—ask about past suicide behavior

Family history

1. Any family history of suicidal behavior

2. Marital history and status, children, and current level of social support within family

3. Any disruptors, social losses, or social strains within family and resilience (how well are they able to handle these social issues?), looking for perceived hopelessness in correcting any social disruptions, and perception of self as important to the family unit which taps perceived burdensomeness or thwarted belongingness

4. Childhood and general style of parenting looking for attachment history and indications of child abuse

Psychosocial history

1. Current social field, including friends and other social contacts and any recent social stressors or losses

2. Social media presence

3. Legal history such as DUIs or incarceration

Items in boldface are content areas to be covered for initial interview.

4. Any history of trauma either as a victim, witness, or perpetrator

5. Current employment and financial status, employment history, education level

6. Recent stressful events or chronic stressors and resilience (how well have they responded to these events?)

7. Sexual orientation

8. Cultural identity and any cultural strains

9. (if applicable) Religious participation and centers of meaning or belief system (life-protecting and life-promoting beliefs, and religious coping style)

10. Friends who have attempted suicide

Health history, including current medical conditions and current medications

1. Current medical conditions and medications and any recent changes

2. (if applicable) Functional limitations, chronic pain, sleep habits (insomnia or nightmares)

Substance history—including substance abuse and use of prescription, alternative, or over-the-counter medications

Mental status exam

1. Expand on mental status and look for disordered thinking such as cognitive rigidity, absolutist thinking, ruminations, or failures at thought suppression

2. Look for psychological strengths including commitments to others

3. Behaviors in treatment including openness, willingness to ask for help, any perception of self-stigma, receptiveness to comments, connection with psychotherapist

Risk factors for self-harm—see information listed above

REFERENCES

Abdollahi, A., Abu Talib, M., Yaacob, S. N., & Ismail, Z. (2015). The role of hardiness in decreasing stress and suicidal ideation in a sample of undergraduate students. *Journal of Humanistic Psychology, 55,* 202–222. http://dx.doi.org/ 10.1177/0022167814543952

Abrutyn, S., & Mueller, A. S. (2014). Are suicidal behaviors contagious in adolescence? Using longitudinal data to examine suicide suggestion. *American Sociological Review, 79,* 211–227. http://dx.doi.org/10.1177/0003122413519445

Al-Mosaiwi, M., & Johnstone, T. (2018). In an absolute state: Elevated use of absolutist words is a marker specific to anxiety, depression, and suicidal ideation. *Clinical Psychological Science, 6,* 529–542. http://dx.doi.org/10.1177/ 2167702617747074

Alavi, N., Reshetukha, T., Prost, E., Antoniak, K., & Groll, D. (2017). Assessing suicide risk: What is commonly missed in the emergency room? *Journal of Psychiatric Practice, 23,* 82–91. http://dx.doi.org/10.1097/PRA.0000000000000216

Alderson, M., Parent-Rocheleau, X., & Mishara, B. (2015). Critical review on suicide among nurses. *Crisis, 36,* 91–101. http://dx.doi.org/10.1027/0227-5910/ a000305

Alonzo, D., Moravec, C., & Kaufman, B. (2017). Individuals at risk for suicide: Mental health clinicians' perspectives on barriers to and facilitators of treatment engagement. *Crisis, 38,* 158–167. http://dx.doi.org/10.1027/0227-5910/a000427

American Association of Suicidology. (n.d.). *Core competencies for the assessment and management of individuals at risk for suicide.* Retrieved from http://www. suicidology.org/Portals/14/docs/Training/RRSR_Core_Competencies.pdf

American Psychological Association. (2007). Record keeping guidelines. *American Psychologist, 62,* 993–1004. http://dx.doi.org/10.1037/0003-066X.62.9.993

American Psychological Association. (2017). *Ethical principles of psychologists and code of conduct* (2002, Amended June 1, 2010, and January 1, 2017). Retrieved from http://www.apa.org/ethics/code/index.aspx

Andreasson, K., Krogh, J., Wenneberg, C., Jessen, H. K., Krakauer, K., Gluud, C., . . . Nordentoft, M. (2016). Effectiveness of dialectical behavior therapy versus collaborative assessment and management of suicidality treatment for reduction of self-harm in adults with borderline personality traits and disorder—a randomized observer-blinded clinical trial. *Depression and Anxiety, 33,* 520–530.

Andriessen, K., Rahman, B., Draper, B., Dudley, M., & Mitchell, P. B. (2017). Prevalence of exposure to suicide: A meta-analysis of population-based studies. *Journal of Psychiatric Research, 88,* 113–120. http://dx.doi.org/10.1016/j.jpsychires.2017.01.017

Anestis, M. D. (2016). Prior suicide attempts are less common in suicide decedents who died by firearms relative to those who died by other means. *Journal of Affective Disorders, 189,* 106–109. http://dx.doi.org/10.1016/j.jad.2015.09.007

Anestis, M. D., Butterworth, S. E., & Houtsma, C. (2018). Perceptions of firearms and suicide: The role of misinformation in storage practices and openness to means safety measures. *Journal of Affective Disorders, 227,* 530–535. http://dx.doi.org/10.1016/j.jad.2017.11.057

Anestis, M. D., Joiner, T., Hanson, J. E., & Gutierrez, P. M. (2014). The modal suicide decedent did not consume alcohol just prior to the time of death: An analysis with implications for understanding suicidal behavior. *Journal of Abnormal Psychology, 123,* 835–840. http://dx.doi.org/10.1037/a0037480

Anestis, M. D., Law, K. C., Jin, H., Houtsma, C., Khazem, L. R., & Assavedo, B. L. (2017). Treating the capability for suicide: A vital and understudied frontier in suicide prevention. *Suicide and Life-Threatening Behavior, 47,* 523–537. http://dx.doi.org/10.1111/sltb.12311

Anestis, M. D., Moberg, F. B., & Arnau, R. C. (2014). Hope and the interpersonal-psychological theory of suicidal behavior: Replication and extension of prior findings. *Suicide and Life-Threatening Behavior, 44,* 175–187. http://dx.doi.org/10.1111/sltb.12060

Aronson, K. R., Kyler, S. J., Love, L., Morgan, N. R., & Perkins, D. F. (2017). Spouse and family functioning before and after a Marine's suicide: Comparisons to deaths by accident and in combat. *Military Psychology, 29,* 294–306. http://dx.doi.org/10.1037/mil0000156

Artenie, A. A., Bruneau, J., Zang, G., Lespérance, F., Renaud, J., Tremblay, J., & Jutras-Aswad, D. (2015). Associations of substance use patterns with attempted suicide among persons who inject drugs: Can distinct use patterns play a role? *Drug and Alcohol Dependence, 147,* 208–214. http://dx.doi.org/10.1016/j.drugalcdep.2014.11.011

Association of State and Provincial Psychology Boards. (2017). *Competencies expected of psychologists at the point of licensure.* Retrieved from https://cdn.ymaws.com/www.asppb.net/resource/resmgr/guidelines/2017_ASPPB_Competencies_Expe.pdf

Austin, A. E., van den Heuvel, C., & Byard, R. W. (2013). Physician suicide. *Journal of Forensic Sciences, 58*(Suppl. 1), S91–S93. http://dx.doi.org/10.1111/j.1556-4029.2012.02260.x

Baba Neal, S. (2017). The impact of a client's suicide. *Transactional Analysis Journal, 47,* 173–185. http://dx.doi.org/10.1177/0362153717711701

Baddeley, J., & Pennebaker, J. W. (2011). The expressive writing method. In L. L'Abate & G. G. Sweeny (Eds.), *Research on writing approaches in mental health* (pp. 85–92). Bingley, England: Emerald Group. http://dx.doi.org/10.1163/9780857249562_007

Bagge, C. L., Littlefield, A. K., & Glenn, C. R. (2017). Trajectories of affective response as warning signs for suicide attempts: An examination of the 48 hours prior to a recent suicide attempt. *Clinical Psychological Science, 5,* 259–271. http://dx.doi.org/10.1177/2167702616681628

Bakhiyi, C. L., Calati, R., Guillaume, S., & Courtet, P. (2016). Do reasons for living protect against suicidal thoughts and behaviors? A systematic review of the literature. *Journal of Psychiatric Research, 77,* 92–108. http://dx.doi.org/10.1016/j.jpsychires.2016.02.019

Balint, M. (1964). *The doctor, his patient and the illness.* London, England: Pitman Medical.

Barlow, M. R., Goldsmith Turow, R. E., & Gerhart, J. (2017). Trauma appraisals, emotion regulation difficulties, and self-compassion predict posttraumatic stress symptoms following childhood abuse. *Child Abuse & Neglect, 65,* 37–47. http://dx.doi.org/10.1016/j.chiabu.2017.01.006

Bastiampillai, T., Sharfstein, S. S., & Allison, S. (2016). Increase in US suicide rates and the critical decline in psychiatric beds. *JAMA, 316,* 2591–2592. http://dx.doi.org/10.1001/jama.2016.16989

Bastin, C., Harrison, B. J., Davey, C. G., Moll, J., & Whittle, S. (2016). Feelings of shame, embarrassment and guilt and their neural correlates: A systematic review. *Neuroscience and Biobehavioral Reviews, 71,* 455–471. http://dx.doi.org/10.1016/j.neubiorev.2016.09.019

Bateman, A., & Fonagy, P. (2009). Randomized controlled trial of outpatient mentalization-based treatment versus structured clinical management for borderline personality disorder. *The American Journal of Psychiatry, 166,* 1355–1364. http://dx.doi.org/10.1176/appi.ajp.2009.09040539

Bateman, A., & Fonagy, P. (2019). A randomized controlled trial of mentalization-based intervention (MBT-FACTS) for families of people with borderline personality disorder. *Personality Disorders, 12,* 70–79. http://dx.doi.org/10.1037/per0000298

Bearse, J. L., McMinn, M. R., Seegobin, W., & Free, K. (2013). Barriers to psychologists seeking mental health care. *Professional Psychology: Research and Practice, 44,* 150–157. http://dx.doi.org/10.1037/a0031182

Beauchamp, T. L., & Childress, J. (1994). *Principles of biomedical ethics* (4th ed.). New York, NY: Oxford University Press.

Beauchamp, T. L., & Childress, J. (2009). *Principles of biomedical ethics* (6th ed.). New York, NY: Oxford University Press.

Beck, A. T. (1991). *Beck Scale Suicide Ideation.* San Antonio, TX: Pearson.

Beck, A. T. (1993). *Beck Hopelessness Scale.* San Antonio, TX: Pearson.

Beck, A. T., Steer, R. A., & Brown, G. K. (1996). *Beck Depression Inventory–II.* San Antonio, TX: Pearson.

Bedics, J. D., Atkins, D. C., Harned, M. S., & Linehan, M. M. (2015). The therapeutic alliance as a predictor of outcome in dialectical behavior therapy versus non-behavioral psychotherapy by experts for borderline personality disorder. *Psychotherapy, 52,* 67–77. http://dx.doi.org/10.1037/a0038457

Bell, C. M., Ridley, J. A., Overholser, J. C., Young, K., Athey, A., Lehmann, J., & Phillips, K. (2018). The role of perceived burden and social support in suicide and depression. *Suicide and Life-Threatening Behavior, 48,* 87–94. http://dx.doi.org/10.1111/sltb.12327

Bennett, B., Knapp, S., Harris, E., Bricklin, P., VandeCreek, L., & Younggren, J. (2006). *Assessing and managing risk in psychological practice*. Washington, DC: APAIT.

Berman, A. L. (2018). Risk factors proximate to suicide and suicide risk assessment in the context of denied suicide ideation. *Suicide and Life-Threatening Behavior, 48*, 340–352. http://dx.doi.org/10.1111/sltb.12351

Berman, A. L., & Silverman, M. M. (2014). Suicide risk assessment and risk formulation part II: Suicide risk formulation and the determination of levels of risk. *Suicide and Life-Threatening Behavior, 44*, 432–443. http://dx.doi.org/10.1111/sltb.12067

Berman, A. L., & Silverman, M. M. (2017). How to ask about suicide? A question in need of an empirical answer. *Crisis, 38*, 213–216. http://dx.doi.org/10.1027/0227-5910/a000501

Bernert, R. A., Turvey, C. L., Conwell, Y., & Joiner, T. E., Jr. (2014). Association of poor subjective sleep quality with risk for death by suicide during a 10-year period: A longitudinal, population-based study of late life. *JAMA Psychiatry, 71*, 1129–1137. http://dx.doi.org/10.1001/jamapsychiatry.2014.1126

Betz, M. E., Kautzman, M., Segal, D. L., Miller, I., Camargo, C. A., Jr., Boudreaux, E. D., & Arias, S. A. (2018). Frequency of lethal means assessment among emergency department patients with a positive suicide risk screen. *Psychiatry Research, 260*, 30–35. http://dx.doi.org/10.1016/j.psychres.2017.11.038

Betz, M. E., & Wintemute, G. J. (2015). Physician counseling on firearm safety: A new kind of cultural competence. *JAMA, 314*, 449–450. http://dx.doi.org/10.1001/jama.2015.7055

Bhugra, D. (2013). Cultural values and self-harm. *Crisis, 34*, 221–222. http://dx.doi.org/10.1027/0227-5910/a000209

Biddle, L., Derges, J., Mars, B., Heron, J., Donovan, J. L., Potokar, J., . . . Gunnell, D. (2016). Suicide and the Internet: Changes in the accessibility of suicide-related information between 2007 and 2014. *Journal of Affective Disorders, 190*, 370–375. http://dx.doi.org/10.1016/j.jad.2015.10.028

Blakey, S. M., Wagner, H. R., Naylor, J., Brancu, M., Lane, I., Sallee, M., . . . the VA Mid-Atlantic MIRECC Workgroup. (2018). Chronic pain, TBI, and PTSD in military veterans: A link to suicidal ideation and violent impulses? *The Journal of Pain, 19*, 797–806. http://dx.doi.org/10.1016/j.jpain.2018.02.012

Blume-Marcovici, A. C., Stolberg, R. A., & Khademi, M. (2013). Do therapists cry in therapy? The role of experience and other factors in therapists' tears. *Psychotherapy, 50*, 224–234. http://dx.doi.org/10.1037/a0031384

Bogdanowicz, K. M., Stewart, R., Chang, C. K., Downs, J., Khondoker, M., Shetty, H., . . . Hayes, R. D. (2016). Identifying mortality risks in patients with opioid use disorder using brief screening assessment: Secondary mental health clinical records analysis. *Drug and Alcohol Dependence, 164*, 82–88. http://dx.doi.org/10.1016/j.drugalcdep.2016.04.036

Bohnert, A. S. B., Roeder, K. M., & Ilgen, M. A. (2011). Suicide attempts and overdoses among adults entering addictions treatment: Comparing correlates in a U.S. national study. *Drug and Alcohol Dependence, 119*, 106–112. http://dx.doi.org/10.1016/j.drugalcdep.2011.05.032

Bolton, I., & Mitchell, C. (1984). *My son . . . my son: A guide to healing after death, loss or suicide*. Atlanta, GA: Bolton Press.

Bongar, B., & Sullivan, G. (2013). *The suicidal patient: Clinical and legal standards of care* (3rd ed.). Washington, DC: American Psychological Association. http://dx.doi.org/10.1037/14184-000

Bonnewyn, A., Shah, A., Bruffaerts, R., Schoevaerts, K., Rober, P., Van Parys, H., & Demyttenaere, K. (2014). Reflections of older adults on the process preceding their suicide attempt: A qualitative approach. *Death Studies, 38*, 612–618. http://dx.doi.org/10.1080/07481187.2013.835753

Borschmann, R., Oram, S., Kinner, S. A., Dutta, R., Zimmerman, C., & Howard, L. M. (2017). Self-harm among adult victims of human trafficking who accessed secondary mental health services in England. *Psychiatric Services, 68*, 207–210. http://dx.doi.org/10.1176/appi.ps.201500509

Brady, J. L., Guy, J. D., Polestra, P. L., & Brokaw, B. F. (1999). Vicarious traumatization, spirituality, and the treatment of sexual abuse survivors: A national study of women psychotherapists. *Professional Psychology: Research and Practice, 30*, 386–393. http://dx.doi.org/10.1037/0735-7028.30.4.386

Brausch, A. M., & Perkins, N. M. (2018). Nonsuicidal self-injury and disordered eating: Differences in acquired capability and suicide attempt severity. *Psychiatry Research, 266*, 72–78. http://dx.doi.org/10.1016/j.psychres.2018.05.021

Breen, A., Blankley, K., & Fine, J. (2017). The efficacy of prazosin for the treatment of posttraumatic stress disorder nightmares in U.S. military veterans. *Journal of the American Association of Nurse Practitioners, 29*, 65–69. http://dx.doi.org/10.1002/2327-6924.12432

Brent, D. A., Poling, K. D., & Goldstein, T. R. (2011). *Treating depressed and suicidal adolescents: A clinician's guide*. New York, NY: Guilford Press.

Britton, P. C., Bryan, C. J., & Valenstein, M. (2016). Motivational interviewing for restriction counseling with patients at risk for suicide. *Cognitive and Behavioral Practice, 23*, 51–61. http://dx.doi.org/10.1016/j.cbpra.2014.09.004

Brown, L. A., Contractor, A., & Benhamou, K. (2018). Posttraumatic stress disorder clusters and suicidal ideation. *Psychiatry Research, 270*, 238–245. http://dx.doi.org/10.1016/j.psychres.2018.09.030

Bryan, C. J., Bryan, A. O., May, A. M., & Klonsky, E. D. (2015). Trajectories of suicide ideation, nonsuicidal self-injury, and suicide attempts in a nonclinical sample of military personnel and veterans. *Suicide and Life-Threatening Behavior, 45*, 315–325. http://dx.doi.org/10.1111/sltb.12127

Bryan, C. J., Garland, E. L., & Rudd, M. D. (2016). From impulse to action among military personnel hospitalized for suicide risk: Alcohol consumption and the reported transition from suicidal thought to behavior. *General Hospital Psychiatry, 41*, 13–19. http://dx.doi.org/10.1016/j.genhosppsych.2016.05.001

Bryan, C. J., Grove, J. L., & Kimbrel, N. A. (2017). Theory-driven models of self-directed violence among individuals with PTSD. *Current Opinion in Psychology, 14*, 12–17. http://dx.doi.org/10.1016/j.copsyc.2016.09.007

Bryan, C. J., Mintz, J., Clemans, T. A., Leeson, B., Burch, T. S., Williams, S. R., . . . Rudd, M. D. (2017). Effect of crisis response planning vs. contracts for safety on suicide risk in U.S. Army Soldiers: A randomized clinical trial. *Journal of Affective Disorders, 212*, 64–72. http://dx.doi.org/10.1016/j.jad.2017.01.028

Bryan, C. J., & Rozek, D. C. (2018). Suicide prevention in the military: A mechanistic perspective. *Current Opinion in Psychology, 22*, 27–32. http://dx.doi.org/10.1016/j.copsyc.2017.07.022

Bryan, C. J., & Rudd, M. D. (2006). Advances in the assessment of suicide risk. *Journal of Clinical Psychology, 62*, 185–200. http://dx.doi.org/10.1002/jclp.20222

Bryan, C. J., & Rudd, M. D. (2018). *Brief cognitive-behavioral therapy for suicide prevention.* New York, NY: Guilford Press.

Bryan, C. J., Rudd, M. D., Peterson, A. L., Young-McCaughan, S., & Wertenberger, E. G. (2016). The ebb and flow of the wish to live and the wish to die among suicidal military personnel. *Journal of Affective Disorders, 202*, 58–66. http://dx.doi.org/10.1016/j.jad.2016.05.049

Bryan, C. J., Stone, S. L., & Rudd, M. D. (2011). A practical, evidence-based approach for means-restriction counseling with suicidal patients. *Professional Psychology: Research and Practice, 42*, 339–346. http://dx.doi.org/10.1037/a0025051

Bush, N. E., Smolenski, D. J., Denneson, L. M., Williams, H. B., Thomas, E. K., & Dobscha, S. K. (2017). A virtual hope box: Randomized controlled trial of a smartphone app for emotional regulation and coping with distress. *Psychiatric Services, 68*, 330–336. http://dx.doi.org/10.1176/appi.ps.201600283

Buysse, D. J., Rush, A. J., & Reynolds, C. F., III. (2017). Clinical management of insomnia disorder. *Journal of the American Medical Association, 318*, 1973–1974. http://dx.doi.org/10.1001/jama.2017.15683

Calati, R., & Courtet, P. (2016). Is psychotherapy effective for reducing suicide attempt and non-suicidal self-injury rates? Meta-analysis and meta-regression of literature data. *Journal of Psychiatric Research, 79*, 8–20. http://dx.doi.org/10.1016/j.jpsychires.2016.04.003

Calati, R., Courtet, P., & Lopez-Castroman, J. (2018). Refining suicide prevention: A narrative review on advances in psychotherapeutic tools. *Current Psychiatry Reports, 20*, 14. http://dx.doi.org/10.1007/s11920-018-0876-0

Calati, R., Ferrari, C., Brittner, M., Oasi, O., Olié, E., Carvalho, A. F., & Courtet, P. (2019). Suicidal thoughts and behaviors and social isolation: A narrative review of the literature. *Journal of Affective Disorders, 245*, 653–667. http://dx.doi.org/10.1016/j.jad.2018.11.022

Campbell, G., Bruno, R., Darke, S., Shand, F., Hall, W., Farrell, M., & Degenhardt, L. (2016). Prevalence and correlates of suicidal thoughts and suicide attempts in people prescribed pharmaceutical opioids for chronic pain. *The Clinical Journal of Pain, 32*, 292–301. http://dx.doi.org/10.1097/AJP.0000000000000283

Canadian Psychological Association. (2017). *Canadian code of ethics for psychologists.* Retrieved from https://www.cpa.ca/docs/File/Ethics/CPA_Code_2017_4thEd.pdf

Capron, D. W., & Schmidt, N. B. (2016). Development and randomized trial evaluation of a novel computer-delivered anxiety sensitivity intervention. *Behaviour Research and Therapy, 81*, 47–55. http://dx.doi.org/10.1016/j.brat.2016.04.001

Carrara, B. S., & Ventura, C. A. A. (2018). Self-stigma, mentally ill persons and health services: An integrative review of literature. *Archives of Psychiatric Nursing, 32*, 317–324. http://dx.doi.org/10.1016/j.apnu.2017.11.001

Carter, G., Milner, A., McGill, K., Pirkis, J., Kapur, N., & Spittal, M. J. (2017). Predicting suicidal behaviours using clinical instruments: Systematic review and meta-analysis of positive predictive values for risk scales. *The British Journal of Psychiatry, 210*, 387–395. http://dx.doi.org/10.1192/bjp.bp.116.182717

Cassiello-Robbins, C., Wilner, J. G., Peters, J. R., Bentley, K. H., & Sauer-Zavala, S. (2019). Elucidating the relationships between shame, anger, and self-destructive behaviors: The role of aversive responses to emotions. *Journal of Contextual Behavioral Science, 12,* 7–12. http://dx.doi.org/10.1016/j.jcbs.2018.12.004

Castonguay, L. G. (2013). Psychotherapy outcome: An issue worth re-revisiting 50 years later. *Psychotherapy, 50,* 52–67. http://dx.doi.org/10.1037/a0030898

Castonguay, L. G., Boswell, J. F., Constantino, M. J., Goldfried, M. R., & Hill, C. E. (2010). Training implications of harmful effects of psychological treatments. *American Psychologist, 65,* 34–49. http://dx.doi.org/10.1037/a0017330

Center for Collegiate Mental Health. (2018). *2017 annual report.* Retrieved from https://ccmh.psu.edu/files/2018/02/2017_CCMH_Report-1r4m88x.pdf

Centers for Disease Control and Prevention. (2016). *Ten leading causes of death by age group, United States—2014.* Retrieved from http://www.cdc.gov/injury/images/lc-charts/leading_causes_of_death_age_group_2014_1050w760h.gif

Chamberlain, S. R., Redden, S. A., & Grant, J. E. (2017). Associations between self-harm and distinct types of impulsivity. *Psychiatry Research, 250,* 10–16. http://dx.doi.org/10.1016/j.psychres.2017.01.050

Chambless, D. L., Allred, K. M., Chen, F. F., McCarthy, K. S., Milrod, B., & Barber, J. P. (2017). Perceived criticism predicts outcome of psychotherapy for panic disorder: Replication and extension. *Journal of Consulting and Clinical Psychology, 85,* 37–44. http://dx.doi.org/10.1037/ccp0000161

Chang, E. C., Lian, X., Yu, T., Qu, J., Zhang, B., Jia, W., . . . Hirsch, J. K. (2015). Loneliness under assault: Understanding the impact of sexual assault on the relation between loneliness and suicidal risk in college students. *Personality and Individual Differences, 72,* 155–159. http://dx.doi.org/10.1016/j.paid.2014.09.001

Chang, E. C., Yu, T., Najarian, A. S.-M., Wright, K. M., Chen, W., Chang, O. D., . . . Hirsch, J. K. (2017). Understanding the association between negative life events and suicidal risk in college students: Examining self-compassion as a potential mediator. *Journal of Clinical Psychology, 73,* 745–755. http://dx.doi.org/10.1002/jclp.22374

Cheavens, J. S., Cukrowicz, K. C., Hansen, R., & Mitchell, S. M. (2016). Incorporating resilience factors into the interpersonal theory of suicide: The role of hope and self-forgiveness in an older adult sample. *Journal of Clinical Psychology, 72,* 58–69. http://dx.doi.org/10.1002/jclp.22230

Chemtob, C. M., Bauer, G. B., Hamada, R. S., Pelowski, S. R., & Muraoka, M. Y. (1989). Patient suicide: Occupational hazard for psychologists and psychiatrists. *Professional Psychology: Research and Practice, 20,* 294–300. http://dx.doi.org/10.1037/0735-7028.20.5.294

Chesin, M. S., Benjamin-Phillips, C. A., Keilp, J., Fertuck, E. A., Brodsky, B. S., & Stanley, B. (2016). Improvements in executive attention, rumination, cognitive reactivity, and mindfulness among high-suicide risk patients participating in adjunct mindfulness-based cognitive therapy: Preliminary findings. *Journal of Alternative and Complementary Medicine, 22,* 642–649. http://dx.doi.org/10.1089/acm.2015.0351

Cheung, G., Merry, S., & Sundram, F. (2015). Late-life suicide: Insight on motives and contributors derived from suicide notes. *Journal of Affective Disorders, 185,* 17–23. http://dx.doi.org/10.1016/j.jad.2015.06.035

Choi, N. G., DiNitto, D. M., Marti, C. N., & Segal, S. P. (2017). Adverse childhood experiences and suicide attempts among those with mental and substance use disorders. *Child Abuse & Neglect, 69,* 252–262. http://dx.doi.org/10.1016/j.chiabu.2017.04.024

Christakis, N. A., & Fowler, J. H. (2009). *Connected: The surprising power of our social network and how they shape our lives.* New York, NY: Little, Brown & Co.

Christensen, H., Batterham, P. J., Mackinnon, A. J., Donker, T., & Soubelet, A. (2014). Predictors of the risk factors for suicide identified by the interpersonal-psychological theory of suicidal behaviour. *Psychiatry Research, 219,* 290–297. http://dx.doi.org/10.1016/j.psychres.2014.05.029

Chu, C., Buchman-Schmitt, J. M., Stanley, I. H., Hom, M. A., Tucker, R. P., Hagan, C. R., . . . Joiner, T. E. (2017). The interpersonal theory of suicide: A systematic review and meta-analysis of a decade of cross-national research. *Psychological Bulletin, 143,* 1313–1345. http://dx.doi.org/10.1037/bul0000123

Chu, C., Klein, K. M., Buchman-Schmitt, J. M., Hom, M. A., Hagan, C. R., & Joiner, T. E. (2015). Routinized assessment of suicide risk in clinical practice: An empirically informed update. *Journal of Clinical Psychology, 71,* 1186–1200. http://dx.doi.org/10.1002/jclp.22210

Chu, C., Walker, K. L., Stanley, I. H., Hirsch, J. K., Greenberg, J. H., Rudd, M. D., & Joiner, T. E. (2018). Perceived problem-solving deficits and suicidal ideation: Evidence for the explanatory roles of thwarted belongingness and perceived burdensomeness in five samples. *Journal of Personality and Social Psychology, 115,* 137–160. http://dx.doi.org/10.1037/pspp0000152

Chu, J., Chi, K., Chen, K., & Leino, A. (2014). Ethnic variations in suicidal ideation and behaviors: A prominent subtype marked by nonpsychiatric factors among Asian Americans. *Journal of Clinical Psychology, 70,* 1211–1226. http://dx.doi.org/10.1002/jclp.22082

Chu, J., Khoury, O., Ma, J., Bahn, F., Bongar, B., & Goldblum, P. (2017). An empirical model and ethnic differences in cultural meanings via motives for suicide. *Journal of Clinical Psychology, 73,* 1343–1359. http://dx.doi.org/10.1002/jclp.22425

Chu, J. P., Goldblum, P., Floyd, R., & Bongar, B. (2010). The cultural theory and model of suicide. *Applied & Preventive Psychology, 14,* 25–40. http://dx.doi.org/10.1016/j.appsy.2011.11.001

Chu, J. P., Hoeflein, B. T. R., Gadinsky, N., Goldblum, P., Bongar, B., Heyne, G. M., & Skinta, M. D. (2017). Innovations in the practice of culturally competent suicide risk management. *Practice Innovations, 2,* 66–79. http://dx.doi.org/10.1037/pri0000044

Chung, D. T., Ryan, C. J., & Large, M. M. (2016). Commentary: Adverse experiences in psychiatric hospitals might be the cause of some postdischarge suicides. *Bulletin of the Menninger Clinic, 80,* 371–375. http://dx.doi.org/10.1521/bumc.2016.80.4.371

Clark, J. L., Algoe, S. B., & Green, M. C. (2018). Social network sites and well-being: The role of social connection. *Current Directions in Psychological Science, 27,* 32–37. http://dx.doi.org/10.1177/0963721417730833

Conner, K. R., Bagge, C. L., Goldston, D. B., & Ilgen, M. A. (2014). Alcohol and suicidal behavior: What is known and what can be done. *American Journal of Preventive Medicine, 47*(Suppl. 2), S204–S208. http://dx.doi.org/10.1016/j.amepre.2014.06.007

Cook, T. B., & Davis, M. S. (2012). Assessing legal strains and risk of suicide using archived court data. *Suicide and Life-Threatening Behavior, 42,* 495–506. http://dx.doi.org/10.1111/j.1943-278X.2012.00107.x

Coope, C., Donovan, J., Wilson, C., Barnes, M., Metcalfe, C., Hollingworth, W., . . . Gunnell, D. (2015). Characteristics of people dying by suicide after job loss, financial difficulties and other economic stressors during a period of recession (2010–2011): A review of coroners' records. *Journal of Affective Disorders, 183,* 98–105. http://dx.doi.org/10.1016/j.jad.2015.04.045

Corrigan, P. W., Sheehan, L., Al-Khouja, M. A., & the Stigma of Suicide Research Group. (2017). Making sense of the public stigma of suicide: Factor analysis of its stereotypes, prejudices, and discriminations. *Crisis, 38,* 351–359. http://dx.doi.org/10.1027/0227-5910/a000456

Coster, J., & Schwebel, M. (1997). Well-functioning in professional psychologists. *Professional Psychology: Research and Practice, 28,* 5–13. http://dx.doi.org/10.1037/0735-7028.28.1.5

Coughlan, K., Tata, P., & MacLeod, A. K. (2017). Personal goals, well-being and deliberate self- harm. *Cognitive Therapy and Research, 41,* 434–443. http://dx.doi.org/10.1007/s10608-016-9769-x

Coupland, C., Hill, T., Morriss, R., Arthur, A., Moore, M., & Hippisley-Cox, J. (2015). Antidepressant use and risk of suicide and attempted suicide or self harm in people aged 20 to 64: Cohort study using a primary care database. *BMJ: British Medical Journal, 350,* h517. http://dx.doi.org/10.1136/bmj.h517

Cramer, R. J., Johnson, S. M., McLaughlin, J., Rausch, E. M., & Conroy, M. A. (2013). Suicide risk assessment training for psychology doctoral programs: Core competencies and a framework for training. *Training and Education in Professional Psychology, 7,* 1–11. http://dx.doi.org/10.1037/a0031836

Cristea, I. A., Gentili, C., Cotet, C. D., Palomba, D., Barbui, C., & Cuijpers, P. (2017). Efficacy of psychotherapies for borderline personality disorder: A systematic review and meta- analysis. *JAMA Psychiatry, 74,* 319–328. http://dx.doi.org/10.1001/jamapsychiatry.2016.4287

Crowder, M. K., & Kemmelmeier, M. (2018). Cultural differences in shame and guilt as understandable reasons for suicide. *Psychological Reports, 121,* 396–429. http://dx.doi.org/10.1177/0033294117728288

Crump, C., Sundquist, K., Winkleby, M. A., & Sundquist, J. (2013). Mental disorders and risk of accidental death. *The British Journal of Psychiatry, 203,* 297–302. http://dx.doi.org/10.1192/bjp.bp.112.123992

Currier, J. M., Smith, P. N., & Kulhman, S. (2017). Assessing the unique role of religious coping in suicidal behavior among U.S. Iraq and Afghanistan veterans. *Psychology of Religion and Spirituality, 9,* 118–123. http://dx.doi.org/10.1037/rel0000055

Czyz, E. K., Horwitz, A. G., Eisenberg, D., Kramer, A., & King, C. A. (2013). Self-reported barriers to professional help seeking among college students at elevated risk for suicide. *Journal of American College Health, 61,* 398–406. http://dx.doi.org/10.1080/07448481.2013.820731

Czyz, E. K., Horwitz, A. G., & King, C. A. (2016). Self-rated expectations of suicidal behavior predict future suicide attempts among adolescent and young adult psychiatric emergency patients. *Depression and Anxiety, 33,* 512–519. http://dx.doi.org/10.1002/da.22514

D'Agata, M. T., & Holden, R. R. (2018). Self-concealment and perfectionist self-presentation in concealment of psychache and suicidal ideation. *Personality and Individual Differences, 125,* 56–61. http://dx.doi.org/10.1016/j.paid.2017.12.034

Davis, D. E., Hook, J. N., McAnnally-Linz, R., Choe, E., & Placeres, V. (2017). Humility, religion, and spirituality: A review of the literature. *Psychology of Religion and Spirituality, 9,* 242–253. http://dx.doi.org/10.1037/rel0000111

Dazzi, T., Gribble, R., Wessely, S., & Fear, N. T. (2014). Does asking about suicide and related behaviours induce suicidal ideation? What is the evidence? *Psychological Medicine, 44,* 3361–3363. http://dx.doi.org/10.1017/S0033291714001299

Dlugos, R., & Friedlander, M. (2001). Passionately committed psychotherapists: A qualitative study of their experiences. *Professional Psychology: Research and Practice, 32,* 298–304. http://dx.doi.org/10.1037/0735-7028.32.3.298

Dodson, T. S., & Beck, J. G. (2017). Posttraumatic stress disorder symptoms and attitudes about social support: Does shame matter? *Journal of Anxiety Disorders, 47,* 106–113. http://dx.doi.org/10.1016/j.janxdis.2017.01.005

Dolsen, M. R., Cheng, P., Arnedt, J. T., Swanson, L., Casement, M. D., Kim, H. S., . . . Deldin, P. J. (2017). Neurophysiological correlates of suicidal ideation in major depressive disorder: Hyperarousal during sleep. *Journal of Affective Disorders, 212,* 160–166. http://dx.doi.org/10.1016/j.jad.2017.01.025

Dorociak, K. E., Rupert, P. A., & Zahniser, E. (2017). Work life, well-being, and self-care across the professional lifespan of psychologists. *Professional Psychology: Research and Practice, 48,* 429–437. http://dx.doi.org/10.1037/pro0000160

Draper, B., Krysinska, K., Snowdon, J., & De Leo, D. (2018). Awareness of suicide risk and communication between health care professionals and next-of-kin of suicides in the month before suicide. *Suicide and Life-Threatening Behavior, 48,* 449–458. http://dx.doi.org/10.1111/sltb.12365

Drouin, K. (2017). *The sentence.* Washington, DC: American Association of Suicidology. Retrieved from https://www.suicidology.org/Portals/14/docs/Writing%20Contest/2017/2017Winner%20List.pdf?ver=2017-08-29-211745-243

Druss, B. G., & Walker, E. R. (2011, February). Mental disorders and medical comorbidity. *Research Synthesis Report 21.* Princeton, NJ: Robert Wood Johnson Foundation.

Dueweke, A. R., Rojas, S. M., Anastasia, E. A., & Bridges, A. J. (2017). Can brief behavioral health interventions reduce suicidal and self-harm ideation in primary care patients? *Families, Systems, & Health, 35,* 376–381. http://dx.doi.org/10.1037/fsh0000287

Dufort, M., Stenbacka, M., & Gumpert, C. H. (2015). Physical domestic violence exposure is highly associated with suicidal attempts in both women and men. Results from the National Public Health Survey in Sweden. *European Journal of Public Health, 25,* 413–418. http://dx.doi.org/10.1093/eurpub/cku198

Dunkley, C., Borthwick, A., Bartlett, R., Dunkley, L., Palmer, S., Gleeson, S., & Kingdon, D. (2018). Hearing the suicidal patient's emotional pain. *Crisis, 39,* 267–274. http://dx.doi.org/10.1027/0227-5910/a000497

Dunster-Page, C., Haddock, G., Wainwright, L., & Berry, K. (2017). The relationship between therapeutic alliance and patient's suicidal thoughts, self-harming behaviours and suicide attempts: A systematic review. *Journal of Affective Disorders, 223,* 165–174. http://dx.doi.org/10.1016/j.jad.2017.07.040

Edwards, S. J., & Sachman, M. D. (2010). No-suicide contracts, no-suicide agreements, and no-suicide assurances: A study of their nature, utilization, perceived effectiveness, and potential to cause harm. *Crisis, 31,* 290–302. http://dx.doi.org/10.1027/0227-5910/a000048

Ehret, A. M., Joormann, J., & Berking, M. (2018). Self-compassion is more effective than acceptance and reappraisal in decreasing depressed mood in currently and formerly depressed individuals. *Journal of Affective Disorders, 226,* 220–226. http://dx.doi.org/10.1016/j.jad.2017.10.006

Ellis, B. J., Bianchi, J., Griskevicius, V., & Frankenhuis, W. E. (2017). Beyond risk and protective factors: An adaption-based approach to resilience. *Perspectives on Psychological Science, 12,* 561–587. http://dx.doi.org/10.1177/1745691617693054

Ellis, T. E., & Newman, C. F. (1996). *Choosing to live: How to defeat suicide through cognitive therapy.* Oakland, CA: New Harbinger.

Epstein, R. M., & Hundert, E. M. (2002). Defining and assessing professional competence. *JAMA, 287,* 226–235. http://dx.doi.org/10.1001/jama.287.2.226

Erlangsen, A., Stenager, E., & Conwell, Y. (2015). Physical diseases as predictors of suicide in older adults: A nationwide, register-based cohort study. *Social Psychiatry and Psychiatric Epidemiology, 50,* 1427–1439. http://dx.doi.org/10.1007/s00127-015-1051-0

Ewing, E. S., Diamond, G., & Levy, S. (2015). Attachment-based family therapy for depressed and suicidal adolescents: Theory, clinical model and empirical support. *Attachment & Human Development, 17,* 136–156. http://dx.doi.org/10.1080/14616734.2015.1006384

Fässberg, M. M., Cheung, G., Canetto, S. S., Erlangsen, A., Lapierre, S., Lindner, R., . . . Wærn, M. (2016). A systematic review of physical illness, functional disability, and suicidal behaviour among older adults. *Aging & Mental Health, 20,* 166–194. http://dx.doi.org/10.1080/13607863.2015.1083945

Feigelman, W., Cerel, J., McIntosh, J. L., Brent, D., & Gutin, N. (2018). Suicide exposures and bereavement among American adults: Evidence from the 2016 General Social Survey. *Journal of Affective Disorders, 227,* 1–6. http://dx.doi.org/10.1016/j.jad.2017.09.056

Fine, C. (2000). *No time to say goodbye: Surviving the suicide of a loved one.* New York, NY: Broadway Books.

Fink, M. (2014). What was learned: Studies by the consortium for research in ECT (CORE) 1997–2011. *Acta Psychiatrica Scandinavica, 129,* 417–426. http://dx.doi.org/10.1111/acps.12251

Fink-Miller, E. L., & Nestler, L. M. (2018). Suicide in physicians and veterinarians: Risk factors and theories. *Current Opinion in Psychology, 22,* 23–26. http://dx.doi.org/10.1016/j.copsyc.2017.07.019

Fogarty, A. S., Spurrier, M., Player, M. J., Wilhelm, K., Whittle, E. L., Shand, F., . . . Proudfoot, J. (2018). Tensions in perspectives on suicide prevention between men who have attempted suicide and their support networks: Secondary analysis of qualitative data. *Health Expectations, 21,* 261–269. http://dx.doi.org/10.1111/hex.12611

Follette, V. M., Polusny, M. M., & Milbeck, K. (1994). Mental health and law enforcement professionals: Trauma history, psychological symptoms, and impact of providing services to child sexual abuse survivors. *Professional Psychology: Research and Practice, 25,* 275–282. http://dx.doi.org/10.1037/0735-7028.25.3.275

Fowler, J. C. (2012). Suicide risk assessment in clinical practice: Pragmatic guidelines for imperfect assessments. *Psychotherapy, 49,* 81–90. http://dx.doi.org/10.1037/a0026148

Fowler, K. A., Jack, S. P. D., Lyons, B. H., Betz, C. J., & Petrosky, E. (2018). Surveillance for violent deaths—National Violent Death Reporting System, 18 states, 2014. *MMWR: Morbidity and Mortality Weekly Report—Surveillance Summaries, 67,* 1–36. http://dx.doi.org/10.15585/mmwr.ss6702a1

Frankfurt, S., & Frazier, P. (2016). A review of research on moral injury in combat veterans. *Military Psychology, 28,* 318–330. http://dx.doi.org/10.1037/mil0000132

Franklin, J. C., Ribeiro, J. D., Fox, K. R., Bentley, K. H., Kleiman, E. M., Huang, X., . . . Nock, M. K. (2017). Risk factors for suicidal thoughts and behaviors: A meta-analysis of 50 years of research. *Psychological Bulletin, 143,* 187–232. http://dx.doi.org/10.1037/bul0000084

Freedenthal, S. (2018). *Helping the suicidal person: Tips and techniques for professionals.* New York, NY: Routledge.

Friedman, H. S., & Martin, L. R. (2011). *The longevity project: Surprising discoveries for health and long life from the landmark eight-decade study.* New York, NY: Penguin.

Friedman, M. J. (2014). Suicide risk among soldiers: Early findings from the Army Study to Assess Risk and Resilience in Servicemembers (Army STARRS). *JAMA Psychiatry, 71,* 487–489. http://dx.doi.org/10.1001/jamapsychiatry.2014.24

Fritzsche, A., Schlier, B., Oettingen, G., & Lincoln, T. M. (2016). Mental contrasting with implementation intentions increases goal-attainment in individuals with mild to moderate depression. *Cognitive Therapy and Research, 40,* 557–564. http://dx.doi.org/10.1007/s10608-015-9749-6

Fuller-Thomson, E., Baird, S. L., Dhrodia, R., & Brennenstuhl, S. (2016). The association between adverse childhood experiences (ACEs) and suicide attempts in a population-based study. *Child: Care, Health and Development, 42,* 725–734. http://dx.doi.org/10.1111/cch.12351

Furuno, T., Nakagawa, M., Hino, K., Yamada, T., Kawashima, Y., Matsuoka, Y., . . . Hirayasu, Y. (2018). Effectiveness of assertive case management on repeat self-harm in patients admitted for suicide attempt: Findings from ACTION-J study. *Journal of Affective Disorders, 225,* 460–465. http://dx.doi.org/10.1016/j.jad.2017.08.071

Gall, T. L., & Guirguis-Younger, M. (2013). Religious and spiritual coping: Current theory and research. In K. I. Pargament, J. J. Exline, & J. W. Jones (Eds.), *APA handbook of psychology, religion, and spirituality* (Vol. 1, pp. 349–364). Washington, DC: American Psychological Association. http://dx.doi.org/10.1037/14045-019

Galynker, I. (2018). *The suicidal crisis: Clinical guide to the assessment of imminent suicide risk.* New York, NY: Oxford University Press.

Gamarra, J. M., Luciano, M. T., Gradus, J. L., & Wiltsey Stirman, S. (2015). Assessing variability and implementation fidelity of suicide prevention safety planning in a regional VA Healthcare system. *Crisis, 36,* 433–439. http://dx.doi.org/10.1027/0227-5910/a000345

Gawande, A. (2009). *The checklist manifesto: How to get things right.* New York, NY: Henry Holt.

Gearing, R. E., & Alonzo, D. (2018). Religion and suicide: New findings. *Journal of Religion and Health, 57,* 2478–2499. http://dx.doi.org/10.1007/s10943-018-0629-8

George-Levi, S., Vilchinsky, N., Tolmacz, R., Khaskiaa, A., Mosseri, M., & Hod, H. (2016). "It takes two to take": Caregiving style, relational entitlement, and medication adherence. *Journal of Family Psychology, 30,* 743–751. http://dx.doi.org/10.1037/fam0000203

Germer, C. K., & Neff, K. D. (2013). Self-compassion in clinical practice. *Journal of Clinical Psychology, 69,* 856–867. http://dx.doi.org/10.1002/jclp.22021

Ghahramanlou-Holloway, M., Neely, L. L., & Tucker, J. (2015). Treating risk for self-directed violence in inpatient settings. In C. J. Bryan (Ed.), *Cognitive behavior therapy for preventing suicide attempts: A guide to brief treatments across clinical settings* (pp. 91–109). New York, NY: Routledge.

Gill, I. J. (2012). An identity theory perspective on how trainee clinical psychologists experience the death of a patient by suicide. *Training and Education in Professional Psychology, 6,* 151–159. http://dx.doi.org/10.1037/a0029666

Glombiewski, J. A., & Rief, W. (2013). Nonadherence to medications [Letter to the editor]. *JAMA, 310,* 1505–1506.

Goldstein, A., & Gvion, Y. (2019). Socio-demographic and psychological risk factors for suicidal behavior among individuals with anorexia and bulimia nervosa: A systematic review. *Journal of Affective Disorders, 245,* 1149–1167. http://dx.doi.org/10.1016/j.jad.2018.12.015

Goodyear, R. K., & Rodolfa, E. (2012). Negotiating the complex ethical terrain of clinical supervision. In S. J. Knapp, M. C. Gottlieb, M. M. Handelsman, & L. D. VandeCreek (Eds.), *APA handbook of ethics in psychology* (Vol. 2, pp. 261–275). Washington, DC: American Psychological Association. http://dx.doi.org/10.1037/13272-013

Gordon, R. (1997, February). Handling transference and countertransference issues with difficult patients. *The Pennsylvania Psychologist, 57,* 19–20, 24.

Gray, J. S., & McCullagh, J. A. (2014). Suicide in Indian country: The continuing epidemic in rural Native American communities. *Journal of Rural Mental Health, 38,* 79–86. http://dx.doi.org/10.1037/rmh0000017

Griffiths, A. W., Wood, A. M., & Tai, S. (2018). The prospective role of defeat and entrapment in caregiver burden and depression amongst formal caregivers. *Personality and Individual Differences, 120,* 24–31. http://dx.doi.org/10.1016/j.paid.2017.08.026

Griffiths, J. J., Zarate, C. A., Jr., & Rasimas, J. J. (2014). Existing and novel biological therapeutics in suicide prevention. *American Journal of Preventive Medicine, 47*(Suppl. 2), S195–S203. http://dx.doi.org/10.1016/j.amepre.2014.06.012

Gutheil, T. G., & Schetky, D. (1998). A date with death: Management of time-based and contingent suicidal intent. *The American Journal of Psychiatry, 155,* 1502–1507. http://dx.doi.org/10.1176/ajp.155.11.1502

Guthrie, E., Kapur, N., Mackway-Jones, K., Chew-Graham, C., Moorey, J., Mendel, E., . . . Tomenson, B. (2001). Randomised controlled trial of brief psychological intervention after deliberate self poisoning. *BMJ, 323,* 135–138. http://dx.doi.org/10.1136/bmj.323.7305.135

Gysin-Maillart, A., Schwab, S., Soravia, L., Megert, M., & Michel, K. (2016). A novel brief therapy for patients who attempt suicide: A 24-months follow-up randomized controlled study of the Attempted Suicide Short Intervention Program (ASSIP). *PLoS Medicine, 13*(3), e1001968. http://dx.doi.org/10.1371/journal.pmed.1001968

Hagan, C. R., Podlogar, M. C., Chu, C., & Joiner, T. E. (2015). Testing the interpersonal theory of suicide: The moderating role of hopelessness. *International Journal of Cognitive Therapy, 8,* 99–113. http://dx.doi.org/10.1521/ijct.2015.8.2.99

Haines, S. J., Gleeson, J., Kuppens, P., Hollenstein, T., Ciarrochi, J., Labuschagne, I., . . . Koval, P. (2016). The wisdom to know the difference: Strategy-situation fit in emotional regulation in daily life is associated with well-being. *Psychological Science, 27*, 1651–1659. http://dx.doi.org/10.1177/0956797616669086

Han, B., Kott, P. S., Hughes, A., McKeon, R., Blanco, C., & Compton, W. M. (2016). Estimating the rates of deaths by suicide among adults who attempt suicide in the United States. *Journal of Psychiatric Research, 77*, 125–133. http://dx.doi.org/10.1016/j.jpsychires.2016.03.002

Han, B., McKeon, R., & Gfroerer, J. (2014). Suicidal ideation among community-dwelling adults in the United States. *American Journal of Public Health, 104*, 488–497. http://dx.doi.org/10.2105/AJPH.2013.301600

Han, J., Batterham, P. J., Calear, A. L., & Randall, R. (2018). Factors influencing professional help-seeking for suicidality: A systematic review. *Crisis, 39*, 175–196. http://dx.doi.org/10.1027/0227-5910/a000485

Harford, T. C., Yi, H.-Y., & Grant, B. F. (2014). Associations between childhood abuse and interpersonal aggression and suicide attempt among U.S. adults in a national study. *Child Abuse & Neglect, 38*, 1389–1398. http://dx.doi.org/10.1016/j.chiabu.2014.02.011

Harris, K. M., & Goh, M. T.-T. (2017). Is suicide assessment harmful to participants? Findings from a randomized controlled trial. *International Journal of Mental Health Nursing, 26*, 181–190. http://dx.doi.org/10.1111/inm.12223

Harris, L. (2018). *To call myself beloved*. Washington, DC: American Association of Suicidology. Retrieved from https://www.suicidology.org/Portals/14/docs/Writing%20Contest/2018%20Winners/QuinnettAwardWinners2018V2.pdf

Harris, R. (2008). *The happiness trap*. Boston, MA: Trumpeter.

Hawkins, D. N., & Booth, A. (2005). Unhappily ever after: Effects of long-term low-quality marriages on well-being. *Social Forces, 84*, 451–471. http://dx.doi.org/10.1353/sof.2005.0103

Hawkins, K. A., Hames, J. L., Ribeiro, J. D., Silva, C., Joiner, T. E., & Cougle, J. R. (2014). An examination of the relationship between anger and suicide risk through the lens of the interpersonal theory of suicide. *Journal of Psychiatric Research, 50*, 59–65. http://dx.doi.org/10.1016/j.jpsychires.2013.12.005

Hayes, J. A., McAleavey, A. A., Castonguay, L. G., & Locke, B. D. (2016). Psycho-therapists' outcomes with White and racial/ethnic minority clients: First, the good news. *Journal of Counseling Psychology, 63*, 261–268. http://dx.doi.org/10.1037/cou0000098

Hayes, J. A., Owen, J., & Bieschke, K. J. (2015). Therapist differences in symptom change with racial/ethnic minority clients. *Psychotherapy, 52*, 308–314. http://dx.doi.org/10.1037/a0037957

Hedegaard, H., Curtin, S. C., & Warner, M. (2016). Age-adjusted suicide rates for females and males by method—National Vital Statistics System, United States, 2000 and 2014. *MMWR: Morbidity and Mortality Weekly Report, 65*, 503. http://dx.doi.org/10.15585/mmwr.mm6519a7

Hedegaard, H., Curtin, S. C., & Warner, M. (2018). *Suicide mortality in the United States 1999–2017* (NCHS Data Brief No. 330). Hyattsville, MD: National Center for Health Statistics.

Heilbron, N., Compton, J. S., Daniel, S. S., & Goldston, D. B. (2010). The problematic label of suicide gesture: Alternatives for clinical research and practice. *Professional Psychology: Research and Practice, 41*, 221–227. http://dx.doi.org/10.1037/a0018712

Heintzelman, S. J., & King, L. A. (2014). Life is pretty meaningful. *American Psychologist, 69*, 561–574. http://dx.doi.org/10.1037/a0035049

Henriques, G. R., Wenzel, A., Brown, G. K., & Beck, A. T. (2005). Suicide attempters' reaction to survival as a risk factor for eventual suicide. *American Journal of Psychotherapy, 162*, 2180–2182. http://dx.doi.org/10.1176/appi.ajp.162.11.2180

Hewer, M. (2015). Data "salvation" for suicide research. *Observer Magazine, 28*(7), 17–18.

Hollingsworth, D. W., Cole, A. B., O'Keefe, V., Tucker, R. P., Story, C. R., & Wingate, L. R. (2017). Experiencing racial microaggressions influences suicidal ideation through perceived burdensomeness in African Americans. *Journal of Counseling Psychology, 64*, 104–111. http://dx.doi.org/10.1037/cou0000177

Hom, M. A., & Joiner, T. E. (2017). Predictors of treatment attrition among adult outpatients with clinically significant suicidal ideation. *Journal of Clinical Psychology, 73*, 88–98. http://dx.doi.org/10.1002/jclp.22318

Hom, M. A., Joiner, T. E., & Bernert, R. A. (2016). Limitations of a single-item assessment of suicide attempt history: Implications for standardized suicide risk assessment. *Psychological Assessment, 28*, 1026–1030. http://dx.doi.org/10.1037/pas0000241

Hom, M. A., Stanley, I. H., Gutierrez, P. M., & Joiner, T. E., Jr. (2017). Exploring the association between exposure to suicide and suicide risk among military service members and veterans. *Journal of Affective Disorders, 207*, 327–335. http://dx.doi.org/10.1016/j.jad.2016.09.043

Hom, M. A., Stanley, I. H., & Joiner, T. E., Jr. (2015). Evaluating factors and interventions that influence help-seeking and mental health service utilization among suicidal individuals: A review of the literature. *Clinical Psychology Review, 40*, 28–39. http://dx.doi.org/10.1016/j.cpr.2015.05.006

Hom, M. A., Stanley, I. H., Podlogar, M. C., & Joiner, T. E., Jr. (2017). "Are you having thoughts of suicide?" Examining experiences with disclosing and denying suicidal ideation. *Journal of Clinical Psychology, 73*, 1382–1392. http://dx.doi.org/10.1002/jclp.22440

Hom, M. A., Stanley, I. H., Rogers, M. L., Gallyer, A. J., Dougherty, S. P., Davis, L., & Joiner, T. E. (2018). Investigating the iatrogenic effects of repeated suicidal ideation screening on suicidal and depression symptoms: A staggered sequential study. *Journal of Affective Disorders, 232*, 139–142. http://dx.doi.org/10.1016/j.jad.2018.02.022

Homaifar, B. Y., Bahraini, N., Silverman, M. M., & Brenner, L. A. (2012). Executive functioning as a component of suicide risk assessment: Clarifying its role in standard clinical applications. *Journal of Mental Health Counseling, 34*, 110–120. http://dx.doi.org/10.17744/mehc.34.2.r70331307tx03871

Hottes, T. S., Bogaert, L., Rhodes, A. E., Brennan, D. J., & Gesink, D. (2016). Lifetime prevalence of suicide attempts among sexual minority adults by study sampling strategies: A systematic review and meta-analysis. *American Journal of Public Health, 106*, e1–e12. http://dx.doi.org/10.2105/AJPH.2016.303088

Husky, M., Olié, E., Guillaume, S., Genty, C., Swendsen, J., & Courtet, P. (2014). Feasibility and validity of ecological momentary assessment in the investigation of suicide risk. *Psychiatry Research, 220*, 564–570. http://dx.doi.org/10.1016/j.psychres.2014.08.019

Iliceto, P., & Fino, E. (2015). Beck Hopelessness Scale (BHS): A second order confirmatory factor analysis. *European Journal of Psychological Assessment, 31*, 31–37. http://dx.doi.org/10.1027/1015-5759/a000201

Ivanova, E., Yaakoba-Zohar, N., Jensen, D., Cassoff, J., & Knäuper, B. (2016). Acceptance and commitment therapy and implementation intentions increase exercise enjoyment and long-term exercise behavior among low-active women. *Current Psychology, 35*, 108–114. http://dx.doi.org/10.1007/s12144-015-9349-3

Jahn, D. R., Quinnett, P., & Ries, R. (2016). The influence of training and experience on mental health practitioners comfort working with suicidal individuals. *Professional Psychology: Research and Practice, 47*, 130–138. http://dx.doi.org/10.1037/pro0000070

James, K., & Stewart, D. (2018). Blurred boundaries—A qualitative study of how acts of self-harm and attempted suicide are defined by mental health practitioners. *Crisis, 39*, 247–254. http://dx.doi.org/10.1027/0227-5910/a000491

Jergensen, K. (2018). Practice what you preach: An exploration of DBT therapists personal skill utilization in burnout prevention. *Clinical Social Work Journal, 46*, 187–199.

Jobes, D. A. (2012). The Collaborative Assessment and Management of Suicidality (CAMS): An evolving evidence-based clinical approach to suicidal risk. *Suicide and Life-Threatening Behavior, 42*, 640–653. http://dx.doi.org/10.1111/j.1943-278X.2012.00119.x

Jobes, D. A. (2016). *Managing suicidal behavior: A collaborative approach* (2nd ed.). New York, NY: Guilford Press.

Jobes, D. A., & Ballard, E. (2011). The therapist and the suicidal patient. In K. Michel & D. A. Jobes (Eds.), *Building a therapeutic alliance with the suicidal patient* (pp. 51–61). Washington, DC: American Psychological Association. http://dx.doi.org/10.1037/12303-003

Jobes, D. A., Rudd, M. D., Overholser, J. C., & Joiner, T. E. (2008). Ethical and competent care of suicidal patients: Contemporary challenges, new developments, and considerations for clinical practice. *Professional Psychology: Research and Practice, 39*, 405–413. http://dx.doi.org/10.1037/a0012896

Johnson, S. (2010). *Where good ideas come from*. New York, NY: Penguin.

Johnson, W. B., Barnett, J. E., Elman, N. S., Forrest, L., & Kaslow, N. J. (2012). The competent community: Toward a vital reformulation of professional ethics. *American Psychologist, 67*, 557–569. http://dx.doi.org/10.1037/a0027206

Johnson, W. B., Bertschinger, M., Snell, A. K., & Wilson, A. (2014). Secondary trauma and ethical obligations for military psychologists: Preserving compassion and competence in the crucible of combat. *Psychological Services, 11*, 68–74. http://dx.doi.org/10.1037/a0033913

Johnson, W. B., Elman, N. S., Forrest, L., Robiner, W. N., Rodolfa, E., & Schaffer, J. B. (2008). Addressing professional competence problems in trainees: Some ethical considerations. *Professional Psychology: Research and Practice, 39*, 589–599. http://dx.doi.org/10.1037/a0014264

Joiner, T. E. (2005). *Why people die by suicide*. Cambridge, MA: Harvard University Press.

Joiner, T. E. (2010). *Myths about suicide*. Cambridge, MA: Harvard University Press.

Joiner, T. E., Jr., Buchman-Schmitt, J. M., & Chu, C. (2017). Do undiagnosed suicide decedents have symptoms of a mental disorder? *Journal of Clinical Psychology, 73*, 1744–1752. http://dx.doi.org/10.1002/jclp.22498

Joiner, T. E., Hom, M. A., Rogers, M. L., Chu, C., Stanley, I. H., Wynn, G. H., & Gutierrez, P. M. (2016). Staring down death: Is abnormally slow blink rate a clinically useful indicator of suicide risk? *Crisis, 37*, 212–217. http://dx.doi.org/10.1027/0227-5910/a000367

Joiner, T. E., Ribeiro, J. D., & Silva, C. (2012). Nonsuicidal self-injury, suicidal behavior, and their co-occurrence as viewed through the lens of the interpersonal theory of suicide. *Current Directions in Psychological Science, 21*, 342–347. http://dx.doi.org/10.1177/0963721412454873

Joiner, T. E., Jr., Steer, R. A., Brown, G., Beck, A. T., Pettit, J. W., & Rudd, M. D. (2003). Worst-point suicidal plans: A dimension of suicidality predictive of past suicide attempts and eventual death by suicide. *Behaviour Research and Therapy, 41*, 1469–1480. http://dx.doi.org/10.1016/S0005-7967(03)00070-6

Joiner, T. E., Van Orden, K. A., Witte, T. K., & Rudd, M. D. (2009). *The interpersonal theory of suicide: Guidance for working with suicidal clients.* Washington, DC: American Psychological Association. http://dx.doi.org/10.1037/11869-000

Joint Commission. (2016). Directing and treating suicidal ideation in all settings. *Sentinel Event Alert, 56*, 1–7.

Jordan, J. T., & McNiel, D. E. (2018). Characteristics of a suicide attempt predict who makes another attempt after hospital discharge: A decision-tree investigation. *Psychiatric Research, 268*, 317–322. http://dx.doi.org/10.1016/j.psychres.2018.07.040

Kahneman, D. (2011). *Thinking fast and slow.* New York, NY: Farrar, Straus & Giroux.

Kallert, T. W., Glöckner, M., & Schützwohl, M. (2008). Involuntary vs. voluntary hospital admission. A systematic literature review on outcome diversity. *European Archives of Psychiatry and Clinical Neuroscience, 258*, 195–209. http://dx.doi.org/10.1007/s00406-007-0777-4

Kapur, N., Cooper, J., O'Connor, R. C., & Hawton, K. (2013). Non-suicidal self-injury v. attempted suicide: New diagnosis or false dichotomy? *The British Journal of Psychiatry, 202*, 326–328. http://dx.doi.org/10.1192/bjp.bp.112.116111

Kavalidou, K., Smith, D. J., & O'Connor, R. C. (2017). The role of physical and mental health multimorbidity in suicidal ideation. *Journal of Affective Disorders, 209*, 80–85. http://dx.doi.org/10.1016/j.jad.2016.11.026

Kazan, D., Calear, A. L., & Batterham, P. J. (2016). The impact of intimate partner relationships on suicidal thoughts and behaviours: A systematic review. *Journal of Affective Disorders, 190*, 585–598. http://dx.doi.org/10.1016/j.jad.2015.11.003

Kegler, S. R., Stone, D. M., & Holland, K. M. (2017). Trends in suicide by level of urbanization—United States, 1999–2015. *MMWR: Morbidity and Mortality Weekly Report, 66*, 270–273. http://dx.doi.org/10.15585/mmwr.mm6610a2

Kessler, R. C., Borges, G., & Walters, E. E. (1999). Prevalence of and risk factors for lifetime suicide attempts in the National Comorbidity Survey. *Archives of General Psychiatry, 56*, 617–626. http://dx.doi.org/10.1001/archpsyc.56.7.617

Keyes, C. L. (2007). Promoting and protecting mental health as flourishing: A complementary strategy for improving national mental health. *American Psychologist, 62*, 95–108. http://dx.doi.org/10.1037/0003-066X.62.2.95

Khaw, K.-T. (2008). *Rose's strategy of preventive medicine.* New York, NY: Oxford University Press.

Khazem, L. R. (2018). Physical disability and suicide: Recent advancements in understanding and future directions for consideration. *Current Opinion in Psychology, 22*, 18–22. http://dx.doi.org/10.1016/j.copsyc.2017.07.018

Kiekens, G., Hasking, P., Boyes, M., Claes, L. Mortier, P., Auergbach, R. P., . . . Bruffaerts, R. (2018). The association between non-suicidal self-injury and first onset suicidal thoughts and behaviors. *Journal of Affective Disorders, 239*, 171–179. http://dx.doi.org/10.1016/j.jad.2018.06.013

Kirtley, O. J., O'Carroll, R. E., & O'Connor, R. C. (2016). Pain and self-harm: A systematic review. *Journal of Affective Disorders, 203*, 347–363. http://dx.doi.org/10.1016/j.jad.2016.05.068

Kitchener, K. (1984). Intuition, critical evaluation and ethical principles: The foundations for ethical decisions in counseling and psychology. *The Counseling Psychologist, 12*, 43–55. http://dx.doi.org/10.1177/0011000084123005

Kleespies, P. M. (2014). *Decision making in behavioral emergencies: Acquiring skill in evaluating and managing high-risk patients.* Washington, DC: American Psychological Association. http://dx.doi.org/10.1037/14337-000

Kleespies, P. M. (2017). Future directions and conclusions. In P. M. Kleespies (Ed.), *The Oxford handbook of behavioral health emergencies and crisis* (pp. 549–556). New York, NY: Oxford University Press.

Kleespies, P. M., AhnAllen, C. G., Knight, J. A., Presskreischer, B., Barrs, K. L., Boyd, B. L., & Dennis, J. P. (2011). A study of self-injurious and suicidal behavior in a veteran population. *Psychological Services, 8*, 236–250. http://dx.doi.org/10.1037/a0024881

Kleespies, P. M., & Dettmer, E. L. (2000). The stress of patient emergencies for the clinician: Incidence, impact, and means of coping. *Journal of Clinical Psychology, 56*, 1353–1369. http://dx.doi.org/10.1002/1097-4679(200010)56:10<1353::AID-JCLP7>3.0.CO;2-3

Kleespies, P. M., Efe, B., & Ametrano, R. M. (2017). When negative events happen: Dealing with the stress. In P. M. Kleespies (Ed.), *The Oxford handbook of behavioral health emergencies and crisis* (pp. 531–549). New York, NY: Oxford University Press.

Kleiman, E. M., Coppersmith, D. D. L., Millner, A. J., Franz, P. J., Fox, K. R., & Nock, M. K. (2018). Are suicidal thoughts reinforcing? A preliminary real-time monitoring study on the potential affect regulation function of suicidal thinking. *Journal of Affective Disorders, 232*, 122–126. http://dx.doi.org/10.1016/j.jad.2018.02.033

Kleiman, E. M., Law, K. C., & Anestis, M. D. (2014). Do theories of suicide play well together? Integrating components of the hopelessness and interpersonal psychological theories of suicide. *Comprehensive Psychiatry, 55*, 431–438. http://dx.doi.org/10.1016/j.comppsych.2013.10.015

Kleiman, E. M., Liu, R. T., & Riskind, J. H. (2014). Integrating the interpersonal psychological theory of suicide into the depression/suicidal ideation relationship: A short-term prospective study. *Behavior Therapy, 45*, 212–221. http://dx.doi.org/10.1016/j.beth.2013.10.007

Kleiman, E. M., & Nock, M. K. (2018). Real-time assessment of suicidal thoughts and behaviors. *Current Opinion in Psychology, 22*, 33–37. http://dx.doi.org/10.1016/j.copsyc.2017.07.026

Kleiman, E. M., Turner, B. J., Fedor, S., Beale, E. E., Huffman, J. C., & Nock, M. K. (2017). Examination of real-time fluctuations in suicidal ideation and its risk factors: Results from two ecological momentary assessment studies. *Journal of Abnormal Psychology, 126*, 726–738. http://dx.doi.org/10.1037/abn0000273

Klimo, G. F., Daum, W. J., Brinker, M. R., McGuire, E., & Elliott, M. N. (2000). Orthopedic medical malpractice: An attorney's perspective. *American Journal of Orthopedics, 29*, 93–97.

Klonsky, E. D., & May, A. M. (2015). The three-step theory (3ST): A new theory of suicide rooted in the "ideation-to-action" framework. *International Journal of Cognitive Therapy, 8*, 114–129. http://dx.doi.org/10.1521/ijct.2015.8.2.114

Klonsky, E. D., Qiu, T., & Saffer, B. Y. (2017). Recent advances in differentiating suicide attempters from suicide ideators. *Current Opinion in Psychiatry, 30*, 15–20. http://dx.doi.org/10.1097/YCO.0000000000000294

Klonsky, E. D., Saffer, B. Y., & Bryan, C. J. (2018). Ideation-to-action theories of suicide: A conceptual and empirical update. *Current Opinion in Psychology, 22*, 38–43. http://dx.doi.org/10.1016/j.copsyc.2017.07.020

Knapp, S. (2016). *The assessment, management and treatment of suicidal patients: An abbreviated course.* Harrisburg, PA: Pennsylvania Psychological Association.

Knapp, S. (2017, May). Competence with suicidal patients: Helping good psychologists become even better. *The Pennsylvania Psychologist, 77*, 1, 7.

Knapp, S. (2018, November). Psychologists and suicide: What if it happened to your patient? *The Pennsylvania Psychologist, 78*, 4.

Knapp, S., Dirks, J., & Magee, J. A. (1982). Act 143 and the rate of involuntary psychiatric commitments. *Journal of Mental Health Administration, 9*, 113–114.

Knapp, S., & Gavazzi, J. (2012, April). Can checklists help reduce treatment failures? *The Pennsylvania Psychologist, 72*, 8–9.

Knapp, S. J., Gottlieb, M. C., & Handelsman, M. M. (2015). *Ethical dilemmas in psychotherapy: Positive approaches to decision making.* Washington, DC: American Psychological Association. http://dx.doi.org/10.1037/14670-000

Knapp, S., Gottlieb, M. C., & Handelsman, M. M. (2017). Some ethical considerations in paid peer consultations in health care. *Journal of Health Service Psychology, 43*, 20–25.

Knapp, S., & Schur, B. (2019, February). Ten questions to promote excellence when working with patients with suicidal thoughts. *The Pennsylvania Psychologist, 79*(2), 1–3, 5–7.

Knapp, S., & VandeCreek, L. (2004). A principle-based interpretation of the 2002 American Psychological Association ethics code. *Psychotherapy: Theory, Research, Practice, Training, 41*, 247–254. http://dx.doi.org/10.1037/0033-3204.41.3.247

Knapp, S., & VandeCreek, L. (2012). Disciplinary actions by a state board of psychology: Do gender and association membership matter? In G. Neimeyer & J. Taylor (Eds.), *Continuing professional development and lifelong learning: Issues, impacts and outcomes* (pp. 155–158). Hauppauge, NY: NOVA Science.

Knapp, S., VandeCreek, L., & Fingerhut, R. (2017). *Practical ethics: A positive approach* (3rd ed.). Washington, DC: American Psychological Association.

Knapp, S., Younggren, J., VandeCreek, L., Harris, E., & Martin, J. (2013). *Assessing and managing risk in psychological practice: An individualized approach* (2nd ed.). Rockville, MD: The Trust.

Koffel, E., Kroenke, K., Bair, M. J., Leverty, D., Polusny, M. A., & Krebs, E. E. (2016). The bidirectional relationship between sleep complaints and pain: Analysis of data from a randomized trial. *Health Psychology, 35*, 41–49. http://dx.doi.org/10.1037/hea0000245

Kraus, D. R., Bentley, J. H., Alexander, P. C., Boswell, J. F., Constantino, M. J., Baxter, E. E., & Castonguay, L. G. (2016). Predicting therapist effectiveness from their own practice-based evidence. *Journal of Consulting and Clinical Psychology, 84*, 473–483. http://dx.doi.org/10.1037/ccp0000083

Kraus, D. R., Castonguay, L., Boswell, J. F., Nordberg, S. S., & Hayes, J. A. (2011). Therapist effectiveness: Implications for accountability and patient care. *Psychotherapy Research, 21*, 267–276. http://dx.doi.org/10.1080/10503307.2011.563249

Kye, S.-Y., & Park, K. (2017). Suicidal ideation and suicidal attempts among adults with chronic diseases: A cross-sectional study. *Comprehensive Psychiatry, 73*, 160–167. http://dx.doi.org/10.1016/j.comppsych.2016.12.001

Kyung-Sook, W., SangSoo, S., Sangjin, S., & Young-Jeon, S. (2018). Marital status integration and suicide: A meta-analysis and meta-regression. *Social Science & Medicine, 197*, 116–126. http://dx.doi.org/10.1016/j.socscimed.2017.11.053

Lambert, M. J., & Shimokawa, K. (2011). Collecting client feedback. *Psychotherapy, 48*, 72–79. http://dx.doi.org/10.1037/a0022238

Large, M., Kaneson, M., Myles, N., Myles, H., Gunaratne, P., & Ryan, C. (2016). Meta-analysis of longitudinal cohort studies of suicide risk assessment among psychiatric patients: Heterogeneity in results and lack of improvement over time. *PLoS One, 11*(6), e0156322. http://dx.doi.org/10.1371/journal.pone.0156322

Large, M., Ryan, C., Walsh, G., Stein-Parbury, J., & Patfield, M. (2014). Nosocomial suicide. *Australasian Psychiatry, 22*, 118–121. http://dx.doi.org/10.1177/1039856213511277

Law, K. C., & Tucker, R. P. (2018). Repetitive negative thinking and suicide: A burgeoning literature with need for further exploration. *Current Opinion in Psychology, 22*, 68–72. http://dx.doi.org/10.1016/j.copsyc.2017.08.027

LeBouthillier, D. M., McMillan, K. A., Thibodeau, M. A., & Asmundson, G. J. G. (2015). Types and number of traumas associated with suicidal ideation and suicide attempts in PTSD: Findings from a U.S. nationally representative sample. *Journal of Traumatic Stress, 28*, 183–190. http://dx.doi.org/10.1002/jts.22010

Lee, E., & Kealy, D. (2014). Revisiting Balint's innovation: Enhancing capacity in collaborative mental health care. *Journal of Interprofessional Care, 28*, 466–470. http://dx.doi.org/10.3109/13561820.2014.902369

Lee, K. (2017, July/August). Psychology students protect thyselves: What graduate students need to know about professional liability, student insurance, and safeguarding their careers. *Monitor on Psychology, 48*(7), 58–60.

Leitzel, J., & Knapp, S. (2017). *Survey of members of the Pennsylvania Psychological Association.* Unpublished data.

Linehan, M. (1993). *Cognitive-behavioral treatment of borderline personality disorder.* New York, NY: Guilford Press.

Linehan, M. M., Korslund, K. E., Harned, M. S., Gallop, R. J., Lungu, A., Neacsiu, A. D., . . . Murray-Gregory, A. M. (2015). Dialectical behavior therapy for high suicide risk in individuals with borderline personality disorder: A randomized clinical trial and component analysis. *JAMA Psychiatry, 72*, 475–482. http://dx.doi.org/10.1001/jamapsychiatry.2014.3039

Liotta, M., Mento, C., & Settineri, S. (2015). Seriousness and lethality of attempted suicide: A systematic review. *Aggression and Violent Behavior, 21*, 97–109. http://dx.doi.org/10.1016/j.avb.2014.12.013

Littlewood, D., Kyle, S. D., Pratt, D., Peters, S., & Gooding, P. (2017). Examining the role of psychological factors in the relationship between sleep problems and suicide. *Clinical Psychology Review, 54,* 1–16. http://dx.doi.org/10.1016/j.cpr.2017.03.009

Liu, D. W. Y., Fairweather-Schmidt, A. K., Burns, R., Roberts, R. M., & Anstey, K. J. (2016). Psychological resilience provides no independent protection from suicide risk. *Crisis, 37,* 130–139. http://dx.doi.org/10.1027/0227-5910/a000364

Lizardi, D., Dervic, K., Grunebaum, M. F., Burke, A. K., Mann, J. J., & Oquendo, M. (2008). The role of moral objections to suicide in the assessment of suicidal patients. *Journal of Psychiatric Research, 42,* 815–821. http://dx.doi.org/10.1016/j.jpsychires.2007.09.007

Lizardi, D., Grunebaum, M. F., Burke, A., Stanley, B., Mann, J. J., Harkavy-Friedman, J., & Oquendo, M. (2011). The effect of social adjustment and attachment style on suicidal behaviour. *Acta Psychiatrica Scandinavica, 124,* 295–300. http://dx.doi.org/10.1111/j.1600-0447.2011.01724.x

Lockwood, D. N. (2018, August). *Firearms and behavioral emergencies: Ethical and legal considerations for lethal means restrictions.* Paper presented at the annual convention of the American Psychological Association, San Francisco, CA.

Louzon, S. A., Bossarte, R., McCarthy, J. F., & Katz, I. R. (2016). Does suicidal ideation as measured by the PHQ-9 predict suicide among VA patients? *Psychiatric Services, 67,* 517–522. http://dx.doi.org/10.1176/appi.ps.201500149

Luxton, D. D., O'Brien, K., Pruitt, L. D., Johnson, K., & Kramer, G. (2014). Suicide risk management during clinical telepractice. *International Journal of Psychiatry in Medicine, 48,* 19–31. http://dx.doi.org/10.2190/PM.48.1.c

Ma, J., Batterham, P. J., Calear, A. L., & Han, J. (2016). A systematic review of the predictions of the interpersonal-psychological theory of suicidal behavior. *Clinical Psychology Review, 46,* 34–45. http://dx.doi.org/10.1016/j.cpr.2016.04.008

Mackelprang, J. L., Karle, J., Reihl, K. M., & Cash, R. E. (2014). Suicide intervention skills: Graduate training and exposure to suicide among psychology trainees. *Training and Education in Professional Psychology, 8,* 136–142. http://dx.doi.org/10.1037/tep0000050

Maeschalck, C. L., & Barfknecht, L. R. (2017). Using client feedback to inform treatment. In D. S. Prescott, C. L. Maeshalck, & D. S. Miller (Eds.), *Feedback informed treatment in clinical practice: Reaching for excellence* (pp. 53–77). Washington, DC: American Psychological Association. http://dx.doi.org/10.1037/0000039-004

Maltsberger, J. T., & Buie, D. H. (1974). Countertransference hate in the treatment of suicidal patients. *Archives of General Psychiatry, 30,* 625–633. http://dx.doi.org/10.1001/archpsyc.1974.01760110049005

Maslach, C., & Jackson, S. E. (1981). The measurement of experienced burnout. *Journal of Occupational Behaviour, 2,* 99–113. http://dx.doi.org/10.1002/job.4030020205

Mattisson, C., Bogren, M., Brådvik, L., & Horstmann, V. (2015). Mortality of subjects with mood disorders in the Lundby community cohort: A follow-up over 50 years. *Journal of Affective Disorders, 178,* 98–106. http://dx.doi.org/10.1016/j.jad.2015.02.028

May, A. M., & Klonsky, E. D. (2016). What distinguishes suicide attempters from suicide ideators? A meta-analysis of potential factors. *Clinical Psychology: Science and Practice, 23,* 5–20. http://dx.doi.org/10.1111/cpsp.12136

McCloskey, M. S., & Ammerman, B. A. (2018). Suicidal behavior and aggression-related disorders. *Current Opinion in Psychology, 22,* 54–58. http://dx.doi.org/10.1016/j.copsyc.2017.08.010

McGuffin, P., Perroud, N., Uher, R., Butler, A., Aitchison, K. J., Craig, I., . . . Farmer, A. (2010). The genetics of affective disorder and suicide. *European Psychiatry, 25*, 275–277. http://dx.doi.org/10.1016/j.eurpsy.2009.12.012

McKeon, R. (2009). *Suicide behavior.* Cambridge, MA: Hogrefe & Huber.

McLaughlin, J., O'Carroll, R. E., & O'Connor, R. C. (2012). Intimate partner abuse and suicidality: A systematic review. *Clinical Psychology Review, 32*, 677–689. http://dx.doi.org/10.1016/j.cpr.2012.08.002

Medalie, L., & Cifu, A. S. (2017). Management of chronic insomnia disorder in adults. *JAMA, 317*, 762–763. http://dx.doi.org/10.1001/jama.2016.19004

Medeiros, T. L. (2017). *The wicked awesome wish list.* Washington, DC: American Association of Suicidology. Retrieved from https://www.suicidology.org/Portals/14/docs/Writing%20Contest/2017/2017Winner%20List.pdf?ver8□2017-08-29-211745-243

Meerwijk, E. L., Parekh, A., Oquendo, M. A., Allen, I. E., Franck, L. S., & Lee, K. A. (2016). Direct versus indirect psychosocial and behavioural interventions to prevent suicide and suicide attempts: A systematic review and meta-analysis. *The Lancet Psychiatry, 3*, 544–554. http://dx.doi.org/10.1016/S2215-0366(16)00064-X

Meichenbaum, D. (2005). 35 years of working with suicidal patients: Lessons learned. *Canadian Psychology, 46*, 64–72. http://dx.doi.org/10.1037/h0087006

Melonas, J. M. (2011). Patients at risk for suicide: Risk management and patient safety considerations to protect the patient and the physician. *Innovations in Clinical Neuroscience, 8*(3), 45–49.

Meyer, D. J. (2012). Split treatment: Coming of age. In R. Simon & R. E. Hales (Eds.), *Textbook of suicide assessment and management* (2nd ed., pp. 263–279). Washington, DC: American Psychiatric Association.

Mezuk, B., Lohman, M., Leslie, M., & Powell, V. (2015). Suicide risk in nursing homes and assisted living facilities: 2003–2011. *American Journal of Public Health, 105*, 1495–1502. http://dx.doi.org/10.2105/AJPH.2015.302573

Mezuk, B., Rock, A., Lohman, M. C., & Choi, M. (2014). Suicide risk in long-term care facilities: A systematic review. *International Journal of Geriatric Psychiatry, 29*, 1198–1211. http://dx.doi.org/10.1002/gps.4142

Michaels, M. S., Balthrop, T., Nadorff, M. R., & Joiner, T. E. (2017). Total sleep time as a predictor of suicidal behaviour. *Journal of Sleep Research, 26*, 732–738. http://dx.doi.org/10.1111/jsr.12563

Michel, K. (2011). General aspects of therapeutic alliance. In K. Michel & D. A. Jobes (Eds.), *Building a therapeutic alliance with the suicidal patient* (pp. 13–28). Washington, DC: American Psychological Association. http://dx.doi.org/10.1037/12303-001

Miller, M. (2012). Preventing suicide by preventing lethal injury: The need to act on what we already know. *American Journal of Public Health, 102*(Suppl. 1), e1–e3. http://dx.doi.org/10.2105/AJPH.2012.300662

Miller, M., Azrael, D., & Hemenway, D. (2006). Belief in the inevitability of suicide: Results from a national survey. *Suicide and Life-Threatening Behavior, 36*, 1–11. http://dx.doi.org/10.1521/suli.2006.36.1.1

Miller, M., & Hemenway, D. (2008). Guns and suicide in the United States. *The New England Journal of Medicine, 359*, 989–991. http://dx.doi.org/10.1056/NEJMp0805923

Miller, W. R., & Rollnick, S. (2013). *Motivational interviewing: Helping people change* (3rd ed.). New York, NY: Guilford Press.

Min, J.-A., Lee, C.-U., & Chae, J.-H. (2015). Resilience moderates the risk of depression and anxiety symptoms on suicidal ideation in patients with depression and/or anxiety disorders. *Comprehensive Psychiatry, 56*, 103–111. http://dx.doi.org/10.1016/j.comppsych.2014.07.022

Mishara, B. L., & Weisstub, D. N. (2010). Resolving ethical dilemmas in suicide prevention: The case of telephone helpline rescue policies. *Suicide and Life-Threatening Behavior, 40*, 159–169.

Mitchell, A. M., & Terhorst, L. (2017). PTSD symptoms in survivors bereaved by the suicide of a significant other. *Journal of the American Psychiatric Nurses Association, 23*, 61–65. http://dx.doi.org/10.1177/1078390316673716

Monahan, J., Vesselinov, R., Robbins, P. C., & Appelbaum, P. S. (2017). Violence to others, violent self-victimization, and violent victimization by others among persons with a mental illness. *Psychiatric Services, 68*, 516–519. http://dx.doi.org/10.1176/appi.ps.201600135

Montross Thomas, L. P., Palinkas, L. A., Meier, E. A., Iglewicz, A., Kirkland, T., & Zisook, S. (2014). Yearning to be heard: What veterans teach us about suicide risk and effective interventions. *Crisis, 35*, 161–167. http://dx.doi.org/10.1027/0227-5910/a000247

Mörch, C. M., Côté, L. P., Corthésy-Blondin, L., Plourde-Léveillé, L., Dargis, L., & Mishara, B. L. (2018). The Darknet and suicide. *Journal of Affective Disorders, 241*, 127–132. http://dx.doi.org/10.1016/j.jad.2018.08.028

Morrison, L. L., & Downey, D. L. (2000). Racial differences in self-disclosure of suicidal ideation and reasons for living: Implications for training. *Cultural Diversity & Ethnic Minority Psychology, 6*, 374–386. http://dx.doi.org/10.1037/1099-9809.6.4.374

Mortier, P., Demyttenaere, K., Auerbach, R. P., Cuijpers, P., Green, J. G., Kiekens, G., . . . Bruffaerts, R. (2017). First onset of suicidal thoughts and behaviours in college. *Journal of Affective Disorders, 207*, 291–299. http://dx.doi.org/10.1016/j.jad.2016.09.033

Muris, P., & Petrocchi, N. (2017). Protection or vulnerability? A meta-analysis of the relations between the positive and negative components of self-compassion and psychopathology. *Clinical Psychology & Psychotherapy, 24*, 373–383. http://dx.doi.org/10.1002/cpp.2005

Murrie, D. C., & Kelley, S. (2017). Evaluating and managing the risk of violence in clinical practice with adults. In P. Kleespies (Ed.), *The Oxford handbook of behavioral emergencies and crises* (pp. 126–145). New York, NY: Oxford University Press.

Myers, D. G. (2008). *Psychology*. New York, NY: Worth.

Nadorff, M. R., Lambdin, K. K., & Germain, A. (2014). Pharmacological and non-pharmacological treatments for nightmare disorder. *International Review of Psychiatry, 26*, 225–236. http://dx.doi.org/10.3109/09540261.2014.888989

National Center for Health Statistics. (2017). *Health: United States, 2016*. Hyattsville, MD: Author.

National Institute of Mental Health. (2018). *Suicide*. Retrieved from https://www.nimh.nih.gov/health/statistics/suicide.shtml

NCQA. (2017). *Follow-up after hospitalization for mental illness*. Retrieved from http://www.ncqa.org/report-cards/health-plans/state-of-health-care-quality/2017-table-of-contents/follow-up

Nock, M. K., Hwang, I., Sampson, N. A., & Kessler, R. C. (2010). Mental disorders, comorbidity and suicidal behavior: Results from the National Comorbidity Survey Replication. *Molecular Psychiatry*, *15*, 868–876. http://dx.doi.org/10.1038/mp.2009.29

Nock, M. K., Park, J. M., Finn, C. T., Deliberto, T. L., Dour, H. J., & Banaji, M. R. (2010). Measuring the suicidal mind: Implicit cognition predicts suicidal behavior. *Psychological Science*, *21*, 511–517. http://dx.doi.org/10.1177/0956797610364762

Norcross, J. C., & Lambert, M. J. (2018). Psychotherapy relationships that work III. *Psychotherapy*, *55*, 303–315. http://dx.doi.org/10.1037/pst0000193

Norcross, J. C., Prochaska, J. O., & DiClemente, C. C. (1986). Self-change of psychological distress: Laypersons' vs. psychologists' coping strategies. *Journal of Clinical Psychology*, *42*, 834–840. http://dx.doi.org/10.1002/1097-4679(198609)42:5<834::AID-JCLP2270420527>3.0.CO;2-A

Norcross, J. C., & Wampold, B. E. (2011). Evidence-based therapy relationships: Research conclusions and clinical practices. *Psychotherapy*, *48*, 98–102. http://dx.doi.org/10.1037/a0022161

O'Connor, R. C., & Portzky, G. (2018). The relationship between entrapment and suicidal behavior through the lens of the integrated motivational-volitional model of suicidal behavior. *Current Opinion in Psychology*, *22*, 12–17. http://dx.doi.org/10.1016/j.copsyc.2017.07.021

O'Connor, R. C., Smyth, R., & Williams, J. M. G. (2015). Intrapersonal positive future thinking predicts repeat suicide attempts in hospital-treated suicide attempters. *Journal of Consulting and Clinical Psychology*, *83*, 169–176. http://dx.doi.org/10.1037/a0037846

O'Connor, S. S., Comtois, K. A., Atkins, D. C., & Kerbrat, A. H. (2017). Examining the impact of suicide attempt function and perceived effectiveness in predicting reattempt for emergency medicine patients. *Behavior Therapy*, *48*, 45–55. http://dx.doi.org/10.1016/j.beth.2016.05.004

Orri, M., Perret, L. C., Turecki, G., & Geoffroy, M.-C. (2018). Association between irritability and suicide-related outcomes across the life-course. Systematic review of both community and clinical studies. *Journal of Affective Disorders*, *239*, 220–233. http://dx.doi.org/10.1016/j.jad.2018.07.010

Ortíz-Gómez, L. D., López-Canul, B., & Arankowsky-Sandoval, G. (2014). Factors associated with depression and suicide attempts in patients undergoing rehabilitation for substance abuse. *Journal of Affective Disorders*, *169*, 10–14. http://dx.doi.org/10.1016/j.jad.2014.07.033

Overholser, J. C., Braden, A., & Dieter, L. (2012). Understanding suicide risk: Identification of high-risk groups during high-risk times. *Journal of Clinical Psychology*, *68*, 349–361. http://dx.doi.org/10.1002/jclp.20859

Owen-Smith, A., Bennewith, O., Donovan, J., Evans, J., Hawton, K., Kapur, N., . . . Gunnell, D. (2014). "When you're in the hospital, you're in a sort of bubble." Understanding the high risk of self-harm and suicide following psychiatric discharge: A qualitative study. *Crisis*, *35*, 154–160. http://dx.doi.org/10.1027/0227-5910/a000246

Pargament, K. I. (2007). *Spiritually oriented psychotherapy*. New York, NY: Guilford Press.

Paris, J., & Zweig-Frank, H. (2001). A 27-year follow-up of patients with borderline personality disorder. *Comprehensive Psychiatry*, *42*, 482–487. http://dx.doi.org/10.1053/comp.2001.26271

Park, C. L., Currier, J. M., Harris, J. I., & Slattery, J. M. (2017). *Trauma, meaning and spirituality: Translating research into clinical practice*. Washington, DC: American Psychological Association. http://dx.doi.org/10.1037/15961-000

Park, J., Goode, J., Tompkins, K. A., & Swift, J. K. (2016). Clinical errors that can occur in the treatment decision-making process in psychotherapy. *Psychotherapy, 53*, 257–261. http://dx.doi.org/10.1037/pst0000066

Patient Assistance Programs for Prescription Drugs. (n.d.). Retrieved from https://www.webmd.com/healthy-aging/patient-assistance-programs-for-prescription-drugs#1

Peteet, J. R., Maytal, G., & Rokni, H. (2010). Unimaginable loss: Contingent suicidal ideation in family members of oncology patients. *Psychosomatics, 51*, 166–170. http://dx.doi.org/10.1016/S0033-3182(10)70677-0

Peterson, J., Skeem, J., & Manchak, S. (2011). If you want to know, consider asking: How likely is it that patients will hurt themselves in the future? *Psychological Assessment, 23*, 626–634. http://dx.doi.org/10.1037/a0022971

Phillips, J. A., & Hempstead, K. (2017). Differences in U.S. suicide rates by educational attainment, 2000–2014. *American Journal of Preventive Medicine, 53*(4), e123–e130. http://dx.doi.org/10.1016/j.amepre.2017.04.010

Pietrzak, R. H., Goldstein, M. B., Malley, J. C., Rivers, A. J., Johnson, D. C., & Southwick, S. M. (2010). Risk and protective factors associated with suicidal ideation in veterans of Operations Enduring Freedom and Iraqi Freedom. *Journal of Affective Disorders, 123*, 102–107. http://dx.doi.org/10.1016/j.jad.2009.08.001

Pitman, A. L., Stevenson, F., Osborn, D. P. J., & King, M. B. (2018). The stigma associated with bereavement by suicide and other sudden deaths: A qualitative interview study. *Social Science & Medicine, 198*, 121–129. http://dx.doi.org/10.1016/j.socscimed.2017.12.035

Plante, T. (2014). Four steps to improve religious/spiritual cultural competence in professional psychology. *Spirituality in Clinical Practice, 1*, 288–292. http://dx.doi.org/10.1037/scp0000047

Podlogar, M. C., Rogers, M. L., Chiurliza, B., Hom, M. A., Tzoneva, M., & Joiner, T. (2016). Who are we missing? Nondisclosure in online suicide risk screening questionnaires. *Psychological Assessment, 28*, 963–974. http://dx.doi.org/10.1037/pas0000242

Poindexter, E. K., Mitchell, S. M., Jahn, D. R., Smith, P. N., Hirsch, J. K., & Cukrowicz, K. C. (2015). PTSD symptoms and suicide ideation: Testing the conditional indirect effects of thwarted interpersonal needs and using substances to cope. *Personality and Individual Differences, 77*, 167–172. http://dx.doi.org/10.1016/j.paid.2014.12.043

Pompili, M., Girardi, P., Tatarelli, G., & Tatarelli, R. (2006). Suicidal intent in single-car accident drivers: Review and new preliminary findings. *Crisis, 27*, 92–99. http://dx.doi.org/10.1027/0227-5910.27.2.92

Pope, K. S., & Tabachnick, B. G. (1993). Therapists' anger, hate, fear, and sexual feelings: National survey of therapist responses, client characteristics, critical events, formal complaints and training. *Professional Psychology: Research and Practice, 24*, 142–152. http://dx.doi.org/10.1037/0735-7028.24.2.142

Qin, P. (2011). The impact of psychiatric illness on suicide: Differences by diagnosis of disorders and by sex and age of subjects. *Journal of Psychiatric Research, 45*, 1445–1452. http://dx.doi.org/10.1016/j.jpsychires.2011.06.002

Quinnett, P. (2018). The role of clinician fear in interviewing suicidal patients. *Crisis*. Advance online publication. http://dx.doi.org/10.1027/0227-5910/a000555

Racine, M. (2018). Chronic pain and suicide risk: A comprehensive review. *Progress in Neuro-Psychopharmacology & Biological Psychiatry, 87*, 269–280. http://dx.doi.org/10.1016/j.pnpbp.2017.08.020

Ramsay, J., & Newman, C. F. (2005). After the attempt: Maintaining the therapeutic alliance following a patient's suicide attempt. *Suicide and Life-Threatening Behavior, 35*, 413–424. http://dx.doi.org/10.1521/suli.2005.35.4.413

Reitzel, L. R., Burns, A. B., Repper, K. K., Wingate, L. R., & Joiner, T. E. (2004). The effect of therapist availability on the frequency of patient-initiated between-session contact. *Professional Psychology: Research and Practice, 35*, 291–296. http://dx.doi.org/10.1037/0735-7028.35.3.291

Rhoades, G. K., Kamp Dush, C. M., Atkins, D. C., Stanley, S. M., & Markman, H. J. (2011). Breaking up is hard to do: The impact of unmarried relationship dissolution on mental health and life satisfaction. *Journal of Family Psychology, 25*, 366–374. http://dx.doi.org/10.1037/a0023627

Ribeiro, J. D., Bender, T. W., Buchman, J. M., Nock, M. K., Rudd, M. D., Bryan, C. J., . . . Joiner, T. E., Jr. (2015). An investigation of the interactive effects of the capability for suicide and acute agitation on suicidality in a military sample. *Depression and Anxiety, 32*, 25–31. http://dx.doi.org/10.1002/da.22240

Ribeiro, J. D., Bender, T. W., Selby, E. A., Hames, J. L., & Joiner, T. E. (2011). Development and validation of a brief self-report measure of agitation: The Brief Agitation Measure. *Journal of Personality Assessment, 93*, 597–604. http://dx.doi.org/10.1080/00223891.2011.608758

Ribeiro, J. D., Bodell, L. P., Hames, J. L., Hagan, C. R., & Joiner, T. E. (2013). An empirically based approach to the assessment and management of suicidal behavior. *Journal of Psychotherapy Integration, 23*, 207–221. http://dx.doi.org/10.1037/a0031416

Ribeiro, J. D., Gutierrez, P. M., Joiner, T. E., Kessler, R. C., Petukhova, M. V., Sampson, N. A., . . . Nock, M. K. (2017). Health care contact and suicide risk documentation prior to suicide death: Results from the Army Study to Assess Risk and Resilience in Servicemembers (Army STARRS). *Journal of Consulting and Clinical Psychology, 85*, 403–408. http://dx.doi.org/10.1037/ccp0000178

Ribeiro, J. D., Silva, C., & Joiner, T. E. (2014). Overarousal interacts with a sense of fearlessness about death to predict suicide risk in a sample of clinical outpatients. *Psychiatry Research, 218*, 106–112. http://dx.doi.org/10.1016/j.psychres.2014.03.036

Rimkeviciene, J., O'Gorman, J., & De Leo, D. (2016). How do clinicians and suicide attempters understand suicide attempt impulsivity? A qualitative study. *Death Studies, 40*, 139–146. http://dx.doi.org/10.1080/07481187.2015.1096314

Roaldset, J. O., & Bjørkly, S. (2010). Patients' own statements of their future risk for violent and self-harm behaviour: A prospective inpatient and post-discharge follow-up study in an acute psychiatric unit. *Psychiatry Research, 178*, 153–159. http://dx.doi.org/10.1016/j.psychres.2010.04.012

Rockett, I. R., Smith, G. S., Caine, E. D., Kapusta, N. D., Hanzlick, R. L., Larkin, G. L., . . . Fraser, D. W. (2014). Confronting death from drug self-intoxication (DDSI): Prevention through a better definition. *American Journal of Public Health, 104*, e49–e55. http://dx.doi.org/10.2105/AJPH.2014.302244

Rockett, I. R., Wang, S., Stack, S., De Leo, D., Frost, J. L., Ducatman, A. M., . . . Kapusta, N. D. (2010). Race/ethnicity and potential suicide misclassification: Window on a minority suicide paradox? *BMC Psychiatry, 10*, Article 35. http://dx.doi.org/10.1186/1471-244X-10-35

Rogers, M. L., Chiurliza, B., Hagan, C. R., Tzoneva, M., Hames, J. L., Michaels, M. S., . . . Joiner, T. E. (2017). Acute suicidal affective disturbance: Factorial structure and initial validation across psychiatric outpatient and inpatient samples. *Journal of Affective Disorders, 211,* 1–11. http://dx.doi.org/10.1016/j.jad.2016.12.057

Rogers, M. L., & Joiner, T. E. (2017). Rumination, suicidal ideation, and suicide attempts: A meta-analytic review. *Review of General Psychology, 21,* 132–142. http://dx.doi.org/10.1037/gpr0000101

Rogers, M. L., & Joiner, T. E. (2018a). Severity of suicidal ideation matters: Reexamining correlates of suicidal ideation using quantile regression. *Journal of Clinical Psychology, 74,* 442–452. http://dx.doi.org/10.1002/jclp.22499

Rogers, M. L., & Joiner, T. E. (2018b). Suicide-specific rumination relates to lifetime suicide attempts above and beyond a variety of other suicide risk factors. *Journal of Psychiatric Research, 98,* 78–86. http://dx.doi.org/10.1016/j.jpsychires.2017.12.017

Rogers, M. L., & Joiner, T. E. (2019). Exploring the temporal dynamics of the interpersonal theory of suicide constructs: A dynamic systems modeling approach. *Journal of Consulting and Clinical Psychology, 87,* 56–66. http://dx.doi.org/10.1037/ccp0000373

Rogers, M. L., Ringer, F. B., & Joiner, T. E. (2018). The association between suicidal ideation and lifetime suicide attempts is strongest at low levels of depression. *Psychiatry Research, 270,* 324–328. http://dx.doi.org/10.1016/j.psychres.2018.09.061

Rogers, M. L., Schneider, M. E., Tucker, R. P., Law, K. C., Anestis, M. D., & Joiner, T. E. (2017). Overarousal as a mechanism of the relation between rumination and suicidality. *Journal of Psychiatric Research, 92,* 31–37. http://dx.doi.org/10.1016/j.jpsychires.2017.03.024

Rogerson, M. D., Gottlieb, M. C., Handelsman, M. M., Knapp, S., & Younggren, J. (2011). Nonrational processes in ethical decision making. *American Psychologist, 66,* 614–623. http://dx.doi.org/10.1037/a0025215

Rojas, S. M., Bujarski, S., Babson, K. A., Dutton, C. E., & Feldner, M. T. (2014). Understanding PTSD comorbidity and suicidal behavior: Associations among histories of alcohol dependence, major depressive disorder, and suicidal ideation and attempts. *Journal of Anxiety Disorders, 28,* 318–325. http://dx.doi.org/10.1016/j.janxdis.2014.02.004

Rosenthal, L. (2016). Incorporating intersectionality into psychology: An opportunity to promote social justice and equity. *American Psychologist, 71,* 474–485. http://dx.doi.org/10.1037/a0040323

Ross, W. D. (1998). What makes right acts right? In J. Rachels (Ed.), *Ethical theory* (pp. 265–285). New York, NY: Oxford University Press. (Original work published 1930)

Rossen, L. M., Hedegaard, H., Khan, D., & Warner, M. (2018). County-level trends in suicide rates in the U.S., 2005–2015. *American Journal of Preventive Medicine, 55,* 72–79. http://dx.doi.org/10.1016/j.amepre.2018.03.020

Rothes, I. A., Scheerder, G., Van Audenhove, C., & Henriques, M. R. (2013). Patient suicide: The experience of Flemish psychiatrists. *Suicide and Life-Threatening Behavior, 43,* 379–394. http://dx.doi.org/10.1111/sltb.12024

Roush, J. F., Brown, S. L., Jahn, D. R., Mitchell, S. M., Taylor, N. J., Quinnett, P., & Ries, R. (2018). Mental health professionals' suicide risk assessment and management practices. *Crisis, 39,* 55–64. http://dx.doi.org/10.1027/0227-5910/a000478

Rubin, N. J., Bebeau, M., Leigh, I. W., Lichtenberg, J. W., Nelson, P., Portnoy, S., . . . Kaslow, N. J. (2007). The competency movement within psychological: An historical perspective. *Professional Psychology: Research and Practice, 38,* 452–462. http://dx.doi.org/10.1037/0735-7028.38.5.452

Rudd, M. D. (2006). Fluid vulnerability theory: A cognitive approach to understanding the process of acute and chronic suicide risk. In T. E. Ellis (Ed.), *Cognition and suicide: Theory, research, and therapy* (pp. 355–368). Washington, DC: American Psychological Association. http://dx.doi.org/10.1037/11377-016

Rudd, M. D. (2012). The clinical risk assessment interview. In R. Simon & R. E. Hales (Eds.), *Textbook of suicide assessment and management* (pp. 57–73). Washington, DC: American Psychiatric Association.

Rudd, M. D., Bryan, C. J., Wertenberger, E. G., Peterson, A. L., Young-McCaughan, S., Mintz, J., . . . Bruce, T. O. (2015). Brief cognitive-behavioral therapy effects on post-treatment suicide attempts in a military sample: Results of a randomized clinical trial with 2-year follow-up. *The American Journal of Psychiatry, 172,* 441–449. http://dx.doi.org/10.1176/appi.ajp.2014.14070843

Rudd, M. D., Cukrowicz, K. C., & Bryan, C. J. (2008). Core competencies in suicide risk assessment and management: Implications for supervisors. *Training and Education in Professional Psychology, 2,* 219–228. http://dx.doi.org/10.1037/1931-3918.2.4.219

Rudd, M. D., Joiner, T., Brown, G. K., Cukrowicz, K., Jobes, D. A., Silverman, M., & Cordero, L. (2009). Informed consent with suicidal patients: Rethinking risks in (and out of) treatment. *Psychotherapy: Theory, Research, & Practice, 46,* 459–468. http://dx.doi.org/10.1037/a0017902

Rudd, M. D., Mandrusiak, M., & Joiner, T. E., Jr. (2006). The case against no-suicide contracts: The commitment to treatment statement as a practice alternative. *Journal of Clinical Psychology, 62,* 243–251. http://dx.doi.org/10.1002/jclp.20227

Rudd, R. A., Seth, P., David, F., & Scholl, L. (2016). Increases in drug and opioid-involved overdose deaths—United States, 2010–2015. *MMWR: Morbidity and Mortality Weekly Report, 65,* 1445–1452. http://dx.doi.org/10.15585/mmwr.mm655051e1

Runeson, B., Odeberg, J., Pettersson, A., Edbom, T., Jildevik Adamsson, I., & Waern, M. (2017). Instruments for the assessment of suicide risk: A systematic review evaluating the certainty of the evidence. *PLoS One, 12*(7), e0180292. http://dx.doi.org/10.1371/journal.pone.0180292

Rupert, P. A., Miller, A. O., & Dorociak, K. E. (2017). Preventing burnout: What does the research tell us? *Professional Psychology: Research and Practice, 46,* 168–174. http://dx.doi.org/10/1037/a0039297

Rutter, P. A., Freedenthal, S., & Osman, A. (2008). Assessing protection from suicidal risk: Psychometric properties of the suicide resilience inventory. *Death Studies, 32,* 142–153. http://dx.doi.org/10.1080/07481180701801295

Ryan, R. M., & Deci, E. I. (2008). A self-determination theory approach to psychotherapy: The motivation basis for effective change. *Canadian Psychology, 49,* 186–193. http://dx.doi.org/10.1037/a0012753

Sachs-Ericsson, N. J., Stanley, I. H., Sheffler, J. L., Selby, E., & Joiner, T. E. (2017). Non-violent and violent forms of childhood abuse in the prediction of suicide attempts: Direct or indirect effects through psychiatric disorders? *Journal of Affective Disorders, 215*, 15–22. http://dx.doi.org/10.1016/j.jad.2017.03.030

Schechter, M. A., & Goldblatt, M. J. (2011). Psychodynamic theory and the therapeutic alliance: Validation, empathy, and genuine relatedness. In K. Michel & D. A. Jobes (Eds.), *Building a therapeutic alliance with the suicidal patient* (pp. 93–107). Washington, DC: American Psychological Association. http://dx.doi.org/10.1037/12303-006

Schmidt, N. B., Norr, A. M., Allan, N. P., Raines, A. M., & Capron, D. W. (2017). A randomized clinical trial targeting anxiety sensitivity for patients with suicidal ideation. *Journal of Consulting and Clinical Psychology, 85*, 596–610. http://dx.doi.org/10.1037/ccp0000195

Schmitz, W. M., Jr., Allen, M. H., Feldman, B. N., Gutin, N. J., Jahn, D. R., Kleespies, P. M., . . . Simpson, S. (2012). Preventing suicide through improved training in suicide risk assessment and care: An American Association of Suicidology Task Force report addressing serious gaps in U.S. mental health training. *Suicide and Life-Threatening Behavior, 42*, 292–304. http://dx.doi.org/10.1111/j.1943-278X.2012.00090.x

Schultz, K. (2018, June). *State board of psychology disciplinary violations: 2007 through 2017.* Poster presented at the annual convention of the Pennsylvania Psychological Association, King of Prussia, PA.

Seda, G., Sanchez-Ortuno, M. M., Welsh, C. H., Halbower, A. C., & Edinger, J. D. (2015). Comparative meta-analysis of prazosin and imagery rehearsal therapy for nightmare frequency, sleep quality, and posttraumatic stress. *Journal of Clinical Sleep Medicine, 11*, 11–22. http://dx.doi.org/10.5664/jcsm.4354

Selby, E. A., Anestis, M. D., & Joiner, T. E. (2008). Understanding the relationship between emotional and behavioral dysregulation: Emotional cascades. *Behaviour Research and Therapy, 46*, 593–611. http://dx.doi.org/10.1016/j.brat.2008.02.002

Shea, S. C. (2011). *The practical art of suicide assessment: A guide for mental health professionals and substance abuse counselors.* New York, NY: Mental Health Press.

Siddaway, A. P., Taylor, P. J., Wood, A. M., & Schulz, J. (2015). A meta-analysis of perceptions of defeat and entrapment in depression, anxiety problems, posttraumatic stress disorder, and suicidality. *Journal of Affective Disorders, 184*, 149–159. http://dx.doi.org/10.1016/j.jad.2015.05.046

Silberman, I. (2005). Religion as a meaning system: Implications for the new millennium. *Journal of Social Issues, 61*, 641–663. http://dx.doi.org/10.1111/j.1540-4560.2005.00425.x

Silva, C., Chu, C., Monahan, K. R., & Joiner, T. E. (2015). Suicide risk among sexual minority college students: A mediated moderation model of sex and perceived burdensomeness. *Psychology of Sexual Orientation and Gender Diversity, 2*, 22–33. http://dx.doi.org/10.1037/sgd0000086

Silverman, J. J., Galanter, M., Jackson-Triche, M., Jacobs, D. G., Lomax, J. W., II, Riba, M. B., . . . the American Psychiatric Association. (2015). The American Psychiatric Association Practice Guidelines for the psychiatric evaluation of adults. *The American Journal of Psychiatry, 172*, 798–802. http://dx.doi.org/10.1176/appi.ajp.2015.1720501

Silverman, M. M. (2014). Suicide risk assessment and suicide risk formulation: Essential components of the therapeutic risk management model. *Journal of Psychiatric Practice, 20*, 373–378. http://dx.doi.org/10.1097/01.pra.0000454784.90353.bf

Simon, G. E., Rutter, C. M., Peterson, D., Oliver, M., Whiteside, U., Operskalski, B., & Ludman, E. J. (2013). Does response on the PHQ-9 Depression Questionnaire predict subsequent suicide attempt or suicide death? *Psychiatric Services, 64,* 1195–1202. http://dx.doi.org/10.1176/appi.ps.201200587

Simon, G. E., Specht, C., & Doederlein, A. (2016). Coping with suicidal thoughts: A survey of personal experience. *Psychiatric Services, 67,* 1026–1029. http://dx.doi.org/10.1176/appi.ps.201500281

Simon, O. R., Swann, A. C., Powell, K. E., Potter, L. B., Kresnow, M. J., & O'Carroll, P. W. (2001). Characteristics of impulsive suicide attempts and attempters. *Suicide and Life-Threatening Behavior, 32*(Suppl. 1), 49–59. http://dx.doi.org/10.1521/suli.32.1.5.49.24212

Simon, R. (1992). *Clinical psychiatry and the law.* Washington, DC: American Psychiatric Press.

Simon, R. I. (2007). Gun safety management with patients at risk for suicide. *Suicide and Life-Threatening Behavior, 37,* 518–526. http://dx.doi.org/10.1521/suli.2007.37.5.518

Simon, R. (2011). *Preventing patient suicide: Clinical assessment and management.* Washington, DC: American Psychiatric Press.

Simons, R. L., Lei, M.-K., Barr, A. B., Beach, S. R. H., Simons, L. G., Gibbons, F. X., & Philibert, P. A. (2018). Discrimination, segregation, and chronic inflammation: Testing the weathering explanation for the poor health of Black Americans. *Developmental Psychology, 54,* 1993–2006. http://dx.doi.org/10.1037/dev0000511

Sinyor, M., Schaffer, A., Nishikawa, Y., Redelmeier, D. A., Niederkrotenthaler, T., Sareen, J., . . . Pirkis, J. (2018). The association between suicide deaths and putatively harmful and protective factors in media reports. *Canadian Medical Association Journal, 190,* E900–E907. http://dx.doi.org/10.1503/cmaj.170698

Smith, A. R., Ribeiro, J. D., Mikolajewski, A., Taylor, J., Joiner, T. E., & Iacono, W. G. (2012). An examination of environmental and genetic contributions to the determinants of suicidal behavior among male twins. *Psychiatry Research, 197,* 60–65. http://dx.doi.org/10.1016/j.psychres.2012.01.010

Smith, A. R., Zuromski, K. L., & Dodd, D. R. (2018). Eating disorders and suicidality: What we know, what we don't know, and suggestions for future research. *Current Opinion in Psychology, 22,* 63–67. http://dx.doi.org/10.1016/j.copsyc.2017.08.023

Smith, N. B., Mota, N., Tsai, J., Monteith, L., Harpaz-Rotem, I., Southwick, S. M., & Pietrzak, R. H. (2016). Nature and determinants of suicidal ideation among U.S. veterans: Results from the National Health and Resilience in Veterans Study. *Journal of Affective Disorders, 197,* 66–73. http://dx.doi.org/10.1016/j.jad.2016.02.069

Snyder, T. (2015). *Slavery and suicide in British North America.* Chicago, IL: University of Chicago Press. http://dx.doi.org/10.7208/chicago/9780226280738.001.0001

Sobelman, S., & Younggren, J. N. (2016). Clinical decision making and risk management. In J. Magnavita (Ed.), *Clinical decision making in mental health practice* (pp. 245–271). Washington, DC: American Psychological Association. http://dx.doi.org/10.1037/14711-010

Soberay, K. A., Monteith, L. L., Dorsey Holliman, B., Gerber, H., Matarazzo, B. B., & Bahraini, N. H. (2016, August). *Risky behaviors and acquired capability for suicide among veterans with military sexual trauma.* Poster presented at the 124th annual convention of the American Psychological Association, Denver, CO.

Spillane, A., Larkin, C., Corcoran, P., Matvienko-Sikar, K., Riordan, F., & Arensman, E. (2017). Physical and psychosomatic health outcomes in people bereaved by suicide compared to people bereaved by other modes of death: A systematic review. *BMC Public Health, 17*, 939. http://dx.doi.org/10.1186/s12889-017-4930-3

Stanley, B., & Brown, G. K. (2012). Safety Planning Intervention: A brief intervention to mitigate suicide risk. *Cognitive and Behavioral Practice, 19*, 256–264. http://dx.doi.org/10.1016/j.cbpra.2011.01.001

Stanley, B., Brown, G. K., Brenner, L. A., Galfalvy, H. C., Currier, G. W., Knox, K. L., . . . Green, K. L. (2018). Comparison of the Safety Planning Intervention with follow-up vs. usual care of suicidal patients treated in the emergency room. *JAMA Psychiatry, 75*, 894–900. http://dx.doi.org/10.1001/jamapsychiatry.2018.1776

Stanley, B., Green, K. L., Ghahramanlou-Holloway, M., Brenner, L. A., & Brown, G. K. (2017). The construct and measurement of suicide-related coping. *Psychiatry Research, 258*, 189–193. http://dx.doi.org/10.1016/j.psychres.2017.08.008

Stanley, I. H., Boffa, J. W., Smith, L. J., Tran, J. K., Schmidt, N. B., Joiner, T. E., & Vujanovic, A. A. (2018). Occupational stress and suicidality among firefighters: Examining the buffering role of distress tolerance. *Psychiatry Research, 266*, 90–96. http://dx.doi.org/10.1016/j.psychres.2018.05.058

Stanley, I. H., Hom, M. A., & Joiner, T. E. (2015). Mental health service use among adults with suicidal ideation, plans, or attempts: Results from a national survey. *Psychiatric Services, 66*, 1296–1302. http://dx.doi.org/10.1176/appi.ps.201400593

Stanley, I. H., Hom, M. A., & Joiner, T. E. (2018). Modifying mental health help-seeking stigma among undergraduates with untreated psychiatric disorders: A pilot randomized trial of a novel cognitive bias modification intervention. *Behaviour Research and Therapy, 103*, 33–42. http://dx.doi.org/10.1016/j.brat.2018.01.008

Stanley, I. H., Hom, M. A., Spencer-Thomas, S., & Joiner, T. E. (2017). Examining anxiety sensitivity as a mediator of the association between PTSD symptoms and suicide risk among women firefighters. *Journal of Anxiety Disorders, 50*, 94–102. http://dx.doi.org/10.1016/j.janxdis.2017.06.003

Stanley, I. H., Rufino, K. A., Rogers, M. L., Ellis, T. E., & Joiner, T. E. (2016). Acute Suicidal Affective Disturbance (ASAD): A confirmatory factor analysis with 1442 psychiatric inpatients. *Journal of Psychiatric Research, 80*, 97–104. http://dx.doi.org/10.1016/j.jpsychires.2016.06.012

Sternlieb, J. (2013, September). A continuum of reflective practices: What, how and why—part 1. *The Pennsylvania Psychologist, 73*, 21.

Sternlieb, J. (2014, October). Self-care has two distinct components. *The Pennsylvania Psychologist, 74*, 4–5.

Stohlmann-Rainey, J. (2017). *Developing power*. Retrieved from https://www.suicidology.org/Portals/14/docs/Writing%20Contest/2017/2017Winner%20List.pdf?ver=2017-08-29-211745-243

Stone, D. M., Luo, F., Ouyang, L., Lippy, C., Hertz, M. F., & Crosby, A. E. (2014). Sexual orientation and suicide ideation, plans, attempts, and medically serious attempts: Evidence from local Youth Risk Behavior Surveys, 2001–2009. *American Journal of Public Health, 104*, 262–271. http://dx.doi.org/10.2105/AJPH.2013.301383

Stone, D. M., Simon, T. R., Fowler, K. A., Kegler, S. R., Yuan, K., Holland, K. M., . . . Crosby, A. E. (2018, June 8). Vital Signs: Trends in state suicide rates—United States, 1999–2016 and circumstances contributing to suicide—27 states, 2015. *MMWR: Morbidity and Mortality Weekly Report, 67*, 617–624. http://dx.doi.org/10.15585/mmwr.mm6722a1

Stroebe, W. (2013). Firearm possession and violent death: A critical review. *Aggression and Violent Behavior, 18*, 709–721. http://dx.doi.org/10.1016/j.avb.2013.07.025

Strosahl, K. D., Hayes, S. C., Wilson, K. G., & Gifford, E. V. (2004). An ACT primer. In S. C. Hayes & K. D. Strosahl (Eds.), *A practical guide to acceptance and commitment therapy* (pp. 31–58). New York, NY: Springer. http://dx.doi.org/10.1007/978-0-387-23369-7_2

Stulz, N., Hepp, U., Gosoniu, D. G., Grize, L., Muheim, F., Weiss, M. G., & Riecher-Rössler, A. (2018). Patient-identified priorities leading to attempted suicide. *Crisis, 39*, 37–46. http://dx.doi.org/10.1027/0227-5910/a000473

Substance Abuse and Mental Health Services Administration. (2013). *Results from the 2013 National Survey on Drug Use and Health: Mental health findings.* Rockville, MD: Author. Retrieved from http://www.samhsa.gov/data/sites/default/files/NSDUHmhfr2013/NSDUHmhfr2013.pdf

Swift, J. K., & Greenberg, R. P. (2015). *Premature termination in psychotherapy: Strategies for engaging clients and improving outcomes.* Washington, DC: American Psychological Association. http://dx.doi.org/10.1037/14469-000

Takahashi, Y. (1997). Culture and suicide: From a Japanese psychiatrist's perspective. *Suicide and Life-Threatening Behavior, 27*, 137–145.

Tal, I., Mauro, C., Reynolds, C. F., III, Shear, M. K., Simon, N., Lebowitz, B., . . . Zisook, S. (2017). Complicated grief after suicide bereavement and other causes of death. *Death Studies, 41*, 267–275. http://dx.doi.org/10.1080/07481187.2016.1265028

Tamura, L. J. (2012). Emotional competence and well-being. In S. Knapp, M. C. Gottlieb, M. M. Handelsman, & L. VandeCreek (Eds.), *APA handbook of ethics in psychology* (Vol. 1, pp. 175–215). Washington, DC: American Psychological Association.

Tangney, J. P., Miller, R. S., Flicker, L., & Barlow, D. H. (1996). Are shame, guilt, and embarrassment distinct emotions? *Journal of Personality and Social Psychology, 70*, 1256–1269. http://dx.doi.org/10.1037/0022-3514.70.6.1256

Tanguturi, Y., Bodic, M., Taub, A., Homel, P., & Jacob, T. (2017). Suicide risk assessment by residents: Deficiencies of documentation. *Academic Psychiatry, 41*, 513–519. http://dx.doi.org/10.1007/s40596-016-0644-6

Taube, D. (2018, November 30). *Clinical, ethical and risk management issues* [Suicidality Webcast].

Teismann, T., Brailovskaia, J., Siegmann, P., Nyhuis, P., Wölter, M., & Willutzki, U. (2018). Dual factor model of mental health: Co-occurrence of positive mental health and suicidal ideation in inpatients and outpatients. *Psychiatry Research, 260*, 343–345. http://dx.doi.org/10.1016/j.psychres.2017.11.085

Teismann, T., Forkmann, T., Brailovskaia, J., Siegmann, P., Glaesmer, H., & Margraf, J. (2018). Positive mental health moderates the association between depression and suicide ideation: A longitudinal study. *International Journal of Clinical and Health Psychology, 18*, 1–7. http://dx.doi.org/10.1016/j.ijchp.2017.08.001

Testa, R. J., Michaels, M. S., Bliss, W., Rogers, M. L., Balsam, K. F., & Joiner, T. (2017). Suicidal ideation in transgender people: Gender minority stress and interpersonal theory factors. *Journal of Abnormal Psychology, 126*, 125–136. http://dx.doi.org/10.1037/abn0000234

Toli, A., Webb, T. L., & Hardy, G. E. (2016). Does forming implementation intentions help people with mental health problems to achieve goals? A meta-analysis of experimental studies with clinical and analogue samples. *British Journal of Clinical Psychology, 55*, 69–90. http://dx.doi.org/10.1111/bjc.12086

Toohey, M. J., & DiGiuseppe, R. (2017). Defining and measuring irritability: Construct clarification and differentiation. *Clinical Psychology Review, 53*, 93–108. http://dx.doi.org/10.1016/j.cpr.2017.01.009

Troister, T., D'Agata, M. T., & Holden, R. R. (2015). Suicide risk screening: Comparing the Beck Depression Inventory-II, Beck Hopelessness Scale, and Psychache Scale in undergraduates. *Psychological Assessment, 27*, 1500–1506. http://dx.doi.org/10.1037/pas0000126

Tucker, R. P., Crowley, K. J., Davidson, C. L., & Gutierrez, P. M. (2015). Risk factors, warning signs, and drivers of suicide: What are they, how do they differ, and why does it matter? *Suicide and Life-Threatening Behavior, 45*, 679–689. http://dx.doi.org/10.1111/sltb.12161

Tucker, R. P., Hagan, C. R., Hill, R. M., Slish, M. L., Bagge, C., Joiner, T. E., & Wingate, L. R. (2018). Empirical extension of the interpersonal theory of suicide: Investigating the role of interpersonal hopelessness. *Psychiatric Research, 259*, 427–432. http://dx.doi.org/10.1016/j.psychres.2017.11.005

Tucker, R. P., Michaels, M. S., Rogers, M. L., Wingate, L. R., & Joiner, T. E., Jr. (2016). Construct validity of a proposed new diagnostic entity: Acute suicidal affective disturbance (ASAD). *Journal of Affective Disorders, 189*, 365–378. http://dx.doi.org/10.1016/j.jad.2015.07.049

Tucker, R. P., Wingate, L. R., O'Keefe, V. M., Hollingsworth, D. W., & Cole, A. B. (2016). An examination of historical loss thinking frequency and rumination on suicidal ideation in American Indian young adults. *Suicide and Life-Threatening Behavior, 46*, 213–222. http://dx.doi.org/10.1111/sltb.12185

Tucker, R. P., Wingate, L. R., O'Keefe, V. M., Slish, M. L., Judah, M. R., & Rhoades-Kerswill, S. (2013). The moderating effect of humor style on the relationship between interpersonal predictors of suicide and suicidal ideation. *Personality and Individual Differences, 54*, 610–615. http://dx.doi.org/10.1016/j.paid.2012.11.023

Turnell, A. I., Fassnacht, D. B., Batterham, P. J., Calear, A. L., & Kyrios, M. (2019). The Self-Hate Scale: Development and validation of a brief measure and its relationship to suicidal ideation. *Journal of Affective Disorders, 245*, 779–787. http://dx.doi.org/10.1016/j.jad.2018.11.047

Twenge, J. M., Joiner, T. E., Rogers, M. L., & Martin, G. N. (2018). Increases in depressive symptoms, suicide-related outcomes, and suicide rates among U.S. adolescents after 2010 and links to increased new media screen time. *Clinical Psychological Science, 6*, 3–17. (Corrigendum published January 14, 2019, *Clinical Psychology Science*) http://dx.doi.org/10.1177/2167702617723376

U.S. Suicide Rates Display Growing Geographic Disparity. (2017). *JAMA, 317*, 1616. http://dx.doi.org/10.1001/jama.2017.4076

Valderrama, J., Miranda, T., & Jeglic, E. (2016). Ruminative subtypes and impulsivity in risk for suicidal behavior. *Psychiatry Research, 236*, 15–21. http://dx.doi.org/10.1016/j.psychres.2016.01.008

Van Orden, K. A., Wiktorsson, S., Duberstein, P., Berg, A. I., Fässberg, M. M., & Waern, M. (2015). Reasons for attempted suicide in later life. *The American Journal of Geriatric Psychiatry, 23,* 536–544. http://dx.doi.org/10.1016/j.jagp.2014.07.003

Van Orden, K. A., Witte, T. K., Cukrowicz, K. C., Braithwaite, S. R., Selby, E. A., & Joiner, T. E., Jr. (2010). The interpersonal theory of suicide. *Psychological Review, 117,* 575–600. http://dx.doi.org/10.1037/a0018697

Vieten, C., Scammell, S., Pilato, R., Ammondson, I., Pargament, K. I., & Lakoff, D. (2013). Spiritual and religious competences for psychologists. *Psychology of Religion and Spirituality, 5,* 129–144. http://dx.doi.org/10.1037/a0032699

Waern, M., Kaiser, N., & Renberg, E. S. (2016). Psychiatrists' experiences of suicide assessment. *BMC Psychiatry, 16,* 440. http://dx.doi.org/10.1186/s12888-016-1147-4

Walfish, S., McAlister, B., O'Donnell, P., & Lambert, M. J. (2012). An investigation of self-assessment bias in mental health providers. *Psychological Reports, 110,* 639–644. http://dx.doi.org/10.2466/02.07.17.PR0.110.2.639-644

Wampold, B. E. (2015). Routine outcome monitoring: Coming of age—with the usual developmental challenges. *Psychotherapy, 52,* 458–462. http://dx.doi.org/10.1037/pst0000037

Wampold, B. E., Baldwin, S. A., Holtforth, M. G., & Imel, Z. E. (2017). What characterizes effective psychotherapists? In L. Castonguay & C. Hill (Eds.), *How and why are some therapists better than others?* (pp. 37–53). Washington, DC: American Psychological Association. http://dx.doi.org/10.1037/0000034-003

Ward-Ciesielski, E. F., Schumacher, J. A., & Bagge, C. L. (2016). Relations between nonsuicidal self-injury and suicide attempt characteristics in a sample of recent suicide attempters. *Crisis, 37,* 310–313. http://dx.doi.org/10.1027/0227-5910/a000400

Ward-Ciesielski, E. F., Wielgus, M. D., & Jones, C. B. (2015). Suicide-bereaved individuals' attitudes toward therapists. *Crisis, 36,* 135–141. http://dx.doi.org/10.1027/0227-5910/a000290

Ward-Ciesielski, E. F., Winer, E. S., Drapeau, C. W., & Nadorff, M. R. (2018). Examining components of emotion regulation in relation to sleep problems and suicide risk. *Journal of Affective Disorders, 241,* 41–48. http://dx.doi.org/10.1016/j.jad.2018.07.065

Webb, K. B. (2011). Care of others and self: A suicidal patient's impact on the psychologist. *Professional Psychology: Research and Practice, 42,* 215–221. http://dx.doi.org/10.1037/a0022752

Webb, R. T., Kontopantelis, E., Doran, T., Qin, P., Creed, F., & Kapur, N. (2012). Risk of self-harm in physically ill patients in UK primary care. *Journal of Psychosomatic Research, 73,* 92–97. http://dx.doi.org/10.1016/j.jpsychores.2012.05.010

Wedig, M. M., Frankenburg, F. R., Bradford Reich, D., Fitzmaurice, G., & Zanarini, M. C. (2013). Predictors of suicide threats in patients with borderline personality disorder over 16 years of prospective follow-up. *Psychiatry Research, 208,* 252–256. http://dx.doi.org/10.1016/j.psychres.2013.05.009

Weingarten, D. (2017, December 6). Why are America's farmers killing themselves in record numbers? *The Guardian.* Retrieved from https://www.theguardian.com/us-news/2017/dec/06/why-are-americas-farmers-killing-themselves-in-record-numbers

Weissberg, N. (2011, June). Working with adult suicidal patients. *The Pennsylvania Psychologist, 71*, 13–14.

Wenzel, A., Brown, G. K., & Beck, A. T. (2009). *Cognitive therapy for suicidal patients: Scientific and clinical applications.* Washington, DC: American Psychological Association. http://dx.doi.org/10.1037/11862-000

Westgate, C. L., Shiner, B., Thompson, P., & Watts, B. V. (2015). Evaluation of veterans' suicide risk with the use of linguistic detection methods. *Psychiatric Services, 66*, 1051–1056. http://dx.doi.org/10.1176/appi.ps.201400283

Whiteside, U. (2016, August 4). *What works in suicide prevention: Perspectives from a clinician with lived experiences in suicidality.* Presentation at the annual meeting of the American Psychological Association, Denver, CO.

Wible, P. (2017). *What I learned from the study of 1,208 physician suicides.* Retrieved from http://www.idealmedicalcare.org/ive-learned-547-doctor-suicides/

Wichers, M., Wigman, J. T. W., & Myin-Germeys, I. (2015). Micro-level affect dynamics in psychopathology viewed from complex dynamical systems theory. *Emotion Review, 7*, 362–367. http://dx.doi.org/10.1177/1754073915590623

Willoughby, T., Heffer, T., & Hamza, C. A. (2015). The link between nonsuicidal self-injury and acquired capability for suicide: A longitudinal study. *Journal of Abnormal Psychology, 124*, 1110–1115. http://dx.doi.org/10.1037/abn0000104

Wingate, L. R., Burns, A. B., Gordon, K. H., Perez, M., Walker, R. L., Williams, F. M., & Joiner, T. E. (2006). Suicide and positive cognitions: Positive psychology applied to the understanding and treatment of suicidal behavior. In T. E. Ellis (Ed.), *Cognition and suicide: Theory, research, and therapy* (pp. 261–283). Washington, DC: American Psychological Association. http://dx.doi.org/10.1037/11377-012

Witte, T. K., Holm-Denoma, J. M., Zuromski, K. L., Gauthier, J. M., & Ruscio, J. (2017). Individuals at high risk for suicide are categorically distinct from those at low risk. *Psychological Assessment, 29*, 382–393. http://dx.doi.org/10.1037/pas0000349

Wolford-Clevenger, C., Febres, J., Elmquist, J., Zapor, H., Brasfield, H., & Stuart, G. L. (2015). Prevalence and correlates of suicidal ideation among court-referred male perpetrators of intimate partner violence. *Psychological Services, 12*, 9–15. http://dx.doi.org/10.1037/a0037338

Wong, Y. J., Vaughan, E. I., Liu, T., & Chang, T. K. (2014). Asian Americans' proportion of life in the United States and suicide ideation: The moderating effects of ethnic subgroups. *Asian American Journal of Psychology, 5*, 237–242. http://dx.doi.org/10.1037/a0033283

Wortzel, H. S., Matarazzo, B., & Homaifar, B. (2013). A model for therapeutic risk management of the suicidal patient. *Journal of Psychiatric Practice, 19*, 323–326. http://dx.doi.org/10.1097/01.pra.0000432603.99211.e8

Wyland, C. L., & Forgas, J. P. (2007). On bad mood and white bears: The effects of mood state on ability to suppress unwanted thoughts. *Cognition and Emotion, 21*, 1513–1524. http://dx.doi.org/10.1080/02699930601063506

Yarborough, B. J. H., Stumbo, S. P., Janoff, S. L., Yarborough, M. T., McCarty, D., Chilcoat, H. D., . . . Green, C. A. (2016). Understanding opioid overdose characteristics involving prescription and illicit opioids: A mixed methods analysis. *Drug and Alcohol Dependence, 167*, 49–56. http://dx.doi.org/10.1016/j.drugalcdep.2016.07.024

Yip, P. S. F., Caine, E., Yousuf, S., Chang, S.-S., Wu, K. C.-C., & Chen, Y.-Y. (2012). Means restriction for suicide prevention. *Lancet, 379*, 2393–2399. http://dx.doi.org/10.1016/S0140-6736(12)60521-2

Youyou, W., Stillwell, D., Schwartz, H. A., & Kosinski, M. (2017). Birds of a feather do flock together: Behavior-based personality-assessment method reveals personality similarity among couples and friends. *Psychological Science, 28,* 276–284. http://dx.doi.org/10.1177/0956797616678187

Yuodelis-Flores, C., & Ries, R. K. (2015). Addiction and suicide: A review. *The American Journal on Addictions, 24,* 98–104. http://dx.doi.org/10.1111/ajad.12185

Zonana, J., Simberlund, J., & Christos, P. (2018). The impact of safety plans in an outpatient clinic. *Crisis, 39,* 304–309. http://dx.doi.org/10.1027/0227-5910/a000495

Zuromski, K. L., Cero, I., & Witte, T. K. (2017). Insomnia symptoms drive changes in suicide ideation: A latent difference score model of community adults over a brief interval. *Journal of Abnormal Psychology, 126,* 739–749. http://dx.doi.org/10.1037/abn0000282

INDEX

ABOUT THE AUTHOR

Samuel J. Knapp, EdD, ABPP, is a licensed psychologist in Pennsylvania, where he worked in community mental health centers in two rural counties delivering psychotherapy and crisis intervention services. Currently, he is the director of professional affairs of the Pennsylvania Psychological Association. He has written or edited 16 books; almost 100 peer-reviewed articles; and almost 500 professional presentations on ethics, suicide prevention, and other issues. He holds a diplomate in counseling psychology from the American Board of Professional Psychology, and he is a fellow of the American Psychological Association Division 31 (State, Provincial and Territorial Psychological Association Affairs).